FRACTURE APHORISMS

1. The saving of life comes first; treat impending asphyxia, hemorrhage, shock, and other life-endangering conditions before treating a fracture.

2. To minimize soft tissue damage and to avoid the conversion of a closed to an open fracture, "splint 'em where they lie" at *first* contact.

3. Examine the injured part for signs of vascular and nerve injuries and record your findings.

4. Eliminate all unnecessary handling of the injured part. Disturb the patient as little as possible.

5. Never deliberately test for crepitus.

6. Make certain that the obvious fracture is the only injury. There may be other fractures or serious soft tissue injuries less apparent. Always x-ray pelvis in presence of major lower limb trauma; always check spine in presence of heel fracture; x-ray should always show both ends of an involved bone.

7. Do not be deceived by the absence of deformity and disability; in many cases of fracture, some ability to use the limb persists.

8. Treat every case of injury as a fracture until it is proved to be otherwise.

9. Obtain roentgenograms in at least two planes and examine them yourself.

10. Reduce the fracture with as little delay as possible. Do not wait for the swelling to go down.

11. Continued severe pain often indicates circulatory impairment and requires immediate attention day or night.

12. In splitting a plaster cast, divide the plaster and the underlying padding down to the skin.

13. Make certain that continuous traction is checked frequently.

14. Immediately activate all joints that are not immobilized for treatment of the fracture.

15. Open fractures are contaminated wounds. Minimize the risk of infection by adequate debridement, delayed closure of the wound as indicated, and immobilization.

16. Treatment should concentrate on assuring future function:

    The chief aim in the treatment of fractures of the upper extremity is to ensure the proper functioning of the hand. Shortening and some malalignment are often acceptable.

    The chief aim in the treatment of fractures of the lower extremity is to ensure painless, stable weight bearing. Malalignment must be prevented, and maintenance of length is desirable.

17. Throughout the treatment of a fracture, focus attention on the patient as a whole as well as on the injured part.

18. Wherever possible, arrange the first visit to the x-ray department to include all indicated procedures (i.e., chest x-ray, cystogram, bone survey, K.U.B.).

Edited by

ALEXANDER J. WALT, M.B., FACS, *Chairman*

Professor and Chairman, Department of Surgery,
Wayne State University School of Medicine,
Detroit Medical Center, Detroit, Michigan

Associate Editors:

LEONARD F. PELTIER
BASIL A. PRUITT, Jr.
DONALD D. TRUNKEY
ROBERT F. WILSON

Early Care of the

THIRD
EDITION

of the

Injured Patient

**COMMITTEE ON TRAUMA
AMERICAN COLLEGE OF SURGEONS**

1982   W. B. SAUNDERS COMPANY

Philadelphia • London • Toronto • Mexico City • Rio de Janeiro • Sydney • Tokyo

W. B. Saunders Company: West Washington Square
Philadelphia, PA 19105

1 St. Anne's Road
Eastbourne, East Sussex BN21 3UN, England

1 Goldthorne Avenue
Toronto, Ontario M8Z 5T9, Canada

Apartado 26370 – Cedro 512
Mexico 4, D.F., Mexico

Rua Coronel Cabrita, 8
Sao Cristovao Caixa Postal 21176
Rio de Janeiro, Brazil

9 Waltham Street
Artarmon, N.S.W. 2064, Australia

Ichibancho, Central Bldg., 22-1 Ichibancho
Chiyoda-Ku, Tokyo 102, Japan

Library of Congress Cataloging in Publication Data

Main entry under title:

Early care of the injured patient.

1. Wounds and injuries – Treatment.   2. Fractures.
   3. Surgical emergencies.   I. Walt, Alexander J.
   II. American College of Surgeons. Committee on Trauma.
   [DNLM: 1. Emergencies.   2. Fracture fixation.
   3. Wounds and injuries – Surgery. WO 700 E12]

RD93.E247 1982   617'.1   81–48149

ISBN 0–7216–1165–6   AACR2

Listed here is the latest translated edition of this book together
with the language of the translation and the publisher.

Spanish (*2nd edition*) – Nueva Editorial Interamericana S.A.
            Mexico 4, D.F., Mexico

German (*2nd edition*) – F. K. Schattauer Verlag,
            Stuttgart, Germany

Early Care of the Injured Patient   ISBN   0-7216-1165-6

Last digit is the print number: 9   8   7   6   5   4   3   2   1

Contributors

JOHN A. BOSWICK, Jr., M.S., M.D., FACS

Professor of Surgery, The University of Colorado Health Sciences Center; Attending Surgeon, Colorado General Hospital, Veterans Administration Hospital, General Rose Hospital, Denver, Colorado

ELI M. BROWN, M.D.

Professor and Chairman, Department of Anesthesiology, Wayne State University School of Medicine; Chairman, Department of Anesthesiology, Sinai Hospital of Detroit; Consultant, Harper-Grace Hospitals, Hutzel Hospital, Detroit Receiving Hospital, Veterans Administration Hospital, Detroit, Michigan

WILLIAM E. DeMUTH, Jr., M.D., FACS

Professor of Surgery, Pennsylvania State University College of Medicine, State College; Attending Surgeon, Milton S. Hershey Medical Center, Hershey, Pennsylvania

THOMAS B. DUCKER, M.D., FACS

Professor and Chairman, Department of Neurosurgery, University of Maryland School of Medicine, Baltimore, Maryland

CLEON W. GOODWIN, M.D.

Chief, Surgical Studies Branch, U.S. Army Institute of Surgical Research, Fort Sam Houston, Texas

ROGER F. JOHNSON, M.D., LL.B.

Assistant Professor in Clinical Psychiatry, University of Colorado Health Sciences Center; Instructor, University of Denver College of Law, Medical-Legal Problems, Denver, Colorado

JESSE B. JUPITER, M.D.

Instructor in Orthopaedic Surgery, Harvard Medical School; Assistant in Orthopaedic Surgery, Massachusetts General Hospital, Boston, Massachusetts

HAROLD E. KLEINERT, M.D., FACS

Clinical Professor of Surgery, University of Louisville School of Medicine; Clinical Professor of Surgery, Indiana University-Purdue University School of Medicine; Director of Hand Surgery Services, University of Louisville Hospitals, Louisville, Kentucky

CHARLES E. LUCAS, M.D., FACS

Professor of Surgery, Wayne State University School of Medicine; Active Staff, Harper-Grace Hospitals, Hutzel Hospital, Detroit Receiving Hospital, Detroit, Michigan

KENNETH L. MATTOX, M.D., FACS

Associate Professor of Surgery, Baylor College of Medicine; Deputy Surgeon-In-Chief and Director of Emergency Surgical Services, Ben Taub General Hospital, Houston, Texas

KENNETH L. MILLER, M.S., C.H.P.

Associate Professor of Radiology, Pennsylvania State University College of Medicine, State College, Pennsylvania

D. S. MULDER, M.D., FRCS(C), FACS

Professor of Surgery, McGill University; Surgeon-in-Chief, Montreal General Hospital, Montreal, Quebec, Canada

LEONARD F. PELTIER, M.D., Ph.D., FACS

Professor of Surgery, Head, Section of Orthopedic Surgery, University of Arizona School of Medicine; Head, Section of Orthopedic Surgery, Arizona Health Sciences Center, Tucson, Arizona

PAUL C. PETERS, M.D., FACS

Professor and Chairman, Division of Urology, The University of Texas Southwestern Medical School; Chief of Service, Parkland Memorial Hospital; Active Attending, Children's Medical Center; Attending, Veterans Administration Medical Center, Medical Arts Hospital; Consultant, Baylor University Medical Center, John Peter Smith Hospital, St. Paul Hospital, Dallas, Texas

BASIL A. PRUITT, Jr., M.D., FACS

Commander and Director, U.S. Army Institute of Surgical Research, Fort Sam Houston, Texas

MARTIN C. ROBSON, M.D., FACS

Professor and Chairman, Section of Plastic and Reconstructive Surgery, University of Chicago, The Pritzker School of Medicine, Chicago, Illinois

JOHN D. SALETTA, M.D., FACS

Clinical Associate Professor of Surgery, Abraham Lincoln School of Medicine, University of Illinois; Attending Surgeon, Cook County Hospital, Senior Active Surgeon, Holy Cross Hospital, Chicago, Illinois

THOMAS G. SAUL, M.D.

Assistant Professor of Neurosurgery, University of Maryland School of Medicine; Attending Neurosurgeon, University of Maryland Hospital, Clinical Director, Neurotrauma Center, Maryland Institute for Emergency Medical Services, Baltimore, Maryland

FRANK A. SCOTT, M.D., FRCS(C), FACS

Assistant Clinical Professor of Surgery, University of Colorado Health Sciences Center; Attending Surgeon, Colorado General Hospital, Veterans Administration Hospital, General Rose Hospital, Denver, Colorado

GEORGE F. SHELDON, M.D., FACS

Professor of Surgery, University of California at San Francisco; Chief, Trauma and Hyperalimentation Services, San Francisco General Hospital; Moffitt-UC Hospital, San Francisco, California

CLIFFORD C. SNYDER, M.D., FACS

Professor and Chairman, Division of Plastic Surgery, University of Utah School of Medicine; Full-time Staff, University Medical Center; Chief of Plastic Surgery, Shriner's Crippled Children's Hospital, Salt Lake City, Utah

DONALD D. TRUNKEY, M.D., FACS

Professor of Surgery, University of California at San Francisco; Chief, Department of Surgery, San Francisco General Hospital, San Francisco, California

FRANKLIN C. WAGNER, Jr., M.D., FACS

Associate Professor of Surgery (Neurosurgery), Yale University School of Medicine, Attending in Surgery (Neurosurgery), Yale-New Haven Hospital, New Haven, Connecticut

ALEXANDER J. WALT, M.B., Ch. B.,
FRCS (C. Eng.), FACS

Professor and Chairman, Department of Surgery, Wayne State University School of Medicine, Detroit, Michigan

ROBERT L. WALTON, M.D.

Assistant Professor of Surgery, Division of Plastic Surgery, University of California, San Francisco; Chief of Plastic and Reconstructive Surgery, San Francisco General Hospital, San Francisco, California

ROBERT J. WHITE, M.D., Ph.D., FACS

Professor and Co-Chairman, Division of Neurological Surgery, Case-Western Reserve University School of Medicine; Director of Neurological Surgery, Cleveland Metropolitan General Hospital, Cleveland, Ohio

ROBERT F. WILSON, M.D., FACS

Professor of Surgery, Director, Thoracic and Cardiovascular Surgery, Wayne State University, School of Medicine; Chief of Surgery, Detroit Receiving Hospital, Detroit, Michigan

Preface

Ever since its formation in 1922, the Committee on Trauma of the American College of Surgeons has had as its central concern the early medical care of the injured patient. Over the years, the Committee has broadened its horizons to encompass development of improved methods of transport, furtherance of rational and expeditious prehospital management of the patient, design and implementation of a variety of educational programs, dissemination of information to the general public of ways to prevent trauma, and development of standards of optimal hospital care. The Committee, through the College, has always been selected to reflect the broad world of surgery and is composed of surgeons from rural and urban areas, from private practice and from the universities, from large and small states, and from all surgical specialties. The essential prerequisites for membership have been a demonstrated interest in the injured patient and a vigorous commitment to trauma at the regional level.

This third edition was commissioned by the Committee on Trauma and has been written by members of the College who are active in the field of trauma. The only exceptions — a physician-lawyer and an anesthesiologist — appropriately reflect the times. An attempt has been made to update the edition of 1976 while preserving the traditional structure of the book. Some chapters are completely new; others have been revised. Since it is often impossible to strip the soft tissues of a revision from the skeleton of the original contribution, direct attribution of chapters to specific authors has been purposely avoided. With this as background, we would like to thank once more all who have contributed to the previous editions that have provided a solid core of continuity.

The chapters on fractures have been completely rewritten and it is a pleasure to single out for special recognition the editorial assistance given by Dr. Andrew Ruoff and Dr. Gerald Shaftan. Virtually every chapter in the book has either been rewritten or has undergone substantial revision. As might be anticipated, the Committee has had the usual difficulty of trying to decide on the boundaries of what constitutes early care, the degree of technical detail to be covered, and the composition of the audience to whom the book is directed. We have chosen to deviate little from what has been deemed in the past to be an invaluable book in the emergency department and in the library of the physician-surgeon who is not ordinarily immersed in the practice of trauma and emergency care. Above all, we have attempted to produce a book that will help us avoid serious errors in the early care of the injured patient.

The Committee would like to depart from custom and dedicate this volume to Oscar Hampton and to Curtis Artz, who have both died since the last edition was published. The Committee on Trauma has not been the same without them for, in their different ways, they served uniquely to spur us on. Some of us think we still hear Oscar Hampton giving sage advice when we encounter difficult problems. This courtly gentleman, fine orthopedic surgeon, decorated soldier, baseball aficionado and most loyal Fellow of the College served as our conscience and our spur for many years. Curt Artz was different but exerted a similar influence. Also a soldier, Curt Artz literally drove us, scattered barrels of new ideas, stimulated us with his unparalleled energy, and served as the indefatigable advocate of the injured patient. Both are greatly missed. We hope they would have approved this new edition.

Notice

This edition has been prepared for the Committee on Trauma of the American College of Surgeons by certain Committee members, other individual Fellows of the College, and nonsurgical consultants to the Committee who have been selected for their special competence in the early care of the injured patient. The College believes that those having responsibility for such patients will find the information to be of value. However, it must be recognized that injured patients present a wide range of complex problems. Accordingly, failure to follow the suggestions of the authors does not necessarily indicate an incorrect approach. The adequacy of care can be assessed only by peers at the level of practice.

Subcommittee on Publications

HARLAN D. ROOT *(chairman)*

MICHAEL W. CHAPMAN

WILLIAM E. DeMUTH, JR.

THOMAS B. DUCKER

GEORGE A. GATES

F. R. C. JOHNSTONE

PAUL C. PETERS

BASIL A. PRUITT, JR.

H. HARLAN STONE

ALEXANDER J. WALT

Contents

Initial Assessment and Management of the Injured Patient

INTRODUCTION

There are several fundamental concepts upon which management of the injured patient is based. These include:

1. Assessment and resuscitation are usually simultaneous procedures, particularly in the patient whose condition is unstable.

2. If the patient's condition remains unstable or deteriorates despite resuscitation, operation and control of hemorrhage become part of the resuscitation.

3. Resuscitation of the trauma patient is often a team effort involving surgeons, emergency physicians, anesthesiologists, and nurses. For the resuscitation to be effective, one person must be "captain of the ship" and direct the resuscitation. This leadership role must be predetermined.

For the purpose of this discussion it will be assumed that the patient's condition is unstable. Time is of the essence, but a more complete assessment leaves less chance for error. The primary goal of the resuscitation is to provide delivery of oxygen to the brain and other vital organs. This requires an intact airway and adequate alveolar ventilation. Once oxygen is delivered to the alveoli, an intact circulation (including pump and volume) is required to deliver oxygen to the brain.

INITIAL EVALUATION

Most modern EMS systems provide notification of the impending arrival of a seriously injured patient. This is extremely valuable and allows the resuscitation team and the trauma surgeon to prepare for arrival of the patient. If cardiopulmonary resuscitation is ongoing when the patient arrives in the emergency department, an orderly transition from field personnel to hospital personnel must be effected. Ideally, the paramedic should remain with the emergency department personnel for as much of

TABLE 1–1. **PRIORITIES IN EVALUATION AND RESUSCITATION OF THE TRAUMA VICTIM**

1. Airway patency and adequate ventilation
2. Cardiovascular adequacy
    a. Pump (treat cardiac arrest or tamponade)
    b. Volume replacement
3. Control of hemorrhage
4. Evaluation of neurological injuries
5. Stabilization of fractures
6. Definitive diagnosis

the resuscitation as possible, providing extra help and gaining the educational experience. If CPR is not being performed, the paramedic or ambulance attendant should immediately give a presentation of the history and all care given at the scene and during transportation.

If the victim has a palpable pulse and is breathing, he should be stripped of his clothing immediately. Provided that there are no contraindications such as suspected neck injury, the victim should be rolled from side to side to make sure that there are no injuries on the back. If there is a possibility of a cervical spinal injury, the neck must be carefully stabilized, particularly if the patient is to be moved at all. The lower extremities should be examined immediately, because cold, pale, and clammy legs indicate that shock is present until proved otherwise. The neck veins should be checked to help determine whether the shock is due to volume, cardiogenic, or preload problems. This quick assessment will allow the surgeon to direct the resuscitation in the most expeditious way. Immediate attention is then turned to the priorities listed in Table 1–1.

AIRWAY

The first maneuver in establishing an airway is to clear the oropharynx. In the unconscious victim, this is best done by inserting the finger into the mouth and sweeping out all of the clots, debris, fragments of bone, teeth, or vomitus that may be present in the upper airway. A tonsil sucker with good suction is invaluable for removing secretions, blood, or vomitus. In the conscious victim, thorough suctioning will usually clear most of the obvious debris. Patients with extensive facial fractures or gunshot wounds causing severe soft tissue injury present complicated problems. Applying a towel clip or noncrushing clamp to the tongue and drawing it forward may help establish an airway in an otherwise hopeless situation. Insertion of nasopharyngeal or oropharyngeal tubes should be reserved for those patients who are unconscious, because they may aggravate or induce vomiting in a conscious or agitated victim.

Maintenance of the airway is best accomplished by lifting the angle of the jaw. If cervical spine injury is suspected, the neck should be moved as little as possible and axial orientation is mandatory. Once the airway has been cleared and is patent, oxygen supplied by nasal tube or mask should be considered. If the patient does not have adequate spontaneous ventilatory movements, an Ambu type of bag and mask should be placed over the nose and mouth and assisted ventilation instituted (see Chapter 3).

Nasotracheal or orotracheal intubation is rarely indicated as a primary means of establishing the airway; however, in the unconscious or critically injured patient, particularly those with severe cardiopulmonary insufficiency, it must be performed promptly. The choice is the physician's and should be governed by the situation. In the patient with a suspected cervical spine injury, orotracheal intubation may cause too much movement of the neck. In such circumstances, nasotracheal intubation or cricothyroidotomy is preferred.

An emergency tracheostomy is almost never required. A cricothyroidotomy is quicker and safer if an airway and ventilation cannot be established rapidly by standard techniques or an endotracheal tube. The most frequent indications include airway problems associated with severe soft tissue injuries of the face and laryngeal fractures or lacerations (see Chapters 3 and 14).

CARDIOVASCULAR

CARDIOVASCULAR PUMP

After oxygen gets to the alveoli, it needs to be transported from the alveoli into the tissues. This requires that the cardiovascular system (including pump and volume) be reasonably intact. Insults that may contribute to pump problems include tension pneumothorax, pericardial tamponade, myocardial lacerations, myocardial contusion, and myocardial infarction.

Tension pneumothorax interferes with preload by shifting the mediastinum, causing compression and distortion of the great veins and decreasing venous return to the heart, thereby compromising oxygen transport. In addition to distended neck veins, physical examination shows respiratory distress, shift of the trachea to the contralateral thorax, ipsilateral percussion tympany, and decreased breath sounds. Tension pneumothorax may be treated temporarily by inserting a large-bore needle into the second intercostal space of the involved hemithorax. Definitive treatment is a tube thoracostomy in the fifth intercostal space in the midaxillary line done as quickly as possible without waiting for a confirmatory x-ray. When a chest tube is inserted without a prior chest x-ray, the finger should be inserted before the chest tube is so as to prevent laceration of a lung held up to the chest wall by adhesions.

Pericardial tamponade can be a life-threatening emergency and the patient may suffer arrest either before or after arrival in the emergency department. The hallmark of diagnosis is that the patient is in shock and has distended neck veins (see Chapter 3). If the patient is hypovolemic, the distended neck veins may not become apparent until intravenous fluids are given. If the tamponade is secondary to penetrating trauma, there is usually an associated penetrating injury in one of the hemithoraces; however, even distant penetrating wounds may transgress the pericardial contents. Although pericardial tamponade is much less common in blunt trauma, it should be suspected, particularly if there is a steering wheel injury, severe anterior chest trauma, or a fractured sternum.

If pericardial tamponade is diagnosed before the patient is in extremis, pericardiocentesis may be helpful in temporarily treating the patient. This is done by inserting a needle in the subxiphoid area (Larrey's point) at a 45-degree angle, aiming for the left shoulder. The V lead of an electrocardiogram clamped to the hub of the needle may assist the clinician in determining the location of the needle. As the needle is advanced, a noisy QRS is obtained that will invert when contact is made with the epicardial surface. Aspiration of as little as 10 ccs of blood may have dramatic results in reversing hypotension.

If the patient arrives in extremis or has a cardiac arrest from tamponade, immediate emergency thoracotomy is indicated. Preparation of the chest with an antiseptic solution is preferred but should not delay the procedure. With the nipple as a guideline, an incision should be made in the fourth intercostal space from the sternal border as far lateral as possible, angling toward the axilla. As soon as the chest is entered, the costal cartilage above and below the incision should be cut in order to improve access. A rib spreader, which should be immediately available in the emergency department, should be positioned and opened wide enough for insertion of two hands. The pericardium is then opened anteriorly and split in a longitudinal fashion, sparing the phrenic nerve as it runs along the lateral aspect. Clots should be quickly evacuated and if the patient still has spontaneous cardiac activity, obvious holes should be controlled by the physician's fingers. A primary repair may be done in the emergency department, avoiding injury to coronary vessels. A more desirable option is to do the definitive repair and closure of the chest in the operating room. If there is no spontaneous cardiac activity, open cardiac massage should be initiated with attempted electrical conversion to normal sinus rhythm when coarse fibrillation is obtained. Coarse fibrillation can be achieved with either cardiac or intravenous epinephrine and correction of pH. If resuscitation is successful, the patient should then be transported to the operating room for definitive care.

Myocardial contusion is usually a sequela of blunt trauma to the chest. The most lethal manifestations occur in the first hour following injury, usually secondary to arrhythmias. These are treated primarily with intravenous lidocaine. If cardiogenic shock becomes a problem, the best treatment is inotropic support with dopamine or dobutamine (see Chapter 3).

Myocardial infarction, particularly in older patients, must always be considered as a possible cause of pump failure after trauma. Conceivably, the patient may have had a myocardial infarction before injury or as a result of the hypotension associated with blood loss. Treatment of a suspected myocardial infarction is directed toward preventing arrhythmias and cardiogenic shock.

CARDIOVASCULAR VOLUME

In all severely injured patients rapid and adequate access to the circulatory system is essential. The most reliable low-risk method is via an intravenous cutdown, either in the long saphenous vein in the ankle or the median antecubital or basilic vein in the arm. An experienced surgeon can usually accomplish this in less than one minute. If the resuscitator is experienced with the techniques, percutaneous insertion of a subclavian, internal jugular, or femoral vein line is acceptable. Ideally, one central line should be available to monitor central venous pressure during resuscitation. One should avoid inserting a line in an extremity if it is the site of obvious injury or if there is a proximal injury; that is, do not use a leg vein if an injury to the inferior vena cava is suspected.

As the first intravenous line is being established, blood should be drawn for typing and crossmatch, hematocrit, and white blood count. Part of the specimen should be reserved to determine electrolytes, BUN, creatinine, amylase, blood sugar, and toxicology, if indicated by later history or subsequent course.

In general, two liters of balanced salt solution can be infused with impunity in the hypovolemic patient. (The choice of fluids is presented in Chapter 2.) The amount of fluid used will vary from patient to patient and should be determined using the indices outlined in Table 1–2. (Also see Chapter 2.)

HEMORRHAGE

The most extreme example of hemorrhage is the patient in cardiac arrest from hypovolemia. In such an instance, the only chance for salvage is immediate emergency thoracotomy and open chest cardiac massage. It is

TABLE 1–2. INDICES OF SUCCESSFUL RESUSCITATION

1. Adequate peripheral perfusion (capillary refill in nail beds <1 sec)
2. Level of consciousness (alert, oriented in non-head injuries)
3. Blood pressure (> 100 systolic)
4. Urine output (> 0.5 cc/kg/hr)
5. Atrial filling pressures (keep between 3–8 Torr)

impossible to resuscitate an empty heart with closed chest massage. The emergency thoracotomy also allows access to the descending aorta that can be controlled with a vascular clamp or, preferably, with the clinician's hand. More of the diminished volume that remains will then be directed to the heart and brain, the two organs critical for survival. As resuscitation progresses and the patient's volume is restored, it is important not to let the left ventricle distend.

Under less extreme circumstances the clinician must be aware of the likely locations of blood loss. Each hemithorax may contain up to two liters of blood. For this reason a chest x-ray is the minimal diagnostic test necessary before the patient is taken to the operating room. This can be extremely helpful to the surgeon in his surgical approach. Another highly suspect area of hidden blood loss is the abdomen. Distention is a late and very unreliable sign. If a patient is in shock and the chest x-ray is normal and there are no other external signs of bleeding, it must be assumed that there is intra-abdominal hemorrhage. The pelvis is considered part of the abdomen and can conceal large amounts of blood. Also, the thigh may contain from four to six units of whole blood after a major fracture or crush injury.

Obvious external bleeding is usually controllable with direct pressure. Tourniquets are rarely indicated except in the case of traumatic amputation. In some circumstances, antishock garments may be useful in temporarily controlling hemorrhage. If the patient arrives in the emergency department with an antishock garment already in place, it is imperative not to remove this until adequate intravenous lines are in place, hypovolemia has been corrected, and the surgeon is ready to treat the specific injury. In general, the antishock garment is best removed in the operating room with the surgeon prepared to treat the injuries definitively.

NEUROLOGICAL

Ideally, a neurological examination should be performed in the field or during transportation to the emergency department. One should definitely be performed as soon as possible after arrival in the emergency department. Repeated clinical examination is the most important assessment of neurological injury and may be all that is required to establish the need for exploratory burr holes and decompressive craniotomy (Table 1–3).

The neurological examination is covered in detail in Chapters 13 and 17. The essentials include assessment of hemispheric function (using a system such as the Glasgow coma scale), brain stem function (as indexed by cranial nerve function, motor activity, and respiration), and spinal cord function (by assessing motor activity, sensation, and bulbocavernous reflex) (see Table 1–3). Cervical spine fractures should be treated by maintaining axial orientation with Gardner-Wells tongs.

TABLE 1–3. CORRELATION BETWEEN CLINICAL SIGNS AND LEVELS OF BRAIN FUNCTION

Anatomic Region	Neurological Sign
Cerebral hemispheres	Verbal responses
	Purposive movements
Brain stem	Reflex motor movements
	1. Decortication
	2. Decerebration
Reticular activating system	Eye opening
Midbrain CN III	Reactive pupils
Pons CN V and VII	Corneal reflex
CN VIII, VI, III, and MLF	Doll's eyes; ice water responses
Medulla	Breathing; blood pressure
Spinal cord	Deep tendon reflexes; bulbocavernous reflex

If the patient's condition stabilizes as a result of resuscitation, further diagnostic tests such as CT scanning or arteriography or both may be warranted. This should be governed by both the clinical course and repeated neurological examination.

FRACTURE MANAGEMENT

Ideally, victims with major fractures should arrive in the emergency department with splints in place. Unsplinted fractures should be splinted as soon as possible after the initial resuscitation, to prevent further blood loss and neurovascular damage, reduce pain, and prevent continued microembolization. Open fractures should be cultured, Gram stained, and wrapped in clean dressings in preparation for irrigation and debridement in the operating room. If the patient's condition stabilizes during resuscitation, x-rays should be obtained of all areas where fractures, dislocations, or deformities are evident or suspected (see Chapter 20).

SUMMARY OF DEFINITIVE DIAGNOSIS

If the patient arrives in an unstable condition and this remains unstable, the only mandatory diagnostic test is a chest x-ray. If the patient arrives in a stable condition or the condition stabilizes after being unstable, definitive diagnostic tests may be used to determine the extent of the injury. The importance of repeated examinations, using the aforementioned guidelines, cannot be overemphasized. Serial hematocrits may be very useful in documenting ongoing bleeding or hidden blood loss.

Similarly, serial white counts may give a clue to peritoneal irritation. Plain films of the abdomen are helpful only in about one third of cases. The most useful evaluation of blunt abdominal trauma is repeated physical examination (see Chapter 10).

In lower chest or abdominal penetrating injuries, when violation of the peritoneum is unproved, peritoneal lavage or local exploration may be a useful diagnostic technique. Peritoneal lavage, however, is most useful in evaluating patients with blunt abdominal trauma, particularly those who are uncooperative, unconscious, paralyzed, or who might be lost to clinical follow-up for some period of time (e.g., those requiring an anesthetic for orthopedic or neurosurgical procedures and those requiring CT scans or arteriography).

If the patient has gross blood at the urethral meatus, a *urethrogram* should be obtained before insertion of a Foley catheter. A urethrogram should also be obtained if resistance is encountered while passing the Foley catheter. If the catheter passes readily and bloody urine is obtained, a *two-view cystogram* should be done. If the cystogram is negative, an intravenous pyelogram is indicated (see Chapter 11). Arteriography is also a useful adjunctive technique in the evaluation of the trauma patient. Table 1–4 lists the indications for arteriography. For further discussion, see chapters dealing with specific injuries.

In summary, the general surgeon is an integral member of the resuscitation team for all trauma patients. In most instances he will be "captain of the ship," directing and taking responsibility for the resuscitation. In addition, he is responsible for obtaining proper consultations and establishing priorities of management for the various injuries. This leadership role is critical and when executed smoothly will often favorably affect outcome.

TABLE 1–4. INDICATIONS FOR ARTERIOGRAPHY FOLLOWING TRAUMA

---

1. Neck injuries — Zones I and III

2. Chest injuries
   a. Mediastinal widening
   b. 1st rib fracture
   c. Deviation of trachea to the right (if no obvious pulmonary problem)

3. Abdominal injuries
   a. Nonvisualization of a kidney by pyelogram
   b. Selected pelvic fractures

4. All penetrating wounds of extremities in proximity to major vessels

5. Dislocation of the knee

6. All fractures associated with abnormal pulses

2

Blood and Fluid Replacement in Shock

Shock is currently defined as a clinical syndrome in which cellular hypoxia is the result or cause of a generalized state of severe circulatory inadequacy that produces alteration of substrate metabolism and accumulation of waste products within the cell. Reflecting these changes, shock is frequently described in terms of hemodynamic, endocrine, metabolic, and cellular consequences. As our understanding of these changes is fundamental to the rational management of the patient in shock, the physiological derangements are outlined as a preface to the section on treatment.

CIRCULATORY SYSTEM IN SHOCK

The complex circulatory response to shock (Fig. 2–1) involves alteration in cardiac function as well as changes due to autoregulation of arterial, venous, and lymphatic conduits. The site of origin of hemorrhage — vein or artery — and the rapidity of blood loss profoundly influence the vascular response. The various causes of shock (Table 2–1) have somewhat different initial hemodynamic responses. Depending on the success of resuscitation, the hemodynamic responses change during therapy.

Studies of hemorrhage in normal men indicate that 10 to 15 percent loss of blood volume is associated with minimal hemodynamic changes. When 15 to 25 percent loss of blood volume occurs, an otherwise healthy individual may remain normotensive unless the loss is very rapid, but the metabolic response to shock will be initiated. When blood loss exceeds 30 to 50 percent of blood volume, hypotension of a profound nature (less than 50 mm of mercury mean blood pressure) occurs with profound metabolic and cellular consequences.

The immediate cardiac and peripheral vascular responses to hemorrhage preserve blood flow to the heart and brain. The kidney, less essential to immediate survival than the heart and brain, is a third priority for

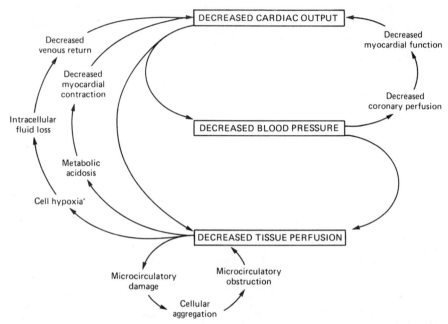

Figure 2-1. Vicious circles in shock. Initiation of the shock syndrome can occur at any point in the cycle. The initiating event may be volume, pressure, flow, or metabolically triggered. (From Dunphy JE and Way LW: Current Diagnosis and Treatment, 4th ed. Los Altos, Lange, 1979, p. 195.)

perfusion. The venous system, which contains 10 to 15 times more blood volume than the arterial system, is significantly involved in this compensatory response. The capacitance blood vessels have *volume* effectors; arteriolar sphincters are *pressure* effectors, and constitute the resistance system. In severe shock (BP<60 mm Hg), the venous system is unable to compensate by increasing blood volume to the heart. Hypovolemic shock is characterized by decreases in (1) pulmonary artery wedge pressure, (2) central venous pressure, (3) diastolic filling of the heart, (4) cardiac stroke volume, and (5) systemic arterial pressure.

Changes in both blood pressure and blood volume stimulate baroreceptors that activate the sympathetic neurohumoral axis. The afferent limb of the neurohumoral axis consists of baroreceptors located in the atrium, carotid and aortic sinuses, and pressure and volume impulses that are received by the hypothalamus and the vasomotor center in the medulla. The efferent arm of the reflex arc is the sympathetic nervous system, which releases catecholamines, as does the adrenal medulla. Catecholamines have inotropic and chronotropic effects on the heart and cause arteriolar vasoconstriction, with consequent reduction of blood flow to the liver and mesenteric vessels.

Clinical signs of diminished blood volume are increased pulse rate,

TABLE 2–1. COMPARISON OF EFFECT AND TYPE OF SHOCK

	Hypovolemic	Septic	Cardiogenic	Neurogenic
Cardiac index	↓ ↑	↑ ↓	↓ ↓	↑
Peripheral resistance	↑	↓	↑	↓ ↓
Venous capacitance	↓ ↓	↓	↑	↑
Blood volume	↓ ↓	↓	↑	→
Core temperature	→ ↓	↑ ↓	→	↓
Metabolic effects	Effect	Cause	→	→
Cellular effects	Late	Cause	→	→

*Most identifiable responses to shock are sequential and may change during resuscitation, i.e., ↑ ↓.

narrowing of pulse pressure, diminution of urine output, and cooling of the skin. Postural hypotension occurs when significant loss (>20 percent blood volume) has occurred. Tachypnea commonly occurs in response to hypovolemia because neural control of respiration is also influenced by blood volume.

In addition to responding to shock, the heart and circulatory system are end organs. "Toxic" factors have been postulated to explain ineffective cardiac function in the late phases of "irreversible" shock when selective vasodilatation occurs. The practicing physician, however, cannot accept so vague a concept as "irreversible shock" as the explanation for the patient's condition, and must constantly seek definite explanations. One contributory factor to this terminal state is often a shock-induced coagulopathy.

ENDOCRINE RESPONSE TO SHOCK

The endocrine response to shock largely functions to conserve extracellular fluid volume. Shock initiates the secretion of catecholamines from the hypothalamus, which stimulates the secretion of hormones of the posterior pituitary gland. Decreased blood flow to the hypothalamus results in increased corticotropin (ACTH) levels. Increased corticotropin stimulates the adrenal cortex to release cortisol, which has salt-retaining, inotropic, and catabolic effects. Antidiuretic hormone (ADH), elaborated by the hypothalamus and posterior pituitary gland, is increased when hypotension, hypovolemia, or lowered serum osmolality occur. Antidiuretic hormone increases water resorption by the nephron. Release of aldosterone in shock by the adrenal gland causes renal retention of salt. The permeability to water of the renal collecting duct is mediated by the hypertonicity of solute (primarily within the renal medulla) by sodium chloride and urea concentrations. High medullary concentrations of solute facilitate the excretion of both urea and potassium, which increase in shock as muscle protein catabolism occurs.

During shock, reflex relaxation of the afferent arterioles decreases renal vascular resistance. When blood pressure falls below 60 mm of mercury, renal autoregulation cannot accommodate the diminished blood flow. Low renal blood flow plus increased aldosterone and antidiuretic hormone secretion in shock, causing salt and water retention, results in a fall in glomerular filtration rate (GFR) and decreased urine volume.

In shock, the kidney releases renin from the juxtaglomerular apparatus, which is converted into angiotension I, and is subsequently converted into angiotension II, a potent vasopressor. When the vasopressor is released, afferent arteriolar constriction occurs and glomerular filtration rate decreases still further. A urine output less than 50 cc/hr in an adult patient in shock is a characteristic response to decreased peripheral perfusion.

METABOLIC AND BIOCHEMICAL EFFECTS OF SHOCK

The shock syndrome is associated with a complex but incompletely understood endocrine response that is probably initiated by the release of catecholamines. The metabolic response to shock (Table 2–2) is associated with conversion of protein, carbohydrate, and fat into energy. Insulin and glucagon levels are elevated in shock and are associated with increased glucose, urea, and free fatty acid values. Moreover, increased glycogenolysis and gluconeogenesis result in an increased glucose pool, with elevation of blood sugar. Lipolysis of fat stores results in an elevation of free fatty acids and triglyceride levels. In spite of increased availability of substrate in shock, as contrasted with normal or starved states, less effective utilization of energy occurs.

Carbohydrate metabolism is profoundly affected by shock (Table 2–3). The aerobic pathway for formation of adenosine triphosphate (ATP) through the tricarboxylic acid (TCA) cycle is the preferred glycolytic pathway under normal conditions. The TCA cycle for formation of ATP from glucose consists of degradation of glucose into three-carbon sugars, which are oxidized to water and carbon dioxide. In liver, adipose tissue, adrenal cortex, thyroid gland, and erythrocytes, five-carbon sugars are

---

TABLE 2–2.   METABOLIC EFFECTS OF SHOCK

- Hyperventilation
- Respiratory alkalosis
- Metabolic acidosis
- Retention of Na, H_2O
- Excretion of nitrogen, P_i, K^+, Mg^{++}, Zn^{++}, S

TABLE 2–3. BIOCHEMICAL EFFECTS OF SHOCK

- Glucose intolerance
- Increased gluconeogenesis
- Glycogenolysis
- Insulin elevation
- Glucagon elevation
- ↑ Synthesis triglycerides, FFA lipoprotein, acute phase protein
- Low inorganic phosphate

aerobically converted into three- and six-carbon sugars, which enter the metabolic pathway through the hexose monophosphate shunt.

When cellular hypoxia occurs, the pyruvate–acetyl CoA enzyme reaction is inhibited and carbohydrate metabolism proceeds through a less efficient anaerobic cycle. Because glucose metabolism is unable to proceed into the TCA cycle, pyruvate is converted to lactate. Acidosis occurs in shock because lactate, acetone, and amino acids accumulate in the serum because of failure to enter aerobic energy pathways.

Protein alterations in shock are characterized by increased liberation from muscle of amino acids and decreased uptake of amino acids by the liver. Mobilization of amino acids provides the major source of glucose for energy following injury through the process of gluconeogenesis. Degradation of amino acids for utilization as energy sources results in increased urinary excretion of nitrogen, zinc, phosphate, potassium, and sulfur. Nitrogen balance and excretion, therefore, are useful clinical indices of metabolic expenditure and the magnitude of injury, reflecting protein degradation.

Lipid metabolism is also significantly altered by low-flow states. Fatty acids and glycerol are normally incorporated into the energy pathway at the pyruvate–acetyl CoA step. Catecholamine elevation in shock initiates lipolysis by accelerating the liberation of triglycerides. Fatty acid release is also enhanced by increased serum levels of thyroid and glucocorticoid in shock. Although fats quantitatively supply more energy than glucose, their utilization in ATP generation may be associated with significant acidosis. Moreover, the stressed patient probably utilizes lipid less effectively than glucose.

THE CELL IN SHOCK

The cellular consequences of shock ultimately determine life or death. When the cell membrane potential falls within the range of −90 millivolts to −60 millivolts, a state approaching "irreversible" shock is reached. In shock of this severity, the cell gains sodium and loses potassium. Even specialized tissues such as skeletal muscle, neurons, and connective tissue are affected by these electrolyte shifts. If shock of this magnitude is rapidly corrected by resuscitation, recovery of the cell is possible.

When electrical activity of the cell is impaired and ion transport is altered by shock, sodium and potassium ATPase pump activity, stimulated by an increase in intramitochondrial sodium, fails. This alteration in cellular membrane transport may be the initiating event in cellular injury. Increased sodium potassium ATPase activity in response to cellular sodium results in degradation of ATP and accumulation of inorganic phosphate. The glycolytic cycle is driven by the need to replenish ATP but is inhibited by the oxygen-dependent pyruvate–acetyl CoA step, during which energy molecules leave the anaerobic glycolytic cycle and enter the aerobic tricarboxylic acid cycle (TCA). The extracellular pH falls because lactate, hydrogen ions, and metabolic waste accumulate during the low-flow state.

Ultrastructural changes associated with shock are probably a result of alteration in the membrane system. Morphologic changes that occur early in the course of severe shock include clumping of nuclear chromatin with dilatation of endoplasmic reticulum as the cell becomes edematous. Polysomes become detached from the membrane of endoplasmic reticulum and are scattered and fragmented in severe shock, an alteration that results in defective protein synthesis. The cell membrane becomes unstable and vesicles are formed as cell death approaches.

SOLUTIONS AVAILABLE FOR TREATMENT OF SHOCK

Regardless of the cause of shock, treatment is broadly directed at timely restoration of circulatory adequacy and efficient oxygen transport, to prevent cell death. The details of resuscitation and monitoring are included in Chapter 3. The response to initial resuscitation and other forms of therapy determine the need for progressive sophistication in monitoring. The ideal fluid for resuscitation of the patient in shock should restore extracellular fluid volume, exchange oxygen for metabolic waste at the cellular level, restore substrate lost in shock, and be free of adverse effects. Because the ideal solution is unavailable, rational fluid resuscitation utilizes available products that approximate the ideal solution (Table 2–4).

TABLE 2–4. **CRYSTALLOID SOLUTIONS**

Isotonic sodium chloride
Hypertonic sodium chloride
Balanced salt solution
1. Ringer's lactate
2. Ringer's acetate
3. Normosol, Plasmolyte, etc.

Although formulas have been developed for the treatment of patients in shock, particularly those with burn shock, the volume of fluid administered is based primarily on response to therapy as determined by physiological monitoring. Although crystalloid solutions are the preferred initial resuscitation fluid, it is incorrect to assume that they are a replacement for blood. Proper resuscitation should proceed in stepwise fashion from initial resuscitation with crystalloid to administration of blood, depending on the evolution of the clinical situation.

A central controversy in the management of shock has been the selection of a colloid or crystalloid solution as the preferred fluid for resuscitation. Both colloid and crystalloid solutions expand the extracellular space and are effective in the treatment of volume loss. Crystalloid solutions are favored for initial resuscitation because they are inexpensive, do not require compatibility testing with the patient, do not transmit infectious disease, and restore ions lost in shock. Although colloid solutions have been thought to have the theoretical advantage of maintaining fluid in the intravascular space and producing less pulmonary interstitial edema, available data from both patient and animal studies suggest that crystalloid solutions are at least as effective as colloid solutions in avoiding pulmonary edema.

A number of crystalloid solutions are available for resuscitation. The pure dextrose solutions are inappropriate in most instances, because they add water and lack ions. Solutions that combine dextrose with electrolytes may be of use if shock is associated with hypoglycemia, as may occur in the terminal phase of septic shock. Most patients with shock, however, have elevated blood sugar values secondary to gluconeogenesis and glycogenolysis, and are not benefited by parenteral administration of glucose.

Saline solutions are unsatisfactory resuscitation fluids because they lack other ions such as potassium and may cause hyperchloremic acidosis if given in large volume or in hypertonic form. In addition, saline solutions administered in large volume result in an excessive sodium load.

Ringer's lactated solution is a popular resuscitation solution containing isotonic quantities of anions and cations. Although it was originally suspected that the lactate in Ringer's might add to the lactic acidosis of shock, it is now known that administered lactate is converted to bicarbonate if liver blood is restored by resuscitation. Second generation electrolyte solutions frequently contain magnesium instead of calcium, and acetate instead of lactate. Acetate is easily metabolized to bicarbonate, but excessive administration may result in metabolic alkalosis. One disadvantage associated with use of a calcium-containing balanced salt solution such as Ringer's lactated solution is the potential of thrombosis formation in the intravenous tubing when one moves from crystalloid to blood administration. When this situation occurs, the calcium in the crystalloid solution partially reverses the anticoagulating effect of citrate, resulting in a blood clot, which may cause coagulopathy, bleeding, or shock or all of these. Consequently, when intravenous solutions containing calcium and possibly magnesium are being administered, the intravenous tubing should be flushed with saline prior to administration of blood products. However, for practical purposes, most balanced salt solutions are acceptable fluids for initiating resuscitation of a patient in shock.

Plasma substitutes are more popular in Europe than in the United States. Dextran, with a molecular weight of 70,000, is available as a plasma expander. Dextran retards platelet aggregation and can be employed as an anticoagulant, if given in excess of 1000 cc. While dextran also lowers blood viscosity, which may be advantageous in patients with shock, it also has some disadvantages. If given in the volume commonly required for resuscitation (>1000 cc), dextran may produce coagulopathy. Also, dextran coats the red blood cell and increases the difficulty of crossmatching blood for transfusion, so blood should be crossmatched *before* dextran is administered.

A number of oxygen-containing solutions are currently under investigation. Stroma-free hemoglobin (SFH) is an oxygen-carrying solution that does not require compatibility testing, and has the potential for being valuable in resuscitation. However, SFH has the disadvantages of a high affinity of hemoglobin for oxygen, and may produce intravascular coagulation. Perfluorochemicals (fluorocarbons) are chemicals that dissolve and carry oxygen within the body after intravenous administration. The chemicals have been administered with safety to human volunteers and have been used in place of blood in clinical situations requiring blood transfusion, as in patients who belong to Jehovah's Witnesses, a religious sect that proscribes receiving blood transfusion. Although perfluorochemicals are experimental drugs requiring an Investigative New Drug (IND) permit, selected approval for use has been granted by the Food and Drug Administration (FDA). The problems associated with the development of perfluorochemicals as blood replacements are (1) slow excretion of the chemicals from the body, (2) the need to keep current preparations frozen to maintain stability, and (3) lack of information about potential long-term effects. In addition, convincing efficacy studies are lacking. It remains to be determined if this family of chemicals has a role in hemotherapy.

AUTOLOGOUS TRANSFUSION

The intraoperative and preoperative salvage of blood for transfusion to the patient has distinct advantages over use of liquid preserved blood as a transfusion product. A patient who receives his own blood avoids the risks of homologous blood, which include isoimmunization, disease transmission, and hemolytic reactions. Although preoperative donation of blood components is currently common practice for elective surgery, it is seldom a practical alternative to banked blood in emergencies.

Autotransfusion, however, is possible in some trauma situations and will probably become more extensively used in the future. More extensive use of autotransfusion will depend on the availability of banked blood and improvement in autotransfusion systems. Nevertheless, simple methods of autotransfusion are already within the scope of most hospitals.

The simplest method of autotransfusion involves the collection of blood from a chest tube and drainage into receptacles containing citrate anticoagulant. When an extensive hemothorax is treated by placement of a chest tube into the pleural space, the chest tube can be temporarily clamped while tubing is attached, which allows the blood to be collected in a sterile bag or bottle containing the anticoagulant. The greatest value, as well as the most appropriate use, of autotransfusion of this nature is in patients with hemothorax exceeding 1000 cc. The collected blood is mixed with anticoagulant and returned to the patient without further processing or filtration while the patient is in the resuscitation area.

Collection of blood from the abdominal cavity, unlike from the thorax, usually requires a suction apparatus to aspirate blood. Hemoperitoneum is frequently associated with intestinal injury and contamination of blood by fecal material. Although intraperitoneal blood and intestinal contents have occasionally been reinfused into the patient without ill effects, it is undesirable to do so. Autotransfusion devices designated to aspirate blood from the operative field and wash it prior to reinfusion are advantageous when blood from the peritoneal cavity is autotransfused.

Although autologous transfusion devices have been used for intraoperative blood salvage for 100 years, the requisites of an ideal autotransfuser have yet to be completely achieved in any currently available apparatus. The characteristics of an ideal autotransfuser are low cost, ease of assembly and operation, rapid return of blood to the patient, and absence of air emboli and coagulopathies. In-line filtration to prevent reinfusion of microaggregates and other debris that could cause embolization or block the reticuloendothelial system is a desirable characteristic also. Red blood cell hemolysis is an undesirable feature of some autotransfusion units that have an extensive air-blood interface. Moreover, some available autotransfusion units require systemic anticoagulation, which is an undesirable requirement when hemorrhage is occurring. Although published reports describing autotransfusion units usually emphasize the simplicity with which the apparatus is employed, the most successful use of such equipment occurs when a skillful technician is available to operate the equipment.

Currently, four intraoperative autologous transfusion systems (ATS) are available that have somewhat different features. The PALL ATS, the Sorenson ATS, and the Haemonetics Cell Saver all operate from wall suction, while the Bentley ATS uses a roller pump to provide suction for intraoperative aspiration of blood. All available systems except the Haemonetics Cell Saver require complete or partial systemic anticoagulation.

All systems except the Haemonetics Cell Saver have been implicated in disseminated intravascular coagulation, whereas air embolism is a problem primarily with the Bentley ATS. The advantage of the Haemonetics Cell Saver over the other systems is that it is designed to wash and concentrate red blood cells. The washing process removes debris and anticoagulant and provides a final product with a high hematocrit. Moreover, it can be used preoperatively to collect and prepare platelets and red cell concentrates. Because the technique involves washing and concentration of red cells, a delay of 10 to 20 minutes is required before intraoperatively collected blood can be reinfused. The greater complexity of the Haemonetics system usually requires for operation of the equipment a technician who is not part of the operating team providing immediate care for the patient. If a hospital has a cardiopulmonary bypass team, the pump technician is the logical person to operate the autotransfusion system.

The advantages of intraoperative autotransfusion are obvious. The patient receives his own blood without the expense and risks involved in homologous blood transfusion, such as transmission of hepatitis and other diseases and transfusion reactions. No compatibility testing is required, and in some instances patients who are Jehovah's Witnesses will accept auto-transfused blood. The advantage of a self-contained blood resource in the event of natural disasters or unavailability of liquid preserved blood is an additional point in favor of autotransfusion systems. Although autotransfusion systems are not as yet used extensively, several centers have had favorable results using available apparatus. It is likely that additional technical advances in the development of such equipment will be accompanied by increased use of autotransfusion units.

BLOOD PRODUCTS AND COLLOID

Modern transfusion therapy is based on the assumption that blood products (Table 2–5) are administered to correct a specific hematological defect. Transfusion of whole blood or components is a graft of tissue from another individual unless the patient is receiving his own blood or that from an identical twin. Liquid preservation of blood at $4°$ C produces changes that are related to the duration of storage. Many of the preservation-related changes that occur during storage, however, are quickly corrected or produce different effects once the blood is received by the patient (Table 2–6).

Most whole blood in the United States is stored at $4°$ C in plastic bags, each of which contains 450 cc of donor blood plus 63 cc of citrate phosphate dextrose (CPD), an anticoagulant. Currently, 21 days of accepted storage life is allowed, although extension to 35 days has been approved by the Food and Drug Administration (FDA) for CPD-adenine preservative.

TABLE 2–5. **COLLOID SOLUTIONS**

A. Blood
    1. Low titer O Negative red cells
    2. Type-specific
    3. Typed and crossed
    4. Washed red cells
    5. Fresh warm blood
B. Plasma and its components
    1. Plasma — fresh frozen
    2. Albumin
    3. Plasmanate
C. Plasma substitutes
    1. Clinical dextran (MW 70,000)
    2. LMW dextran (MW 40,000)
D. Miscellaneous
    1. Stroma-free hemoglobin
    2. Hemacel, etc.
    3. Starch
    4. Fluorocarbons

Whole blood has been the standard product against which clinicians judge and compare the newer products. Red cell concentrates, formerly called packed red blood cells, are whole blood with two thirds of the plasma removed. Various levels of packing are possible; concentrates behave metabolically similarly to whole blood — except that less citrate, antigenic debris, phosphate, potassium, and negative thermal load are present. Washed red blood cells have most of the plasma fraction removed, which eliminates the disadvantages therein, decreases the level of immunization against red cell antigens, and possibly decreases the risk of disease transmission.

Frozen red cells retain the cell characteristics that existed just prior to freezing. For example, if the cells are frozen soon after collection, they function like fresh cells; if frozen near the end of liquid preservation, they retain many of the functional characteristics of older blood, as well as the defects of preservation.

TABLE 2–6. **PROPERTIES OF BLOOD**

	Bag	*Patient*
pH	Acid	Alkali
2,3 DPG	↓	↑
Citrate	↑	→
Phosphate	↑	↓ ↑
Ammonia	↑	→
K+	↑	↓
Platelets	↓	↓
Factor V	↓	↓
Factor VIII	↓	↑
Thermal load	↓	↓

RED CELL COMPONENTS

During liquid preservation, many alterations occur within the red blood cell. In 1966, it was demonstrated that the red blood cell's ability to load and unload oxygen was regulated by organic intraerythrocytic glycolytic intermediates, primarily 2,3 diphosphoglycerate (2,3 DPG). This important end product of red cell metabolism deteriorates to a nearly unmeasurable value by the end of the 21-day storage interval in CPD or ACD preservative. The commonly used preservative citrate phosphate dextrose (CPD) gives red cells approximately two weeks of relatively normal oxygen-carrying capacity. A recently licensed preservative solution, citrate phosphate dextrose–adenine (CPD–adenine), has been approved for 35 days of liquid preservation.

The fall in 2,3 DPG values that occurs at different rates in all citrate preservatives is accompaned by a decrease in the P_{50} of the oxyhemoglobin dissociation curve and an increase in saturation of the red cells.

Blood of extended shelf life contains red cells that have a high affinity of hemoglobin for oxygen and that have impaired ability to release oxygen to tissues.

PLATELETS AND CLOTTING FACTORS

Whole blood stored longer than three days in liquid preservation should be considered devoid of functioning platelets. Platelet concentrates contain 5.5×10^{10} platelets stored in 3 to 15 cc of plasma obtained from a single donor. Currently, platelets can be stored up to 72 hours in CPD, but are usually administered *within* 24 hours of collection. Moreover, storage of platelets at 4° C further impairs platelet function, as cold platelets are less effective in providing hemostasis than warm ones. ABO compatibility between donor and recipient is advisable when transfusing platelets. Compatibility for HL-A type reduces the immunization of the recipient and results in longer platelet survival after infusion. Administration of large numbers of platelets from a single HL-A matched donor can be carried out using techniques adapted from plasmapheresis, which is the most efficient form of platelet therapy. When repeated infusion of platelets is needed, plasmapheresis is the method of choice.

Leukocyte concentrates are being stored in several blood banks for patients with special susceptibility to infection. Current data would indicate little beneficial effect from leukocyte concentrates unless the recipient is markedly neutropenic on a transient level. The use of leukocyte transfusion is a new field still in the developmental phase.

With the exception of the labile Factors V and VIII, clotting factors deteriorate slowly during the storage of whole blood. By the end of the 21-day shelf life, levels of only Factors V and VIII are low enough to have clinical significance. In addition to deteriorating during the storage interval, Factors V and VIII are the products consumed in the process of coagulation, because they are attacked by plasmin. Fibrinogen is a potentially dangerous product with limited indications for use. Cryoprecipitate provides sufficient fibrinogen in an acceptably small volume for most uses with lower risk of transmitting hepatitis than fibrinogen infusion. Factor V is present in normal concentration in fresh frozen plasma (FFP). Factor VIII is present in FFP and in cryoprecipitate in a more concentrated form. Plasma has been removed from the U.S. market because of the high risk of hepatitis and the availability of safer alternatives.

The surgical patient with specific coagulation defects, exclusive of those caused by massive transfusion, is best managed in consultation with a hematologist. The use of FFP and specific clotting factors without documentation of coagulation defects in the usual massively transfused patient is of questionable value.

Both albumin and plasma protein fraction (PPF) are sometimes used to restore colloid osmotic pressure and are administered to expand extracellular fluid volume. Considerable controversy has occurred in recent years regarding the use of these products as opposed to crystalloid solutions. Current evidence suggests that, in most instances, crystalloid solution is preferable, because it is cheaper, equally effective, and with it the need for filters is avoided.

PROBLEMS OF MASSIVE BLOOD TRANSFUSION IN SHOCK

Massive transfusion may be clinically defined in the trauma patient as the infusion of 90 percent or more of the patient's blood volume within a three-hour period. Because blood in liquid preservation develops a "storage lesion," defects in preserved blood assume greater clinical significance in massive transfusion than in low-volume elective transfusion.

Because 2,3 diphosphoglycerate falls to undetectable levels by the end of the storage interval, an exchange transfusion with blood of extended shelf life replaces the patient's circulating blood volume with a red blood cell that has a high affinity of hemoglobin for oxygen. The defective hemoglobin function is accompanied by physiological changes in oxygen transport, such as increased cardiac output and oxygen extraction to meet basal oxygen needs. Because only part of the calculated oxygen utilization in resuscitation can be accounted for by measurable parameters, such as the cardiac output, venous oxygen tension, and P_{50} of the oxyhemoglobin dissociation curve, additional metabolic and circulatory defects in oxygen transport presumably occur.

Recovery of red cell oxygen transport function, as indicated both by the P_{50} of the oxyhemoglobin dissociation curve and by diphosphoglycerate values, is usually complete by 12 to 24 hours after transfusion. It remains unclear if blood containing hemoglobin with a high affinity for oxygen adds to or even significantly fails to correct the cellular hypoxia of shock any less satisfactorily than red cells of lower oxygen affinity.

For practical purposes, no special advantage of fresh blood over blood of longer shelf life can be clearly defined. Because blood available for transfusion can be assumed to lack functional platelets needed to produce the hemostatic plug that initiates blood clotting, the commonest coagulopathy caused by massive transfusion is dilutional thrombocytopenia. Platelet counts are frequently less than 100,000/mm³ in patients with major injury, and functional platelets often are less than 30 percent normal. However, bleeding from dilutional thrombocytopenia seldom occurs unless the platelet count is below 50,000/mm³. Unless low platelet counts are associated with bleeding or unless extensive further transfusion is anticipated, platelet transfusions are unnecessary. When needed, the proper treatment of transfusion-related thrombocytopenia associated with bleeding is administration of 10 platelet packs (fresh platelets removed from 10 donor units), unrefrigerated and less than 72 hours old.

Although levels of Factor V and Factor VIII decline during liquid preservation, massive transfusion is seldom accompanied by bleeding in which low levels of clotting factors are implicated as the cause of defective hemostasis. In fact, Factor VIII values are commonly elevated following massive transfusion as a consequence of increased Factor VIII production after injury. The massively transfused patient, however, may have simultaneous dilution of multiple clotting factors, which, combined with dilutional thrombocytopenia, may result in prolongation of clotting time. Unless associated with bleeding, often observed at the margin of incisions or at venipuncture sites, no specific treatment is required. When clotting time is prolonged and bleeding is present, fresh frozen plasma (FFP) is administered. This is done although specific documentation is lacking that plasma fractions are necessary in massive transfusion, since the primary cause of bleeding in this situation is usually insufficient platelets.

Citrate intoxication is an archaic term that refers to the binding of ionized calcium as a result of massive transfusion of citrate preservatives. The harmful effects of this condition — now known as hypocalcemia — are hypotension, narrowed pulse pressure, and elevated left ventricular end diastolic, pulmonary artery, and central venous pressures. Although commercially available electrodes allow evaluation of ionized calcium, they are technically imperfect and are infrequently used. Because hypocalcemia produces electrocardiographic abnormalities (prolonged Q-T interval), documentation of calcium deficiency is by serial electrocardiograms, which is a marginally satisfactory procedure. In general, most normothermic adults can withstand an infusion of one unit of blood every five minutes without requiring supplemental calcium. Supplemental calcium in the ionized form (calcium chloride) should be administered cautiously, for hypercalcemia may occur and may be fatal if calcium is given in excess. A common practice is to administer one ampule $CaCl_2$ (14.5 mEq) for every five units of blood products, if the rate of administration is greater than five units per hour.

Potassium concentration in stored blood increases to as much as 32 mEq per liter by 21 days of shelf life. Because patients receiving multiple units of blood have increased urinary excretion of potassium, significant hyperkalemia seldom occurs, unless a transfusion rate of 100 to 150 cc per minute is exceeded. Hyperkalemia is mainly a risk in patients with renal failure when hemodialysis and exchange resins are used to control elevated potassium values. Hyperkalemia, associated with hypocalcemia, may significantly alter cardiac function. Hyperkalemia is diagnosed by tall, peaked T-waves on the electrocardiogram, as well as by serum values, and is treated by administration of insulin and glucose.

THERMAL LOAD

Surgical procedures in the thoracic or abdominal cavities frequently result in lower body core temperature, as does blood stored at 4° C when rapidly administered. A decrease in temperature of less than 1° C can greatly increase oxygen consumption and cardiac output by causing shivering. Lowered temperature also increases the affinity of hemoglobin for oxygen, which is additive to the 2,3 DPG and alkalosis-caused increase in the red cell–oxygen affinity. Further temperature decline also impairs platelet function, and may contribute to bleeding complications, which result in increased need for transfusion. Citrate metabolism also suffers due to hypothermia, increasing the potential for hypocalcemia during massive transfusion.

Hypothermia is best prevented by warming the blood before administration, using a coiled tubing in a heating bath. Various commercial varieties of blood warmers are available. Radiant heat warmers offer the potential of instant warming of blood, but they produce hemolysis and are no longer used.

Although stored blood is intrinsically acid with a pH of about 6.4, the early result most often seen in the successfully resuscitated patient is a post-transfusion alkalosis. On metabolic conversion, the sodium citrate in the anticoagulant yields sodium bicarbonate, so that the end result of massive transfusion is not acidosis but alkalosis. Alkalosis initially increases red cell–oxygen affinity, but aids in restoration of 2,3 DPG values by enhancing red cell glycolysis. Post-transfusion alkalosis also causes increased potassium excretion, and is commonly associated with minimal hypokalemia.

MANAGEMENT STRATEGIES BASED ON
CLASSIFICATION OF HEMORRHAGE

The American College of Surgeons' Committee on Trauma has classified hemorrhage as follows:

Class I. Acute blood loss of 15 percent of blood volume, which induces minimal increase in pulse rate and respiration, is usually accompanied by normal blood pressure. Blanching of the nail capillary bed by pressure may be increased, suggesting peripheral vasoconstriction. The "tilt test," i.e., having the patient sit up for over 90 seconds without symptoms of vertigo or pulse drop, is usually tolerated. Examples of situations involving hemorrhage of this magnitude include a blood donation, pronounced epistaxis, most fractures, and minor injuries to solid intra-abdominal organs. Hemorrhage of this magnitude is treated by replacing the volume loss with balanced salt solutions such as Ringer's lactated or Ringer's with acetate. The quantity of crystalloid utilized in this and other instances of hemorrhage is based on the "3:1 rule." Three times as much crystalloid is administered as estimated volume loss because two thirds of the crystalloid infused diffuses into tissues and one third remains in the extracellular fluid space. It is unnecessary to administer blood products to patients with hemorrhage less than 15 percent of blood volume.

Class II. This is a major blood loss in which 20 to 25 percent of the circulating blood volume is lost. Clinical symptoms include tachycardia (> 120/minute), tachypnea (>24 to 30/minute), and hypotension. Hemorrhage of this magnitude is associated with a fall in cardiac output, an increase in peripheral resistance, and a narrowing of pulse pressure. The "tilt test" and the "capillary blanch test" are positive. Usually no diminution in urine output occurs in hemorrhage of this magnitude. Class II hemorrhage commonly occurs in pelvic and long bone fractures, contained vascular injuries, and splenic and liver trauma. Appropriate fluid therapy is with crystalloid solution in which three milliliters of crystalloid are

TABLE 2–7. **PRINCIPLES OF HEMOTHERAPY AND
FLUID RESUSCITATION**

Emergency Department
  Hemothorax — autotransfuse
  Crystalloid
  Type-specific or O Negative blood
Operating Room
  More than 10 units — platelets plus FFP
  Check clot for occurrence, presence retraction
  Use unseparated blood less than 3 days old
  Warm blood
  Blood gases
  ECG — K^+ and CA^{++}

---

administered for every estimated milliliter of blood loss; it is unnecessary to administer blood products to patients with hemorrhage of this magnitude. However, it is commonly unclear if the hemorrhage is controlled and anticipation of further hemorrhage may require transfusion while a patient is prepared for operation. Moreover, pelvic and long bone fractures may be associated with an initial hemorrhage of 25 percent, but continue to bleed over 24 to 48 hours and are best treated by early transfusion of red cell concentrates before more extensive blood loss occurs.

Class III. This is defined as 30 to 40 percent loss of circulating blood volume. All clinical signs and symptoms of shock previously described occur with hemorrhage of this magnitude, including fall in urine volume. Common injuries associated with Class III hemorrhage include splenic and hepatic rupture, vascular and thoracic injuries, and multiple trauma with fractures. Resuscitation begins with crystalloid solutions using the 3:1 rule but includes transfusion of blood products. Appropriate blood products are whole blood or red cell concentrates. If the patient's condition has not stabilized hemodynamically with crystalloid and whole blood is unavailable, red cell concentrates may be suspended in saline solution to lower the viscosity of the red cell concentrate to allow rapid transfusion.

Class IV. This is defined as loss of 40 to 50 percent or more of circulating blood volume. All signs and symptoms associated with lesser degrees of shock are present and accentuated. The patient usually lacks vital signs and is obtunded. Examples of injuries resulting in hemorrhage of this magnitude are uncontained vascular and thoracic injuries, severe injury to the liver, spleen, or kidney, and multiple trauma. Treatment involves the resuscitation plan system outlined in Table 2–7.

Because the magnitude of hemorrhage may be unappreciated on initial examination, diagnosis and treatment, regardless of the apparent "class" of shock, proceed in rapid succession as if all instances of hemorrhage have the potential for Class IV hemorrhage. The response to therapy and identification of the source and potential magnitude of hemorrhage dictate whether resuscitation proceeds beyond crystalloid resuscitation to use of specific blood products.

Initial management involves obtaining as extensive a history as possible, which should include the mechanism of injury and allergies. Physical examination is directed at initial treatment of life-threatening injuries. Cardiac arrhythmias or respiratory distress are immediately assessed and treated. Vital signs, including blood pressure, pulse, respiration, central venous pressure, level of consciousness, and urine output are measured initially and followed at 15-minute intervals until the patient's condition is stable. The adequacy of ventilation is assessed and oxygen is administered through nasal prongs or an endotracheal tube. Obvious bleeding is controlled by compression; tourniquets are used only if compression fails to control hemorrhage.

Vascular access is obtained promptly by two intravenous lines. Large-caliber percutaneous (16-gauge) venous silastic catheters are inserted into accessible arm veins. Frequently an antecubital vein cutdown is used for central venous pressure monitoring and fluid administration. Saphenous vein cutdowns with the insertion of tubing the size of intravenous tubing are useful in severely shocked patients. While venous access is being established, blood is obtained for typing and crossmatch, baseline hemoglobin, hematocrit, sodium, potassium, chloride, blood urea nitrogen, creatinine, and liver function tests. Arterial blood gas measurements (PO_2, CO_2, pH) are obtained. A catheter is placed in the bladder; urine is drained and analyzed. Hourly urine output measurements are performed as part of the monitoring routine.

When vascular access has been obtained, a fluid challenge of balanced salt solution is administered consisting of 200 cc over a 10-minute period, or 1000 cc over one hour, to determine the need for further fluid. If central venous pressure rises and urine output increases, a positive response indicating progress in resuscitation has occurred. If a rapid rise in central venous pressure (8 to 12 cm H_2O at heart level) occurs and does not decrease to normal CVP values (0 to 5 cm H_2O) within 10 minutes, fluid overload or restriction of cardiac output by tamponade, tension pneumothorax, or intrinsic heart disease should be suspected. If fluid overload has occurred, urine output will usually exceed 100 cc/hour and intravenous fluid therapy should be limited. Frequently, continuous fluid therapy is required to maintain urine output at 50 cc/hour.

As fluid therapy proceeds, blood products are prepared to supplement crystalloid for resuscitation. If continued high-volume crystalloid administration is required to maintain vital signs (>5 liters/hour), blood products should be administered. Appropriate use of blood products involves coordination with the blood bank. The initial blood product used if hemothorax is present is autologous whole blood collected from the chest tube into citrate preservative and infused without further processing. More commonly, stored products are employed, such as low-titer O Negative whole blood, the universal donor, which has been safely used in large volume in both civilian and military situations. Recently the Standards Committee of the American Association of Blood Banks has recommended that O Negative whole blood be discontinued as a product dispensed from blood banks. For that reason, in urgent situations in which the time required (45 minutes) for complete type crossmatch would delay transfusion, other hemotherapy options are employed. O Negative red cell concentrates can be diluted with 500 cc of saline solution to lower the viscosity and facilitate transfusion. A preferable plan is to utilize uncrossmatched blood that is type specific because the laboratory testing by slide test requires less than five minutes. Incompatibilities resulting from transfusion of type-specific uncrossmatched blood are usually minor, although delayed hemolytic anemia (7 to 21 days after transfusion), may occur from isoimmunization. Because lives continue to be lost because of the unwilling-ness to use uncrossmatched blood in exsanguinating patients, transfusion should not be delayed while a full crossmatch is completed.

Intraoperatively, a number of decisions need to be made regarding appropriate hemotherapy. The first decision involves an estimate of the amount and type of blood needed to complete the operation. If the patient has received an exchange transfusion (approximately 10 units or more) within a three-hour period, and continued massive transfusion is anticipat-ed, platelets are administered. The ability of the blood to clot is sequentially evaluated by the anesthesiologist's hanging a red-topped tube containing a sample of blood from the patient on the intravenous pole. If a clot is formed, this indicates that platelets are abundant enough to allow the clotting cascade to occur. The clot is then evaluated at 30- to 60-minute intervals for lysis, as consumption coagulopathy may result in bleeding from mismatched blood or tissue procoagulants from the injury. When 10 units have been administered and an additional 10 to 15 units of blood are likely to be required, the senior surgeon should communicate with the blood bank and possibly use unseparated whole blood in CPD preservative, which is less than 72 hours old and preferably warm. No other use of "fresh blood" is considered legitimate. Fresh whole blood including platelets provides all of the needed components. During the normal operating hours of the blood bank, the blood is administered prior to refrigeration to minimize hypothermia.

During convalescence from massive transfusion, patients frequently become anemic. The anemia may be due to excess extracellular fluid volume and may not reflect a true decrease in red cell mass. All patients with anemia after massive transfusion should be evaluated for delayed hemolytic reaction one to two weeks after the transfusion. In addition, they should be evaluated as to whether reticulocytosis is occurring. If the patient is anemic but asymptomatic and producing reticulocytes, no further transfusion therapy is warranted, regardless of the level of anemia.

RECOMMENDED READINGS

1. Gann DS: Endocrine control of plasma protein and volume. Surg Clin N Am 56:1135, 1976.
2. Gump FE et al: The significance of altered gluconeogenesis in surgical catabolism. J Trauma 15(8):704, 1975.
3. Trunkey DD, Sheldon GF: The treatment of shock. *In* Zuidema GD et al (eds): The Man-agement of Trauma. Philadelphia, WB Saunders Co, 1979, pp. 80–101.
4. Hemotherapy in Trauma and Surgery. A Technical Workshop. American Association of Blood Banks, 1979.
5. Hardy JD (ed): Critical Surgical Illness. Philadelphia, WB Saunders Co, 1980.

Chapter

3

Cardiopulmonary Resuscitation (CPR)

Cardiopulmonary resuscitation (CPR) in its broadest sense refers to those measures used to restore effective ventilation and circulation in persons who have sustained sudden, unexpected cessation of these functions. In 1973, a National Conference of Standards for CPR and Emergency Cardiac Care was held, and the principles developed were published in JAMA 227(7):833-868, 1974. Numerous other conferences have been held by the American Heart Association, American Trauma Society, American College of Emergency Physicians, the National Heart and Lung Institute, and the National Academy of Science Research Council on the subject of CPR, resulting in continued evolution in the scope and physiology of the recommended modes of therapy. Although CPR in general connotes forced, assisted ventilation and external cardiac massage, cardiopulmonary resuscitation in the victim of either blunt or penetrating trauma may require additional invasive maneuvers or adjunctive techniques that are ordinarily not applied.

PATHOGENESIS

The common denominator in all cases of cardiac arrest and sudden death is *anoxia*. Causes may include drowning, electrocution, cerebrovascular accident, smoke and gas inhalation, drug and chemical intoxication, head, neck, and upper airway injuries, myocardial infarction and convulsion, or unconsciousness from any cause. Anoxia and cardiac arrest in the patient who sustains trauma may be secondary to hypovolemic shock, cardiac tamponade, tension pneumothorax, massive tracheobronchial injury, fracture of the larynx, air emboli to the coronary arteries, massive air emboli to the right side of the heart, or traumatic asphyxia. The majority of trauma patients who sustain cardiac and respiratory arrest during the transportation and resuscitative phases have massive exsanguinating hemorrhage, obstruction of the airway, and complications of chest injury (tension pneumothorax, etc.) as the most common etiologies.

DEFINITIONS OF DEATH

Many states have a law defining death in terms of loss of cerebral function. Brain death occurs when there is loss of reflexes and spontaneous respiratory effort and when there is no evidence of activity on repeated electroencephalographic examination. Special allowance should be made when a patient is hypothermic or has taken drugs. Concepts of cortical death and cerebral death produce variations in some of the definitions of brain death. Clinical death occurs when there is absence of peripheral pulses, heartbeat, and effective circulation, when pupils are dilated and unresponsive to light, and when ventilation is absent. With absent circulation of oxygenated blood in the normothermic patient, the death of organs varies from organ to organ (three to five minutes for the brain to several hours for muscle mass).

PHYSIOLOGY

In cardiac arrest, hypoxemia rapidly ensues with acidosis, hyperkalemia, and other metabolic factors that can further contribute to disintegration of function. These factors in association with hypovolemia often present in the trauma patient produce a continued cycle resulting in progressive lowering of cardiac output and acidosis, which becomes more and more unresponsive if corrective measures are not taken immediately.

BASIC LIFE SUPPORT

Basic life support consists of emergency first aid procedures including recognition of respiratory and cardiac arrest and immediate institution of CPR. The CPR is continued until the patient recovers sufficiently to be transported or until advanced life support is available.

The advantage of CPR, especially in the patient who has a metabolic or medical cause for cardiac arrest, is that it may be immediately instituted by adequately trained personnel with no special equipment being necessary. Delay in initiating CPR may lead to irreversible hypoxic cerebral damage. Indications for instituting CPR include respiratory arrest, cardiac arrest from ventricular fibrillation, ventricular standstill, or absence of effective circulation for any reason. In the unconscious person, the adequacy or absence of effective ventilation and circulation must be determined immediately. If ventilation alone is inadequate, the establishment of an airway and artificial ventilation may be all that is required. If circulation is ineffective or absent, then artificial circulation must be started in combination with artificial ventilation.

The primary goals of CPR in the trauma patient are (1) establishment of an adequate airway and (2) preservation of existing circulatory dynamics. In general, CPR is most successful after heart attacks, particularly if the cardiac arrest is secondary to arrhythmias. If cardiac arrest is secondary to trauma, CPR is at best temporizing, since the patient almost invariably needs restoration of blood volume and control of hemorrhage.

CONTRAINDICATIONS TO CPR

Although there is widespread enthusiasm for the increasing use of resuscitative skills, CPR should not be attempted in some circumstances, including the following:

1. The victim of penetrating or blunt truncal trauma without pulse or respiration for a protracted period of time (approximately 10 minutes in the absence of hypothermia).
2. The patient with known disseminated, irreversible neoplastic disease or end-stage terminal medical illness.
3. The terminally ill patient who has expressly stated that no resuscitative efforts should be carried out.
4. The trauma victim with irreversible central nervous system injury.
5. Possibly the patient with 100 percent total-body full-thickness burn.

ARTIFICIAL VENTILATION

The basic steps required are maintenance or establishment of an adequate airway and assurance of adequate ventilation.

Ventilatory inadequacy may result from a mechanical obstruction to the airway, e.g., tongue, foreign bodies, vomitus, food, blood, or from respiratory failure. A partially obstructed airway is indicated by:

1. Noisy and labored breathing (stridor).
2. Use of the accessory muscles of breathing (sternomastoids).
3. Soft tissue retraction of the intercostal, supraclavicular, and suprasternal areas.
4. Paradoxical or "seesaw" breathing. Normally in the unobstructed airway, the chest and abdomen rise and fall together. If the airway is partially or completely obstructed and cardiac arrest has not occurred, the chest is sucked in as the abdomen rises.
5. Cyanosis. A circulating reduced hemoglobin level of < 5 gm% is often associated with clinical cyanosis. This is a late sign of hypoxia, especially if the patient is anemic.

Ventilatory failure is noted by minimal or absent chest or abdominal movements and an inability to detect air movement through the mouth or nose.

AIRWAY MANAGEMENT

The most important step for successful resuscitation is immediate opening of the airway. A head tilt is performed by placing one hand under the victim's neck, the other on the forehead. The neck is lifted with one hand and the head is tilted back with the other. This action extends the neck and lifts the tongue off the posterior pharyngeal wall. The head must be maintained in this position. By observing the chest wall and listening at the victim's mouth, the rescuer can rapidly ascertain whether breathing is present or absent. Manipulation of the neck in the head tilt maneuver should be performed with extreme caution in the trauma patient with suspected neck injury.

If breathing does not commence, the rescuer performs four rapid mouth-to-mouth ventilations. The rescuer inhales deeply and applies his widely opened mouth to the victim's mouth and inflates the lungs. The nose must be occluded by pinching during this maneuver.

Adequate inflation can be verified by seeing the chest rise, sensing the resistance or "compliance" of the victim's lungs as they expand, and hearing the escape of air during exhalation.

Mouth-to-nose ventilation may be used if:

1. The mouth is impossible to open.
2. Serious injuries to the mouth are present.
3. Difficulty is experienced in obtaining a good seal with mouth-to-mouth breathing.

In these circumstances, the rescuer keeps the head tilted back with one hand on the forehead while the other hand is used to lift the victim's lower jaw; this closes the victim's lips. The rescuer then inflates the lungs by sealing his lips around the victim's nose and blowing.

Infants and Children. Airway management is similar to that in adults. The larynx in infants and small children lies more anteriorly so that overextension of the neck may obstruct the airway; consequently, the neck should be held in the midposition. The rescuer covers both the mouth and nose with his mouth, uses small puffs of air, and inflates the lungs once every three seconds.

Trauma Patients. If a possibility of neck fracture exists, caution must be exercised to avoid neck extension and all neck movements. The patient's head and neck should be kept in the neutral position. If there is evidence of upper airway obstruction, this can be overcome by two appropriate measures: inserting an oropharyngeal or nasopharyngeal tube, and performing protraction of the mandible (jaw thrust). If mouth-to-mouth respiration is necessary, the triple airway maneuver should be used. This consists of protraction of the jaw and sealing the nose with the rescuer's cheek while giving mouth-to-mouth ventilation.

Within the hospital, a patient with a suspected neck injury can have establishment of an airway through nasotracheal or orotracheal intubation.

Foreign Bodies.   The rescuer should not look for foreign bodies in the airway as an initial step, prior to instituting mouth-to-mouth ventilation. Inability to ventilate with proper neck extension will reveal this situation. If foreign bodies appear to be present, the victim should be rolled on his side away from the rescuer, and the jaw opened with thumb and index finger technique. The index finger of the other hand is used to explore the victim's oropharynx; this will permit identification and removal of large foreign bodies. When skilled personnel are available, direct laryngoscopy is indicated to remove the foreign body with forceps, followed by rapid endotracheal intubation after the victim has been ventilated with high oxygen concentrations from a bag-valve-mask unit. If a laryngoscope is not available, then three or four sharp blows with the heel of the rescuer's hand should be delivered between the victim's shoulder blades. The pharynx should be re-explored and attempts made to ventilate the victim.

The Obstructed Upper Airway.   Back blows as well as abdominal thrusts have been proposed as possible means of removing an obstructing foreign body trapped in the larynx. These incidents of choking are usually associated with ingestion of alcohol. Such an incident may occur in restaurants or at picnics, and is usually treated by nonmedical personnel. The classical signal of distress in patients with an acutely obstructed airway is a sudden clenching of the throat while the patient, still conscious, struggles for air. If back blows or abdominal thrusts are unsuccessful, mechanical removal of the obstructed material should be attempted.

TRACHEOSTOMY AND OTHER FORMS OF SURGICAL INTUBATION

In the prehospital phase, tracheostomy, cricothyroidotomy, cricothyroid membrane puncture and other surgical techniques should not, as a general rule, be attempted by nonsurgeons. Although reports of successful tracheostomy in the prehospital setting appear sporadically, the need for tracheostomy or cricothyroidotomy in the trauma patient, even in the emergency center, is rare. Indications for surgical establishment of the airway in the trauma patient include fracture of the larynx with obstructed airway, mid-face massive fracture with obstructed airway, or respiratory arrest when assisted ventilation cannot be provided through other means (mask and bag, endotracheal intubation, nasotracheal intubation). Except in extremely rare circumstances, surgical establishment of the airway should be performed by trained surgical personnel in the operating room rather than in the emergency center or in the field.

AIRWAY CONTROL TECHNIQUES

Control of the airway may be achieved with or without a technique involving cannulation. The noncannulation technique requires manipulation of the upper airway and on occasion assisted ventilation. Noncannulation control of airway embraces the following:

1. Head tilt
2. Chin lift
3. Forward displacement of the mandible
4. Intermittent positive pressure ventilation
5. Removal of foreign bodies
6. Oropharyngeal and nasopharyngeal mechanical airway devices

Cannulation control of airway may be established by:

1. Esophageal obturator airway
2. Orotracheal intubation
3. Nasotracheal intubation
4. Cricothyroidotomy
5. Transtracheal jet ventilation
6. Tracheostomy

GASTRIC DISTENTION AND ASPIRATION

The most common cause of gastric distention is an inadequate airway. Vomiting is an active reflex act, while regurgitation of stomach contents is a passive phenomenon based on a pressure difference between intragastric contents and the oropharynx, i.e., atmospheric pressure. The latter occurs in cardiopulmonary arrest. Significant aspiration of gastric contents with a pH of 2.5 or less is associated with a mortality of 50 to 60 percent in itself and is a common occurrence in cardiopulmonary arrest. Gross distention can be relieved by applying moderate pressure to the epigastrium. This should be done with the patient turned on his side, so that any gastric contents will drain out of the mouth by gravity.

RECOGNITION OF CARDIAC ARREST

This should take no longer than 10 seconds and requires in the first place only the observation that the victim remains unresponsive when shaken. Cardiac arrest is assumed if large vessel pulse and ventilation are absent and if there is unconsciousness with a deathlike appearance, confirmed by fixed dilated pupils.

In the unwitnessed arrest, the carotid pulse should be checked following four lung ventilations. While one hand tilts the head, the index finger of the other hand locates the victim's larynx and slides into the groove between the trachea and sternomastoid muscle. The carotid is selected over other arterial pulses as the main indicator for the following reasons:

1. Proximity, since the rescuer is at the victim's head.
2. The neck is readily available — no clothing has to be removed.
3. Because the carotids are large central arteries, their pulsation may still occur in low cardiac output states, after other peripheral pulses have disappeared. Femoral artery palpation is an acceptable alternative in hospital patients.

Absence or questionable absence of the carotid pulse is an indication for starting external cardiac compression (ECC). As the heart is compressed between the sternum and vertebral column, blood is ejected from the left ventricle; during relaxation, cardiac filling occurs. Properly performed ECC produces a cardiac output approximately 20 to 33 percent of normal, and must always be accompanied by artificial ventilation.

METHODS OF EXTERNAL CARDIAC COMPRESSION

1. Patient must be in a horizontal position.
2. Elevation of the lower extremities may augment venous return and cardiac output.
3. A firm surface is mandatory. A board or a tray placed under the victim's shoulders and thorax will suffice. If these are not immediately available, ECC should not be delayed, and placing the patient on the floor may be the best (quickest) method.
4. The rescuer places himself close to the victim's side, and locates the tip of xiphoid process. The heel of the hand is placed three fingerbreadths above this in the long axis of the sternum. The other hand is placed over the first one, the rescuer brings his shoulders directly over the victim's sternum, and with his arms and shoulders straight, exerts pressure vertically downward to depress the sternum 1½ to 2 inches in the adult. Compression must be smooth, regular, and uninterrupted. Relaxation immediately follows compression, but the heel of the rescuer's hand should not be removed from the sternum. No "bouncing" should occur.

The rate of ECC for two rescuers is 60/minute, and a ventilation is interposed after each fifth chest compression, giving a 5:1 ratio. Practice on a manikin is essential for all persons who perform CPR.

To maintain proper rate, the person compressing the chest must count loudly, "One–one thousand, two–one thousand" to "five–one thousand." Switching positions between rescuers is important, as properly performed CPR is hard work. This is accomplished by the ventilating rescuer moving to the side of the victim immediately following lung inflation. His hands are placed in the air next to the hands of the chest rescuer. As the chest rescuer removes his hands, usually after the third or fourth compression, the other rescuer finishes the sequence. The former chest rescuer is now at the victim's head, has it properly extended and is ready to inflate the lungs at the completion of the count of "five–one thousand."

The rate of compression of the single rescuer is 80/minute. This rate is necessary to maintain an actual cardiac compression rate of 60/minute while interspersing two rapid lung inflations after each 15 compressions. The single rescuer can maintain the proper rate by counting "one and two and three . . . to fifteen."

Infants and Small Children. In small children, the heel of one hand is used; in infants the tips of the middle and index fingers. The pressure should be exerted at the midsternal area because in children the heart lies higher in the chest than it does in the adult, and the danger of liver laceration is highest in this group. Infants require ½ to ¾ inch of sternal compression; children ¾ to 1½ inch. The compression rate is faster, 80 to 120/minute, and breaths are delivered as rapidly as possible at the completion of every fifth compression. A firm support can be provided by the chest compressor using his other hand under the thorax, or a folded blanket may serve the same purpose. In small infants, an alternative method is to encircle the chest with both hands and compress the midsternum with both thumbs.

Effectiveness of CPR

1. Pulse. The carotid pulse should be checked periodically during CPR to gauge the adequacy of chest compression. It should always be checked when rescuers change positions.

2. Pupils. The reactivity of pupils is the best gauge of the effectiveness of CPR. Pupils that constrict to light and remain small indicate that the cerebral circulation is probably adequate. Widely dilated pupils that are nonresponsive to light indicate that serious hypoxic brain damage is imminent or has already occurred.

3. Color. Peripheral circulation may be evaluated by periodically squeezing the earlobes and noting capillary refill time.

4. Consciousness. The victim may make respiratory or other movements; these suggest adequacy of CPR but do not necessarily mean CPR should be discontinued. On the contrary, efforts should be continued if a definite pulse cannot be detected when ECC is stopped tentatively.

Technique in the Witnessed Arrest

1. Tilt the head, open the airway, and simultaneously feel the carotid pulse.

2. If there is no breathing, give four quick ventilations.

3. If vital signs and ventilation are not restored within seconds, begin single rescuer CPR.

TECHNIQUE IN THE MONITORED PATIENT

This is to be used in patients who have a sudden ventricular fibrillation (VF) or ventricular tachycardia (VT) without an effective pulse.

1. Check the monitor for cardiac rhythm and simultaneously feel for a carotid pulse.
2. If there is VF or VT, administer countershock with 500 watt-seconds from a DC defibrillator.
3. Recheck pulses; if absent, follow with four quick ventilations.
4. Recheck the carotid pulse; if absent, start CPR.

RULES FOR CPR PERFORMANCE

1. CPR should not be interrupted for longer than five seconds because effective circulation falls to zero in that time. The single exception to the rule not to interrupt CPR is an interruption to allow endotracheal intubation. This is an advanced life support measure and should be performed only by experienced personnel, and only after prior initial airway management, and after proper equipment becomes available. It should not take longer than 5 to 10 seconds to intubate the patient.
2. In penetrating wounds about the heart or when there is evidence of recent cardiothoracic surgery, closed chest massage is usually contraindicated and open thoracotomy is generally advisable.
3. Chest compression and relaxation should be smooth, regular, and uninterrupted. Quick jabs increase the possibility of injury to the victim and do not improve cardiac output.
4. In order to perform effective compression, to obtain normal cardiac output and to prevent rescuer fatigue, the rescuer must be high enough above the victim, and vertical pressure on the sternum must be used.
5. Ventilation must be interposed between compressions, but the chest compressor should not break the compression and relaxation rhythm to wait for the lungs to be inflated by the second rescuer.

POTENTIAL PROBLEMS IN CPR

1. Compression of the lower sternum may result in abdominal visceral lacerations.
2. Malposition of the hands on the ribs or lateral instead of vertical compression increases the likelihood of fractured ribs and a flail chest.

3. Other complications include fractured sternum, costochondral separation, pneumothorax, hemothorax, liver lacerations, and fat embolization. These can occur with a properly conducted CPR but are far more likely to occur with improper technique.

ADVANCED LIFE SUPPORT

Airway and Ventilation. Ventilation with rescuer-expired air delivers 16 to 18 percent oxygen. Enrichment with a high inspired oxygen is highly desirable in view of the low cardiac output and the presence of large intrapulmonary shunts. Even in the presence of high inspired oxygen tensions, arterial tensions are often very low.

Bag-Valve-Mask Units (BVMU). These are composed of a self-inflating bag with unidirectional valves, to which a mask is fitted and which is applied over the patient's mouth and nose. The units basically operate by providing unidirectional flow to the patient during bag compression and allow expiration to the atmosphere.

A clear facemask should be used for observation of the patient's mouth for vomitus.

The use of these BVMU's requires training and practice. They should be used with oxygen enrichment whenever possible. With 10 to 15 liters of oxygen added to the units, without a reservoir system, the oxygen concentration never exceeds 40 to 45 percent. BVMU's with reservoir systems provide oxygen concentrations in excess of 70 percent.

BVMU's have several advantages. With them mouth-to-mouth contact is avoided. They enable a high oxygen concentration to be delivered. If properly used, they will deliver a tidal volume of 700 to 1100 ml, and they may be connected to a standard 15 mm endotracheal tube adaptor.

Among disadvantages of BVMU's are that they may not be instantly available, and they provide less tidal volume than does mouth-to-mouth ventilation. A good mask fit and training in proper airway management are essential for their use. A further disadvantage involves mechanical problems that may occur.

MASKS

Various sizes should be available. The rescuer must position himself at the victim's head and extend the neck with jaw protraction. This is accomplished by placing the little finger at the angle of the mandible, the ring finger at the middle of the ramus, and the third finger at the symphysis menti. The index and thumb hold the face mask in position, tightly applied over the nose and mouth. The most effective means of learning this technique is to practice on volunteers.

Oropharyngeal Airways

In patients in whom adequate head and neck positioning have been carried out and ventilation is not possible, an oropharyngeal airway introduced after opening the jaw holds the tongue away from the posterior pharyngeal wall. This ensures an adequate airway, provided that there is no distal obstruction. Oropharyngeal airways should be used only in unconscious patients, since their introduction into conscious or stuporous patients may induce vomiting or laryngospasm. Incorrect placement may displace the tongue into the pharynx and cause complete obstruction of the airway. They should be used only with bag-valve-mask units.

Endotracheal Intubation

Adequate oxygenation with the BVMU should generally be accomplished prior to endotracheal intubation. If the patient is vomiting, endotracheal intubation may be more urgent. This is usually a semielective procedure, although rapid, effective intubation following bag-mask ventilation and high oxygen concentrations is very desirable to avoid aspiration of gastric contents. The vast majority of victims can be effectively ventilated with mouth-to-mouth breathing or BVMU. Experience is needed to achieve rapid intubation, because unskilled and often fruitless attempts at laryngoscopy and intubation are harmful to the patient. The oral route is the most rapid and should be accomplished in under 15 seconds. Decompression of the stomach, which always contains excessive amounts of air, should be carried out routinely via a nasogastric tube following intubation.

Nasotracheal Intubation. In patients with respiratory arrest, in patients with suspected cervical fracture, and in patients with penetrating injuries of the neck in whom there is a cervical hematoma or hematoma at the thoracic outlet, nasotracheal intubation is extremely beneficial and safe. The neck need not be hyperextended. Nasotracheal intubation can be done with the patient awake, without producing gagging, straining, retching, or vomiting. An endotracheal tube of sufficient length, usually 7.0 to 7.5 mm in diameter, is inserted through the nares into the hypopharynx. As the patient breathes, one listens to the respiration and slowly advances the tube. As the tube is just above the cords and at the time of maximum inspiration, the tube is rapidly advanced between the cords and the balloon inflated. This technique is also applicable to patients who are having seizures, patients in diabetic ketoacidosis and others in whom orotracheal intubation is deemed unsatisfactory. Topical anesthesia of the nares and nasopharynx is helpful in the conscious patient.

Esophageal Obturator Airway

This airway consists of a cuffed endotracheal tube mounted through a clear facemask, and modified by a soft plastic obturator blocking the distal orifice. Multiple openings are situated in the upper one third of the tube at the level of the pharynx. This airway is introduced blindly into the esophagus and the cuff is inflated after the mask is sealed over the face. When mouth-to-tube or bag-to-tube ventilation is performed, air or oxygen is discharged through the holes in the pharyngeal tube and passes into the trachea, because the esophagus is blocked. This mitigates against regurgitation of gastric contents and aspiration. An esophageal obturator airway should be used only in comatose patients who are not breathing. This device is being used effectively by well-trained rescue squads in the field but has no place in the hospital.

The tube should be left in place until endotracheal intubation has been accomplished. If it is removed prior to intubation, a rush of gastric contents under pressure may flood the pharynx and be aspirated. Finally, it should be recognized that these tubes may cause esophageal perforation.

Oxygen-Powered Mechanical Breathing Devices

Conventional pressure-cycled ventilators, positive-negative pressure resuscitators, and resuscitator inhalators should not be used with ECC. Cardiac compression triggers termination of the inflation cycle resulting in inadequate or no ventilation.

Time-cycled volume limited devices are effective because they provide adequate instantaneous high flow rates, adequate pressures, and 100 percent oxygen. However, BVMU's are equally effective and are usually available and easy to use.

Automatic Chest Compressions

These are useful for prolonged ECC, such as during transportation. They are not to be used prior to the manual methods. They provide effective ECC, relieve operator fatigue, and simultaneously provide time-cycled volume ventilation with 100 percent oxygen. Disadvantages are that they are expensive, heavy and difficult to move around, are available for adults only, and require extensive training of personnel prior to use.

Internal Cardiac Massage

This is strictly an in-hospital procedure carried out in special circumstances when ECC is ineffective in the intubated patient. A suitably trained physician with the necessary equipment should carry out a thoracotomy through the left fifth intercostal space. The pericardial sac is opened to allow direct manual cardiac compression. The circumstances under which this should be considered include:

1. Penetrating wounds of the heart, internal thoracic injuries, and cardiac tamponade.
2. Chest or spinal deformities.
3. Severe emphysema.
4. Flail chest.
5. Air embolism.
6. Previous cardiac surgery.
7. Hypovolemic cardiac arrest.

Antishock Trousers

Antishock lower extremity and abdominal compression devices have been marketed recently. These devices assist in stabilization of fractures, perhaps decrease bleeding from pelvic fractures, are helpful in stabilizing the condition of patients who must be transported over great distances, and may increase the cardiac afterload with resultant increase in the systemic blood pressure. There is a potential theoretical advantage of a moderate compression of the lower extremity to increase the truncal intravascular volume, but the amount is unknown. The examining physician treating a patient who arrives with antishock trousers placed during the prehospital phase should be cognizant of the fact that these trousers should not be removed until intravascular volume has been restored. Because of marked reduction in the cardiac afterload, hypotension will ensue if the trousers are deflated in the hypovolemic patient.

Electrocardiographic Monitoring

ECG monitoring should be established immediately in the emergency department in patients who present with symptoms and signs suggestive of a myocardial infarction or shock. Most sudden deaths following acute myocardial infarction are due to arrhythmias, and they are particularly likely to occur in the first 24 hours. Early detection and appropriate therapy can avert potentially lethal situations. Advanced life support training must establish the capability of recognizing arrhythmias and prescribing necessary therapy. The most common arrhythmias include:

1. Cardiac standstill (or VA)
2. Bradycardias (cardiac rate < 60/minute)
3. Supraventricular and infraventricular tachycardias (VT)
4. Premature ventricular contractions (PVC)
5. Ventricular fibrillation (VF)
6. Atrioventricular blocks of all degrees
7. Atrial fibrillation and flutter

An ECG is not an index of cardiac output or tissue perfusion.

DEFIBRILLATION

Direct current defibrillators are used that can produce an energy of 400 watt-seconds. Defibrillation produces depolarization of all the myocardial muscle fibers, following which the sinoatrial pacer node may fire normally with the impulse conducted to the ventricles. This will occur only if there is reasonable oxygenation and acid-base status of the muscle. The defibrillator paddles are usually placed one on the left lateral chest wall and one on the left anterior chest wall, just to the left of the sternum.

Electrode paste is applied to the paddles to obtain good skin contact, with care being exercised not to allow the paste to drip over the paddle handles, as this can give the paddle holder the same wattage as the patient. The energy selected will depend on the patient; a wattage of approximately 300 is selected for the initial shock, but if unsuccessful, the full wattage should be used. No longer than five seconds should elapse between cessation of CPR, application of the paddles, electric shock, and recommencement of CPR.

Indications for use of defibrillation in the monitored patient are as described previously. In the unmonitored patient defibrillation is indicated in the presence of ventricular tachycardia without a peripheral pulse, in ventricular fibrillation, and in cases in which it is impossible to be sure whether the heart is in a fine VF or in VA.

INTRAVENOUS INFUSION

Large (14- to 16-gauge) intravenous lines should be started as soon as possible. If a "push-in" cannot be started rapidly, a subclavian or internal jugular "stick" or a peripheral cutdown should be carried out for the administration of drugs and fluids. The recognized complication of pneumothorax following a subclavian "stick" may have a particular morbidity when positive pressure ventilation is used, because tension pneumothorax may result.

DRUGS

Definitive drug therapy is required for almost all cases of cardiopulmonary arrest. Intracardiac injection is used only for the administration of epinephrine. It is beyond the scope of this chapter to cover in detail all the drugs that can be used, and only the common ones are listed in Table 3–1.

Sodium Bicarbonate.   The rationale for giving this drug is to combat the lactic acidosis produced by the cardiopulmonary arrest and to establish a relatively normal pH in the myocardium in the event of arrhythmias. The initial dose is 1 mEq/kg intravenously as soon as the intravenous line is inserted. If ventricular fibrillation is present, defibrillation should be performed. If effective circulation is not re-established, another dose is given. Further administration should be governed by the arterial blood gases and pH. None should be given following the successful restoration of circulation because a profound metabolic alkalosis and hyperosmolarity can occur.

Epinephrine.   Epinephrine causes increased myocardial contractility, elevates perfusion pressure, lowers defibrillation threshold, and, in some instances, restores myocardial contractility in electromechanical dissociation. It can restore electrical activity in cardiac arrest and convert it to ventricular fibrillation when defibrillation may be successful. A dose of at least 1 or 2 ml of a 1:1000 solution is injected into the heart or intravenously and is usually not repeated more than once.

Atropine Sulfate.   This drug enhances atrioventricular conduction, reduces vagal tone, and accelerates cardiac rate in cases of sinus bradycardia. If cardiac rate is < 60/minute, with a systolic blood pressure of < 100, or if a high degree of atrioventricular block exists, 0.5 mg is given intravenously, and it may be repeated to a dose of 2 mg. It is of no value in ventricular bradycardias in the absence of atrial activity.

Lidocaine.   This is an antiarrhythmic drug, and it exerts its effect by increasing the electrical stimulation threshold of the ventricle during diastole. In therapeutic doses, it produces little myocardial depression or change in the systemic arterial pressure and absolute refractory period. It is effective in decreasing ventricular irritability in those patients in whom successful defibrillation repeatedly reverts to ventricular fibrillation. Mul-

TABLE 3–1.   DRUGS USED IN CPR

Sodium bicarbonate	50 ml ampules containing 44.6 mEq
Epinephrine	1 ml of 1:1000 diluted to 10 ml
Atropine sulfate	1 mg/ml
Lidocaine	1% solution for bolus administration 500 mg in 500 ml 5% D/W (1 mg/ml)
Calcium chloride	10% solution

tifocal premature ventricular contractions and episodes of ventricular tachycardias also respond to a bolus of 50 to 100 mg intravenously. A continuous drip of 1 mg/ml given at a rate of 1 to 3 ml/minute may be given following the bolus. It is of no value in cardiac arrest.

Calcium Chloride. This drug increases myocardial contraction, prolongs systole, and enhances ventricular excitability. Sinus node impulse formation is suppressed. The drug should be used with caution and avoided in digitalized patients. Calcium chloride may be useful in restoring electrical rhythm in cardiac arrest in a dose of 2.5 to 5 ml of a 10 percent solution (3.4 to 6.8 mEq Ca^{++}). Large doses are hazardous and must not be mixed with sodium bicarbonate because precipitation will occur.

Other Drugs. Drugs such as dopamine, isoproterenol, metaraminol, propranolol, and steroids may be indicated on occasion, but they are not usually used.

CARE AFTER CPR

As soon as the patient's vital signs are stable, transfer to either the cardiac care unit or intensive care unit is desirable. Transfer should take place with the patient being ventilated on 100 percent oxygen, with a portable monitor attached, accompanied by nurses and a responsible physician. In an advanced life support unit, attention should be given to the following:

1. Central nervous system. The only factors that reduce the incidence of cerebral damage are the rapid restoration of cardiac output, tissue perfusion, oxygenation, and correction of acid-base balance. Decadron, 6 to 8 mg given intravenously, will help to reduce cerebral edema.

2. Circulation. An indwelling arterial line is very useful to monitor arterial pressures. A central venous pressure or a Swan-Ganz flow-directed catheter is of great help in monitoring cardiac function, in determining fluid therapy, and in the administration of vasoactive drugs.

3. Ventilation. The endotracheal tube should not be removed, and the patient should be put on a respirator. Low cardiac output and large intrapulmonary shunts persist for hours and sometimes days following cardiopulmonary arrest. In addition, if a flail chest becomes apparent or concurrent aspiration has occurred during the CPR, days of ventilation will be required. A chest x-ray should be taken after arrival in the unit to assess endotracheal tube position and the state of the lung fields.

INDICATIONS FOR STARTING AND TERMINATING BASIC LIFE SUPPORT

If cardiopulmonary arrest has persisted for longer than 10 minutes prior to the initiation of cardiopulmonary resuscitation, it is extremely unlikely that a satisfactory outcome in terms of the victim's central nervous system status will result. If, however, there is question about the duration of the arrest, the victim should be given the benefit of any doubt. In cardiac arrest occurring outside the hospital, CPR should be started and continued until responsibility is assumed in the emergency department. The physician has an enormous community responsibility in relation to CPR. This responsibility ranges from instruction to quality control of performance on the basis of American Heart Association Standards. The psychomotor skills of CPR require practice at regular intervals on a recording manikin, and the regular training sessions should be part of any program. The medicolegal implications of this are obvious.

SUMMARY

In the Field.   For the trauma patient, cardiopulmonary resuscitation should basically involve rapid assessment, maintenance of airway, insertion of intravenous lines, and rapid transport to a trauma center. In general, external cardiac compression in patients with penetrating thoracic or abdominal trauma or both initiated in the ambulance or prehospital phase some distance from the trauma center rarely results in salvage of the patient.

In the Emergency Center.   For the trauma patient, cardiopulmonary resuscitation in the emergency department involves rapid assessment, stabilization, maintenance of an airway, insertion of large-bore venous cannulae, and preparation of the patient for definitive system and organ repair. The patient who sustains cardiac arrest secondary to penetrating or blunt trauma rarely survives external cardiac massage as the sole means of cardiac resuscitation in the emergency center. For the patient with penetrating thoracic trauma who suffers cardiac arrest or rapid deterioration while in the emergency center, left anterolateral thoracotomy, control of exsanguinating hemorrhage, internal cardiac massage with crossclamping of the descending thoracic aorta, and resuscitation of the heart are more appropriate resuscitative measures. These maneuvers should be performed by trained surgical personnel and should be part of a sequential plan in concert with in-hospital surgical support.

In the patient with penetrating injury or rupture of the thoracic aorta with contained hematoma, care must be taken not to resuscitate the patient to an excessive cardiac output or blood pressure, as the contained hematoma may rupture. Intraoperative and immediate postoperative resuscitation of the trauma patient are beyond the scope of this chapter.

Care of the Wound

All wounds result in tissue injury followed by local and systemic responses that direct the healing of the wound. Wound healing is manifested by various cellular events of which epithelization, collagen synthesis, and contraction are fundamental. Wounds heal at a maximal rate only when they are allowed to do so. The local state of the wound and the general state of the patient are pivotal influences in this regard. Healing is adversely affected by tissue necrosis, foreign bodies, bacteria, hematoma, edema, vascular disease, cutaneous eruptions, radiation injury, and wound tension. Alterations in the body's capacity to respond to injury may also impede healing. Notable examples of these adverse influences include continuing stress, diabetes mellitus, radiation, malnutrition, bleeding disorders, steroids, and chemotherapy.

In order to provide the ideal setting for wound healing, we must eliminate to the extent possible all undesirable influences. Systemic aberrations from normal can be minimized by close monitoring and medications. However, factors such as radiation injury and microvascular disease represent irreversible processes that require special attention such as the transfer of well-vascularized soft tissue into the wound, hyperbaric oxygen therapy (rarely) or, as a last resort, amputation of the affected part.

Initial care of the wound is perhaps the single most decisive influence on healing. By understanding the basic principles of wound management, the surgeon can intercede to provide the best possible chances for a superior result.

WOUND ASSESSMENT

Initial evaluation of the acute wound should include assessment of the mechanism, site, and type of injury, the extent of tissue damage, and the presence of foreign bodies or other contamination.

A careful examination of the wound is imperative for proper management. This should be conducted in a facility equipped with adequate lighting and instruments. Sterile technique and gentle handling of the tissues are mandatory.

45

In all injured patients, priority is given to life-threatening conditions. A thorough history and physical examination is essential, with a careful initial evaluation of the wound to assess the type and extent of injury. The surgeon should avoid causing additional tissue injury or contamination. Gross debris is removed gently. Major hemorrhage should be controlled with direct pressure, precise identification and ligation of the bleeding vessel, application of a pressure dressing, or (rarely) a tourniquet. The wound should then be covered with a sterile dressing until definitive evaluation and management can be effected.

Definitive wound evaluation requires a cooperative patient. In the unruly patient, wound evaluation may be difficult if not impossible. In such situations, it may be necessary to use restraints, sedation, local or general anesthesia, or even to delay the examination until more favorable conditions are present.

The examining physician must ascertain the depth of injury, whether important underlying structures such as nerves, major blood vessels, ducts, ligaments, bones, or joints are involved, and whether or not there is loss of function. The extent of contamination and the presence of foreign bodies must be ascertained as well as the viability of any injured parts.

Consideration must be given to the location of the wound. Deep injuries to the head, neck, and the extremities frequently involve important underlying structures. These complex anatomical areas are not amenable to extensive debridement without major functional or cosmetic loss. Wounds of the chest and abdomen must be evaluated for possible injury to underlying viscera.

Extensive wounds and minor wounds involving major structures are best evaluated and managed in the operating room. Regardless of the type and extent of a wound, however, anesthesia must be provided in order to effect proper evaluation and management.

Wounds may be classified as being tidy or untidy. Tidy wounds from sharp objects such as knives have minimal tissue injury or contamination and can usually be closed. Untidy wounds are characterized by extensive soft tissue injury with or without contamination. These wounds require major intervention to convert them to tidy wounds so that closure can be done.

The predictability of certain injury patterns has given rise to a nomenclature for wound typing, i.e., abrasions, lacerations, contusions, avulsions, amputations, etc. Lacerations are the result of shear forces applied to the skin by sharp bodies. Very little energy is required to produce a laceration and therefore a minimal amount of tissue is injured. The risk of infection of such wounds is low and the general demands for wound healing are easily satisfied.

Tensile forces produce a stretching of the soft tissues. When the tensile force exceeds the elastic yield of the tissue, separation of its parts will occur. This results in traction, avulsion, and tearing types of injuries. The area of energy absorption in the soft tissue is much greater than that seen in simple lacerations, and consequently the extent of tissue injury may be much greater and much more deceptive. Stretch injuries produce intimal damage to blood vessels with subsequent thrombosis and alterations in flow to the injured parts. Nerves, muscles, and ligaments suffer disruption of their structural integrity. In extreme situations, whole units of soft tissue may be separated with compromise of their nerves and blood supplies. The extent of injury in these wounds places more demands upon the biological processes of repair. It also decreases wound defense mechanisms, enhancing the susceptibility to infection.

Compression of soft tissue between two opposing forces often results in the greatest amount of tissue injury. Hemorrhage into the soft tissues is common and leads to ecchymosis and hematoma formation. Edema further complicates repair by reducing capillary blood flow and prolonging the inflammatory response. If the compression force is of sufficient magnitude, actual separation of the skin and soft tissue will occur. This is defined as a "bursting" type of injury. Wounds resulting from compression are in general more susceptible to infection and are slower to heal.

ANESTHESIA

The choice of anesthesia depends upon the status of the patient and the requirements for therapy. A careful sensory and motor examination is performed prior to the administration of any anesthetic. Local anesthesia is employed for most minor wounds. Many local anesthetics are available and vary in terms of safety, potency, and duration of action. Lidocaine hydrochloride is perhaps the safest and most commonly used local anesthetic (see Chapter 7).

Infiltration of the local anesthetic agent is performed gently near the edge of the wound or directly into the wound with a small-gauge needle. The pain experienced with local infiltration is related, in part, to the stretching of sensitive nerve endings in the dermis. This can be overcome by using smaller, more concentrated volumes of anesthetic and slower infiltration rates. It is wise to use the least amount of anesthetic that will provide adequate anesthesia. This is particularly true for facial lacerations in which infiltration distorts important landmarks, making precise matching of the wound edges quite difficult. Infiltration of the anesthetic directly into the wound is relatively painless but carries the risk of spreading potential infection in those wounds that are heavily contaminated.

Acute blood loss in the traumatic wound is ordinarily checked by vasospasm, platelet plugging, and fibrin clot formation. Lidocaine and similar agents cause relaxation of spastic vessels, and if the platelet or fibrin plug is insufficient, bleeding may recur. The addition of epinephrine to the local anesthetic will overcome this tendency. The vasoconstrictive effects of epinephrine also decrease the rate of clearance of the local anesthetic from the wound and thereby prolong its duration of action. To be effective, the concentration of epinephrine should be greater than 1:400,000. At least seven minutes should be allowed for the full vasoconstrictive effect. It is preferable to use fresh vials of 1:1,000 epinephrine diluted with plain lidocaine to achieve reliable vasoconstriction. Premixed solutions of ep-inephrine-containing local anesthetics may become weakened with shelf life.

Although epinephrine has been shown to have little effect on the survival of experimental cutaneous flaps, its use in traumatically elevated skin flaps or in tissues with questionable viability is not recommended. Epinephrine should not be administered in areas in which segmental blood supply is critical, such as the fingers and toes. By nature of its vasoconstrict-ing effect, epinephrine severely compromises local wound defense mech-anisms and its use in heavily contaminated wounds is contraindicated. The systemic side effects of epinephrine should be considered when con-templating its use in patients with heart and vascular disease (see Chapter 7).

PREPARATION OF THE WOUND

HAIR REMOVAL

Wounds in dense hair-bearing areas are difficult to debride and suture. Shaving of the hair adjacent to the wound edge facilitates manage-ment but invites bacterial proliferation and wound infection if the infun-dibulum of the hair follicle is injured. This can be avoided by clipping the hair 1 to 2 mm above the level of the skin. Depilatory agents and special razors equipped with recessed blades will also allow safe removal of the hair without infundibular injury. Care should be exercised to avoid contaminat-ing the wound with the removed hair. Hair in a closed wound acts as a foreign body, inviting infection and compromising the wound healing process. In areas such as the eyebrow, hair removal is not recommended because this destroys critical landmarks and makes accurate alignment of the wound edges difficult. This often leads to notch or step-off deformities in the brow line.

SKIN CLEANSERS

The wound and surrounding skin should be cleansed to remove microflora, gross contaminants, and coagulated blood. In most instances, a simple wash of the open wound with saline will remove 90 percent of the surface bacteria. The use of soaps and detergents is controversial because these may cause tissue injury or interfere with wound defense mechanisms.

SKIN DISINFECTANTS

Skin disinfectants are used to reduce the number of bacteria on the skin surface. Not all wounds require a preoperative skin preparation. For example, tidy wounds of the face are receptive to local skin cleansing with a soap solution followed by a simple wound irrigation. When a skin disinfectant is used, however, it must be nonirritating to the skin and have a rapid onset of action and a broad antimicrobial spectrum. Iodine compounds such as povidone iodine satisfy these requirements and are most commonly used today. The iodine in these compounds is bound, in part, to a nonsurfactant moiety — polyvinylpyrrolidone. Their free iodine content, although low, is highly effective against bacterial activity. If absorbed, however, the bound fractions of these iodine complexes are retained by the body because of the kidney's inability to excrete them. Application of these agents to the open wound in any large quantity is therefore not advisable, as their long-term effects are unknown.

DEBRIDEMENT

Contaminated or devitalized tissue must be excised and mechanically cleansed. Surgical debridement consists of sharply excising those portions of the wound that are devitalized, severely contaminated, or so irregular as to make wound closure impractical. In all cases, it is advantageous to perform debridement with a scalpel. The simplest method of debridement is total excision of the wound, creating a surgically clean wound base. This should be limited to those wounds that do not involve specialized structures.

Complete excision of the wound is advantageous in those regions containing an abundance of soft tissue, such as the trunk and thighs. It is often helpful to pack the wound with gauze, close it with sutures, and excise the entire mass as if it were a tumor, leaving a cuff of normal tissue attached. Care is exercised to avoid exposure of the gauze during the dissection. An alternative method is to close the wound after staining it with a vital dye such as methylene blue, and then to excise the entire area of staining. These methods, while assuring the adequacy of debridement, cannot be applied to wounds containing specialized structures. In these situations, it is best to cleanse the wound mechanically and then perform selective debridement of all grossly nonviable tissue. Under special circumstances, even devascularized tissues should be retained if they serve an important function and can be rendered surgically clean. Examples include the salvaging of contaminated tendons, fascia, and dura. These structures can survive as free grafts if appropriate wound coverage is provided. Other than the sparing of such structures, all nonviable tissues should be removed because they constitute an excellent medium for bacterial growth while inhibiting important leukocyte function.

A reliable test for tissue viability has not been perfected. Irrefutable signs of tissue death such as rigor mortis and putrefaction are usually absent in the acute wound. Therefore, the guidelines for determining tissue viability must be based on careful examination and sound clinical judgment. The potential for survival of an injured part is perhaps of greater importance than its observed state of viability. Direct cellular destruction, such as that encountered in a burn wound, constitutes an irreversible process, necessitating removal of devitalized parts. Crush and blast injuries represent indeterminate areas in which some cells are destroyed and others survive but where the diffuseness of the injury makes precise surgical debridement impossible and for the most part impractical.

The separation of a part from its blood supply will obviously result in necrosis unless that part can be converted to a graft or have its blood supply re-established. Thick segments of tissue, such as muscle or composite flaps of skin and subcutaneous tissue, do not survive well as free grafts and should not be used as such in acute wounds. Avulsed skin, however, if appropriately cleaned, debrided, and defatted, may serve admirably as a free graft. Similarly, amputated parts have an excellent potential for survival if revascularization is feasible.

The potential viability of attached soft tissue parts is related to the extent of injury as well as the vascular supply of the part. Of the latter, venous effluent is critical. Mangled, irregular wound edges imply severe local tissue injury and should be sharply debrided. Traumatically elevated skin flaps should be assessed for capillary refill and the presence of venous congestion. Rapid capillary refill or cyanosis in the flap indicates venous obstruction. If there is a sharp demarcation between normal and abnormal perfusion of the flap, excision of the abnormal portion is indicated. If conditions permit, the excised portion can then be reapplied as a graft. In those situations in which vascular perfusion is uncertain, the intravenous fluorescein dye test has been employed to assess tissue viability. Fluorescein dye fixes to perfused tissues and its presence can be detected as fluorescence under ultraviolet light. Although tissue fluorescence reflects arterial perfusion of a part, it is not an absolute indicator of tissue survivability.

HEMOSTASIS

Prior to wound closure, absolute hemostasis must be effected to prevent hematoma formation and further loss of blood as well as to provide a clear field for precise wound closure. Coagulated blood in the wound serves as an excellent pabulum for bacterial proliferation and increases scar tissue formation. Hematoma is the most common cause of skin graft loss, and its presence beneath a skin flap severely compromises the flap's viability.

Braided, nonabsorbable suture materials such as silk, cotton, or Dacron are poor choices for vascular ligation in the contaminated wound. These materials are very reactive and their presence significantly increases the incidence of wound infection. Monofilamentous synthetics such as polypropylene are perhaps the least reactive suture materials but their low friction coefficient makes them unsuitable as ligatures in most situations. Exceptions are to be found in the repair or suture ligation of major vascular tributaries. Absorbable sutures are commonly used for tying and suture ligation in the acute wound. The synthetic absorbables polyglycolic acid (Dexon) and polyglactin (Vicryl) are advantageous because of their low reactivity and high friction coefficients.

Damped electrical current is effective in coagulating small vessel ends. Monopolar cautery causes approximately three times as much tissue necrosis as does bipolar coagulation. Pinpoint coagulation is preferred, with delivery of the least amount of current needed for vessel thrombosis. Some surgeons use undamped electrical current for cutting tissues during debridement of the acute wound. Although quite effective in diminishing blood loss, cutting current inflicts significant thermal injury to the surrounding tissues, increasing their susceptibility to infection, and is therefore not recommended for wound debridement or hemostasis. Heat, in the form of hot saline compresses, should also be avoided for similar reasons.

Indirect methods for achieving hemostasis in the acute wound include pressure, elevation, and application of vasoconstrictive agents. These methods are, for the most part, effective in the control of diffuse vascular oozing and lymph extravasation. The amount of pressure applied should not be greater than capillary perfusion pressures (30 mm Hg) and the site of pressure should not impede vascular flow to distal parts.

Elevation of the injured part "above the level of the heart" is least damaging to the tissues and markedly diminishes capillary oozing. Caution should be exercised in the elderly patient with arteriosclerotic vascular disease, as elevation of the lower extremity may induce tissue hypoxia.

ANTIBIOTICS

The use of antibiotics in the patient with an acute wound must be based upon the likelihood of infection occurring if the wound is closed. Antibiotics are effective in preventing wound infection only when the bacterial level in the wound is less than 10^9 organisms per gram of tissue. To be effective, the antibiotic must be delivered prior to wound closure in appropriate doses via an appropriate route, and the bacterial contaminants in the wound must be sensitive to it.

Sharp lacerations are markedly resistant to infection, and in most instances will not require antibiotic therapy. Open wounds, by virtue of their inflammatory response and resistance to bacterial dissemination, rarely become infected unless the initial level of contamination is great. Furthermore, the fibrous coagulum in these wounds limits the effectiveness of systemic antibiotics on bacterial contaminants.

The level of bacterial contamination after irrigation and debridement can be detected by quantitative assay. If high levels persist ($\geq 10^5$ organisms per gram of tissue) and the extent of the tissue injury does not mitigate wound closure, an antibiotic is indicated. A Gram stain of the bacteria in the wound is helpful in determining the antibiotic of choice. It must be remembered, however, that wounds containing more than 10^9 bacteria will develop infection regardless of the use of antibiotics.

Even small inoculums of bacteria will result in infection if their presence is accompanied by necrotic debris, a foreign body, or altered tissue defense mechanisms (such as in crush or contused wounds). In these situations, broad-spectrum antibacterial prophylaxis may be advantageous.

In grossly contaminated wounds such as those contaminated by feces, pus, or saliva, wound closure should not be attempted. Antibiotic therapy is indicated to prevent the overwhelming bacterial inoculum from gaining a foothold and to allow the wound to increase its resistance. The choice of antibiotic is based upon the suspected predominance of the bacterial contaminants. In most cases, a mixture of aerobic and anaerobic organisms will be present.

Tetanus prophylaxis should always be considered in traumatic wounds, especially when these are contaminated.

DETERMINANTS OF WOUND CLOSURE

The decision to close a wound is predicated upon many circumstances, of which the level of contamination remains a significant consideration. A "golden period" for wound closure has been advocated for many years and unfortunately reflects our inability to apply general rules to individualized problems. Time allows bacteria to proliferate in the wound. If the bacterial inoculum or colonization reaches a critical level (usually defined as $> 10^5$ organisms per gram of tissue) infection will follow wound closure. Infection is more closely related to the *number* of bacteria present at the time of wound closure than to the *type* of bacteria present. The number of bacteria required to produce an infection is markedly less in the presence of foreign body, tissue necrosis, or diminished local defense mechanisms in the wound. Of the latter, local blood supply is perhaps the most important factor.

Primary closure of the wound is always the ideal goal but this may not be attainable. An open wound invites fibrous tissue proliferation and contraction, both of which may lead to diminished function and unsightly appearance. Infection in the wound, however, will defeat any possible gains from primary closure. The timing of wound closure is therefore a compromise between the likelihood of infection and the ability to provide favorable conditions for closure.

Within three hours of injury, most civilian wounds contain less than 10^5 organisms per gram of tissue. Exceptions are found in bite and other heavily contaminated wounds. Beyond three hours, bacterial proliferation exceeding the critical level is quite variable. The location of a wound and mechanisms of injury are significant factors in this regard. For instance, well-vascularized regions such as the face and scalp are markedly resistant to bacterial invasion compared to the trunk and lower extremities. Simple lacerations with minimal tissue injury and bacterial contamination are likewise less likely to develop critical levels of bacteria early on, compared to crush or heavily contaminated wounds. Inflammation in the acute wound suggests infection, and is therefore a contraindication to closure. Owing to a lag phase that exists between the microscopic and clinical signs of infection, however, the appearance of a wound will not always reflect the number of bacteria present. Other than a high index of suspicion based upon the history and clinical examination, the only reliable method of accurately measuring the amount of bacteria in a wound is by quantitative assay.

QUANTITATIVE ASSAY

Some surgeons believe that quantification of bacteria in the wound should be performed after completion of irrigation and debridement. This will allow the surgeon to assess adequately the results of his intervention and make a reasonable decision regarding the feasibility of wound closure.

Quantitative assay of wound bacteria may be performed via two techniques. The first technique utilizes serial dilutions of bacteria cultured from a known weight of wound biopsy specimen. The levels of bacterial growth can then be identified by colony counting. Results are available within 24 hours of sampling. The applicability of this technique to the acute wound has obvious limitations unless, of course, one chooses to delay wound closure. An alternative technique for quantification of bacteria in the acute wound was developed by Heggers, Robson, and Doran[1] (Table 4–1). The "rapid slide" technique involves direct examination of the tissue sample for bacteria. Information regarding the presence of critical levels of bacteria in the wound can be obtained within 30 minutes of biopsy. The accuracy of this technique approaches 95 percent and the test can be performed by most hospital laboratories equipped with the basic tools for bacteriological assessment.

With appropriate debridement, irrigation, and closure, wounds con-

TABLE 4–1. THE RAPID SLIDE TECHNIQUE FOR ASSESSMENT
OF CRITICAL LEVELS OF WOUND BACTERIA*

1. The surface of the wound biopsy area is cleansed with 70 per cent isopropyl alcohol.
2. The biopsy specimen is obtained with a 3- or 4-mm dermal punch or with a scalpel. No anesthesia is required for an open wound.
3. After the tissue is weighed, flamed, and diluted 1:10 with thioglycolate (1 ml/gm), it is homogenized.
4. Exactly 0.02 ml of the suspension is spread on a glass slide from a 20-lambda Sahli pipette. The inoculum is confined to an area 15 mm in diameter.
5. The slide is oven dried for 15 minutes at 75° C.
6. The slide is stained, using either a Gram stain or the Brown and Brenn modification for tissue staining, to accentuate the gram-negative organisms.
7. The smear is read under 1.8 mm (magnification × 97) objective and all fields are examined for the presence of bacteria.
8. The presence of even a single organism is evidence that the tissue contains a level of bacterial growth greater than 10^5 bacteria per gram of tissue.

*From Heggers JP, Robson RC, and Doran ET: Quantitative assessment of bacterial contamination of open wounds by a slide technique. Trans R Soc Trop Med Hyg 63:532, 1969.

taining less than 10^5 organisms per gram of tissue seldom become infected. In the final analysis, however, the decision to close a wound must be based upon a multitude of factors with consideration given to the type of injury, its location, the level of contamination, and the status of the patient.

MISSING TISSUE

Wounds can also be classified in accordance with the presence or absence of tissue. Major defects resulting from injury or debridement or both will strongly influence the type as well as the timing of wound closure. Primary closure consists of coaptation of the wound edges without tension in a manner favorable for uneventful wound healing. If the wound defect precludes the mechanical ability to effect closure, the surgeon must consider advancing local tissue, applying skin grafts, or transferring well-vascularized flaps into the wound. The coverage of large wounds places additional stresses upon the patient, and should probably be dealt with secondarily.

OBJECTIVES OF REPAIR

Ideally, the ultimate goal of any wound closure is the restoration of function and cosmetic appearance of the injured area. This is best achieved by precise alignment and close apposition of the injured parts, without tension, and without further injury to the already injured tissues. The physical strength of a repaired wound reflects the efficacy of the repair. In this regard, attention should be directed toward repairing those layers of the wound that are responsible for its ultimate strength. Fibrous tissue layers such as fascia and dermis comprise the strongest components of soft tissue; hence their repair will give the best chance for obtaining maximal wound strength and appearance. Materials employed for coaptation of the various layers of the wound must be chosen on the basis of their ability to maintain apposition until the strength of the wound, or its parts, is sufficient to withstand mechanical stress. This depends on the healing capacity of the tissues to be approximated and the condition of the wound at the time of closure. Fascial layers heal slowly and require materials that will maintain tissue apposition for long periods. More vascular tissues such as the epidermis heal faster, are not subjected to as much stress, and therefore require only temporary materials for maintenance of apposition. Consideration must also be given to the reactivity of the materials used and their influence on wound defense mechanisms.

SUTURES

Sutures are the most common materials employed for wound closure. The biological interaction between a suture and the wound is of primary importance with regard to the final result. This is related to the composition of the suture, the quantity of suture material in the wound, and the technique of suture placement.

Two basic categories of suture materials are available: absorbable and nonabsorbable. Absorbable sutures are biodegradable and for the most part lose their tensile strength within 60 days. Gut and synthetic materials are the two major types used for absorbable sutures. Nonabsorbable sutures maintain their tensile strength for periods longer than 50 days. They are classified into three major groups: natural fibers, metallics, and synthetics. As a rule, the synthetic nonabsorbable sutures are least reactive.

Absorbable Sutures

Gut sutures are derived from sheep mucosa or beef serosa and are digested by proteolytic enzymes in the wound. Plain catgut incites an intense inflammatory reaction in the wound and loses its tensile strength within two weeks. Treatment of gut with chromium salts decreases its tissue reactivity and prolongs its tensile strength in the wound. Gut sutures are more rapidly degraded in the presence of infection. Their knot-holding ability is rather inconsistent, although chromic gut seems to be the best in this regard.

The synthetic sutures polyglycolic acid (Dexon) and polyglactin (Vicryl) produce minimal tissue reaction in the wound. They are degraded by hydrolysis and lose 50 percent of their tensile strength in 20 to 30 days. This is comparable to chromic catgut. These materials are not influenced by the presence of infection. The byproducts of their degradation have been shown to have antibacterial activity in the experimental wound. Absorbable materials of this type are superior for use in the acute wound because of their low tissue reactivity. Although similar to silk in their handling characteristics, they do not hold knots quite as well. They are used most commonly for vascular ligation and dermal closure.

Nonabsorbable Sutures

Silk sutures represent the most common type of natural fiber suture. Because silk gradually loses its tensile strength with time, it should be classified as a slowly absorbable suture material. The tissue reactivity of silk is the greatest of all nonabsorbable sutures, and for this reason its use in the acute wound has generally been abandoned.

Stainless steel sutures and metallic clips have been employed for years because of their presumed inertness. However, these materials have been shown to increase significantly the infection rates in contaminated wounds. This is probably due to the mechanical irritation that they cause because of their rigidity as opposed to corrosion degradation. Staples decrease wound closure time; this advantage must be weighed against the increased susceptibility of the wound to infection that they cause. The stiffness of metallic sutures makes tying quite cumbersome and is related to suture size.

Synthetic nonabsorbable sutures are made of Dacron, nylon, polyethylene, and polypropylene. Dacron is a polyester that elicits less tissue reaction than silk. Because of its high friction coefficient, it is difficult to handle as a suture. The friction injury imposed upon the tissues by Dacron can be overcome by coating it with Teflon. However, tissue reactivity to this material is unaltered as a result of this coating.

Nylon exhibits minimal tissue reactivity and its use in contaminated wounds results in diminished wound infection rates. In monofilamentous form, this material will lose approximately 20 percent of its tensile strength within a year. The monofilamentous form of nylon is quite stiff and does not hold knots well. Multifilamentous forms of nylon demonstrate no tensile strength in the wound after six months. This is the result of chemical degradation of the material by the wound. The byproducts of nylon degradation are similar to polyglycolic acid in exhibiting antibacterial activity in the experimental wound.

Polypropylene and polyester materials produce the least reactivity of all suture materials. They maintain their tensile strength indefinitely, and are the suture materials of choice for closure of contaminated wounds.

These materials are used most commonly for fascial and skin closure. They are also advantageous in the repair of vascular, nerve, and tendon injuries. Because of their softer consistency, these materials generally hold knots better than nylon.

The physical configuration of a suture material must be considered when closing a contaminated wound. In braided or multifilamentous materials, bacteria can become sequestered out of reach of inflammatory cells. Monofilamentous materials prevent bacterial sequestration and theoretically should be advantageous for use in a contaminated wound. Experimentally, however, the physical configuration of a suture material plays less of a role in the development of early wound infection than does its chemical composition.

All sutures represent foreign bodies in the wound. The size and the amount of suture material in the wound is closely related to the level of tissue inflammation. For this reason, the smallest size and amount of suture that will adequately produce tissue apposition should be employed. In contaminated wounds, sutures should be avoided unless they are absolutely needed to maintain alignment of these parts.

WOUND TAPES

Sutureless closure of the acute wound is superior in providing the maximum resistance to infection. This is done using various tape materials and results in significantly diminished wound infection rates compared to suture closure. Tape closure is most advantageous in the contaminated wound. It is also useful in superficial tidy wounds and wounds in children and obese patients.

In irregular lacerations and crush injuries, sutures allow for better approximation of the skin edges than do tapes. Moreover, tape only approximates the superficial portion of the wound. This leaves the deeper wound layers more vulnerable to local biomechanical stresses and may result in a weaker and more unsightly scar. In clean wounds, it is sometimes preferable to close the deep layers with suture and then coapt the superficial layers with tape.

To be effective, skin tapes must be strong enough to support the wound edges in close apposition until sufficient healing has occurred. They must have excellent skin adherence and should not macerate the underlying skin surface. Microporous rayon-reinforced wound tapes satisfy these requirements quite well and are used most commonly today. Adherence to the skin is enhanced if all moisture is removed and a defatting agent such as acetone is used. This will allow tape adherence for up to two weeks. Tincture of benzoin is occasionally used to supplement skin adhesiveness. Although benzoin may initially enhance tape adhesion, it is solubilized by skin oils and rapidly loses its adherence capabilities.

DRAINAGE OF THE WOUND

Drains constitute foreign bodies, produce tissue necrosis, and serve as conduits for bacterial contamination of the wound. If sound principles of management have been carefully followed, drains are usually unnecessary in the acute wound. Contrary to popular opinion, drains are rather ineffective in the prevention of hematoma. If oozing cannot be controlled, it is preferable to delay wound closure. Drains, however, are effective in evacuating pus and necrotic exudates. This fact should be considered when contemplating the closure of a contaminated wound.

POSTOPERATIVE WOUND CARE

Postoperative wound care is designed to provide an ideal environment for wound healing. This is accomplished primarily through the use of dressings. A dressing serves primarily one or a combination of seven different functions: protection, immobilization, compression, absorption, debridement, medication, and cosmesis.

Wounds closed by percutaneous sutures are susceptible to surface bacterial invasion for the first 48 hours after closure. During this time, the wound should be protected with sterile dressings or frequent suture line care. If dressings are employed, nonadherent materials (Telfa, vaseline-impregnated gauzes, etc.) are favored because their removal will cause little disturbance of the sutures or coapted wound edges. Suture line care for facial wounds involves frequent, meticulous cleaning with saline or a diluted hydrogen peroxide solution. Cleansing removes the adherent coagulum from the suture-skin junction, decreasing the likelihood of stitch abscess formation. After cleansing, the wound is dressed with an antibiotic cream or ointment.

Taped wounds are very resistant to surface bacterial contamination. They usually require no protection other than that provided by the tape itself. These wounds should be checked frequently to assess for wound drainage beneath the tape. Excessive drainage can cause maceration of the wound edge and provide an excellent pabulum for bacterial proliferation.

Immobilization of the wound enhances its resistance to bacterial proliferation and decreases the lymphatic dissemination of bacteria. By diminishing dynamic forces across the wound, support is given during the critical phases of rapid collagen turnover. Immobilization is accomplished with splints, bulky dressings, or skin tapes. The length of immobilization varies with the demand of the local tissues and the desire to achieve an optimal result. Ideally, immobilization of the wound should be continued until the wound is no longer vulnerable to infection and has gained sufficient strength to withstand the biomechanical stresses of motion and skin tension. For the former, the goal is achieved within a week. The latter generally requires approximately six weeks. Too much immobilization will defeat its possible advantages. For instance, extended immobilization in the elderly may result in permanent joint contractures with marked decrease in function. The advantages of wound immobilization must therefore be critically weighed against its undesirable consequences. Extended immobilization is advantageous for wounds of the face or wherever cosmetic considerations are especially important. Areas such as the jaw line, chin, shoulder, or knee are subjected to excessive static and dynamic stresses and frequently require support for up to three months to achieve an optimal result. Extended wound support is also indicated in patients with neoplasms or immunoincompetence.

Edema is counterproductive to wound healing — it slows down the machinery of repair and increases fibrous tissue proliferation. The wound with minimal edema will show earlier complete healing and return of function.

Elevation of the wound above the level of the heart is the simplest way of limiting the amount of excess tissue fluid in the wound. In the ambulatory patient, however, this may not be practical or reliably accomplished. In certain situations, it is advantageous to apply compression to the wound to subserve the benefits of elevation. This is managed by bulky pressure dressings. It is important to avoid constriction of proximal parts with these dressings because venous and lymphatic congestion will occur as a result of the tourniquet effect. Careful padding of bony prominences, generous use of bulk, and even wrapping is mandatory for the proper placement of a compression dressing. In the hand, it is important to place one or two layers of gauze between the fingers to prevent sweat maceration. Roller gauze or bias-cut stockinette is preferred to elastic bandages; the latter are often too constricting. The finished dressing should sound like a ripe watermelon when thumped.

In extremity injuries, compression dressings should be applied proximally from the most distal point. Tips of toes and fingers should be exposed so that sensibility and capillary refill may be assessed. Continued pain or diminished sensibility necessitates removal of the dressing followed by careful examination of the wound. The compression dressing should not be used in crush injuries or in injuries that may evolve into compartmental syndromes. Although used frequently to diminish postoperative bloody oozing at the operative site, compression dressings should not be employed as substitutes for diligent hemostasis.

Peak wound edema occurs by 48 hours and gradually resolves over the next four to six days. A compression dressing would therefore be beneficial during the first week of healing. Persistent tissue edema beyond seven days suggests inflammation or infection.

In closed wounds, dry dressings are preferable because moist dressings will cause maceration of the skin, inviting bacterial invasion. In the open wound, it is preferable to apply moist dressings to the open wound surface and then back these with dry dressings to achieve a "capillary effect." An exception to this principle is in deep, tunnel-shaped wounds in which surface evaporation is limited, thus diminishing the capillary effect. These wounds are best managed by packing with dry gauze to achieve maximum absorption.

In all instances, absorptive dressings should be composed of tightly woven or spun fabric. Cotton meshes and synthetic equivalents become incorporated into the wound as foreign bodies that incite tissue inflammation and subsequent bacterial proliferation.

Dextran polymers have remarkable hydroscopic properties and serve well as absorbent dressings. They are quite effective in removing bacterial toxins and serous effluents from the wound surface. Wound healing is not significantly altered by their use.

Dressings are frequently used for debridement of the open wound. The traditional wet-to-dry method utilizes avulsion of adherent tissues to remove devitalized remnants from the wound surface. Unfortunately, this method does not discriminate between the viable and nonviable components and results in re-injury of the wound with each dressing change. Although painful and markedly detrimental to the wound healing process, this method is effective if performed properly. Several layers of moist gauze are applied to the wound surface and allowed to dry. After about four hours, the adherent dressing is removed. Moistening the dry dressing prior to removal (as is done by many sympathetic nurses) decreases its adherence to the wound, thereby defeating the effectiveness of debridement.

An alternative to mechanical avulsion debridement is enzymatic debridement. The activity of certain proteolytic enzymes is quite effective in removing particulate necrotic debris and fibrinous coagulum from the wound. A popular enzyme produced by *Bacillus subtilis* (travase) has been shown to cause little injury to the viable wound parts. Another enzyme, collagenase, has recently been introduced as an adjunct to wound debridement but its precise clinical usefulness has yet to be determined.

The most common medicaments used in dressings are antibacterials. Topical antibacterials are employed to control those bacteria that cannot be reached by systemic agents. Necrotic eschar and granulation tissue are their prime targets. Their efficacy is enhanced by their ability to penetrate dead tissues. Sulfamylon and silver sulfadiazine are most effective in this regard. These agents are also useful in partial thickness injuries or marginally viable tissues. By decreasing the potential for bacterial invasion, they diminish the likelihood of full thickness tissue conversion and necrosis. Their use must be monitored closely because excessive amounts may cause acid-base imbalances (Sulfamylon) or leukopenia (silver sulfadiazine). Both agents retard wound epithelization and should be discontinued when the necrotic debris has been removed and the wound bacterial counts are less than 10^6 organisms per gram of tissue.

BIOLOGICAL DRESSINGS

Acute wounds characterized by extensive loss of skin are not readily amenable to immediate closure by flaps or grafts. These defects are easy prey for bacterial invasion and severely tax the machinery of healing by major blood losses of fluid, protein, and other metabolic essentials. Ideally, early closure of the wound is best, but may be impractical from the standpoint of patient tolerance or safety. In these situations, temporary skin substitutes may be beneficial. Biological dressings serve these purposes well by duplicating all the protective functions of skin except permanence.

Many types of biological dressings are available. Pigskin is perhaps the most commonly used because of its ready supply. This dressing is excellent for providing protection of the wound and for diminishing fluid loss, but it is not efficacious in reducing bacterial populations in the wound. Effective reduction of the bacterial counts in a wound requires a "take" of the biological dressing to the wound surface. Human tissues are the only biological dressings that will actually develop a blood supply from human wounds. For these purposes, homograft skin and human fetal membranes are quite advantageous. Cadaver skin is not readily available in most hospitals and is extremely expensive. Amniotic membranes, however, are abundant and provide an excellent source of biological dressings. If placed with their chorionic side facing the wound, they will adhere much like a skin graft. In any case, biological dressings should be removed within 48 hours and fresh dressings reapplied. Keeping the biological dressing on longer will increase its adherence and initiate strong rejection reactions that may be detrimental to wound healing. Homograft and amniotic dressings are effective in reducing wound bacterial counts. In wounds in which the bacterial count exceeds 10^5 organisms per gram of tissue, dressings should be changed every 24 hours.

A major disadvantage of any biological dressing is its inability to prevent bacterial proliferation in the presence of dead tissue or foreign bodies. This may constitute a relative contraindication to its use in the acute wound.

Over the past several years, several synthetic dressings have been introduced that behave similarly to biological dressings in their wound-protection capabilities. Biobrane is a silastic-collagen laminate that has been shown to have excellent adherence to the open wound. When compared to human allograft there is essentially no difference in pain relief, initial adherence, or the ability to keep bacterial counts in the wound below 10^5 organisms per gram of tissue. This and similar synthetics represent a significant breakthrough in the temporary coverage of the open wound. Further investigation is needed to determine the precise role of synthetics in wound management.

SPECIAL WOUNDS

BLAST INJURIES

Wounds resulting from high-velocity missiles and shotgun blasts are among the most severe encountered in the civilian population. Extensive tissue destruction is incurred locally with loss or disruption of the wound parts to form a cavity. Sites distant to the point of impact may be injured as a result of shock waves. The extent of injury in these complex wounds is difficult to assess and primary closure is ill-advised. Initial care is directed to hemostasis, cleansing, and minimal debridement. Repeated explorations staged 24 to 48 hours apart may be employed to remove necrotic or devitalized tissues. Antibiotic prophylaxis is recommended. The wounds are then closed secondarily with priority given to the re-establishment of bony relationships, followed by soft tissue coverage.

DEGLOVING INJURIES

Separation of the skin and subcutaneous tissues from the underlying musculofascial planes constitutes a degloving injury. The determinant of survival in those flaps attached by a pedicle is their circulation. Grossly mangled, contaminated portions should be sharply debrided. Areas of venous congestion and demarcation should likewise be removed. Areas of questionable viability are assessed with fluorescent markers. In intensive degloving injuries, it is often advantageous to remove completely the potentially nonviable but minimally injured parts and reapply them as free grafts after appropriate defatting and debridement. For lesser injuries, the degloved segment should be cleansed, debrided, and carefully repositioned. In all instances, the underlying soft tissues must be appropriately managed. The flap should then be sutured where it lies without tension or stretching. These wounds often cannot be closed primarily. A light compression dressing is employed to obliterate dead space. The returned portions of the degloved skin are closely monitored over the next 72 hours to assess tissue viability as well as infection. A broad-spectrum antimicrobial is helpful in preventing bacterial colonization in marginally viable flaps.

AMPUTATIONS

The chances for survival of an amputated part can be correlated with ischemic injury. Six hours is probably the longest time that a part can be deprived of its blood supply during warm ischemia and still survive. If cooled immediately, the tolerable ischemia time of the amputated part is increased to 12 to 24 hours. This is particularly important when replantation must be delayed for transfer to an appropriate facility (see Chapter 19).

Contraindications to replantation are (1) the presence of significant associated injuries that may be life-threatening, (2) severe degloving or crushing injuries of the amputated part, and (3) major systemic disease.

BITES

Wounds resulting from human and dog bites are heavily contaminated from the outset. Dog bites are sharper, are often located on the face, and are best treated by prompt excision within six hours of injury. If the extent of the wound or time since injury precludes primary closure, these wounds should be irrigated, debrided, and left open.

Human bites are more virulent than dog bites and are commonly located over the knuckles or dorsum of the hand. Despite their rather innocuous initial appearance, these wounds are extremely dangerous. Their propensity for severe necrotizing infection if improperly treated is high. Management includes vigorous irrigation and debridement. Wounds of this type are never closed. The injured part should be elevated, immobilized, and frequently checked to assess for possible spread of infection. It may be advantageous to employ topical antibacterials to reduce local bacterial counts. Signs of necrotizing infection are progressive erythema, blistering, or frank necrosis. If these signs occur, wide debridement of the involved parts is indicated.

In both human and dog bites, antibiotic prophylaxis is recommended as well as aggressive tetanus prophylaxis. In dog bites, one should always be alert to the possibility of rabies infection (see Chapter 23.)

REFERENCE

1. Heggers JP, Robson RC, Doran ET: Quantitative assessment of bacterial contamination of open wounds by a slide technique. Trans R Soc Trop Med Hyg 63:532, 1969.

5

Infection

Infection is the most frequent complication occurring in injured patients. The morbidity and mortality due to sepsis can be minimized only by early surgery, meticulous technique, appropriate use of antibiotics, and timely physiologically directed postoperative care. Traumatic wounds must always be considered contaminated by microorganisms having the potential to cause infection. The consequences of such contamination are related to both microbial and host factors influencing the proliferation and invasive capacity of the microorganisms. These factors include microbial density (the presence of 10^5 or more organisms in a gram of tissue commonly indicates infection) and virulence, tissue viability, local circulation, and immune competence. Wounds may be contaminated by exogenous bacteria with or without associated foreign bodies such as clothing, soil, water, or whatever medium surrounds the wound at the time of injury. Wounds may also be contaminated by bacteria from endogenous sources as may occur with penetrating injuries of the abdominal and thoracic cavities in which there is perforation of the respiratory, alimentary, and genitourinary tracts.

FACTORS THAT PREDISPOSE WOUNDS TO INFECTION

The combination of wounding agent, wound environment, host resistance, and treatment factors determines the consequences of contamination and influences the incidence of infection following injury.

Nature and Velocity of Wounding Agent. The velocity, mass, and configuration of the wounding agent influence the severity and extent of tissue injury. Debridement and wound care are dictated by those factors and involve removal of all nonviable tissue and establishment of adequate drainage. Adequate wound care is important even for innocuous-appearing puncture wounds, which if untreated and undebrided may provide an anaerobic environment favoring the development of tetanus or other clostridial infections.

Density, Type, and Invasive Capacity of Contaminating Bacteria. Infection occurs when the microbial density exceeds host defense capabilities. The mere presence of microorganisms in a wound does not mean that infection will inevitably occur. The presence of 10^5 or more microorganisms per gram of tissue shows good correlation with infection, and the presence of microbes in viable tissue is diagnostic of invasive sepsis. Virulence that can be described in terms of laboratory animal mortality is difficult to define clinically. Invasive capacity is found to vary from organism to organism and from strain to strain. Synergism between different bacteria in the wound may also influence the likelihood and severity of wound infection.

Nature and Location of Wound. Large amounts of devitalized tissue contained in extensive wounds serve as an excellent culture medium for bacteria and other microorganisms. Wounds produced by crushing injuries and associated with heavy contamination are frequently characterized by extensive tissue destruction, severe shock, and early infection. The location of the wound is important because various tissues in the body have differing degrees of resistance to infection.

The amount of devitalized tissue within the wound and the state of the local circulation are especially important, since ischemic or dead tissue invites and supports the growth of microorganisms while healthy tissue with an intact blood supply possesses remarkable capacity to resist invasion and kill microorganisms. Differences in local blood supply also influence treatment, e.g., wounds on the face are usually closed primarily, whereas similar wounds on the foot may be left open or have delayed closure.

Presence of Foreign Bodies. Foreign material may introduce large numbers of microorganisms into the wound and increase the likelihood of infection by eliciting a local inflammatory reaction.

Treatment Factors. Surgical excision of all dead tissue and foreign bodies is of primary importance in reducing the risk of infection. Definitive surgical treatment should be undertaken within six hours after injury if possible. The local treatment of wounds and wound debridement may have to be delayed while general resuscitative measures are carried out in patients with multiple wounds associated with shock or profound hemorrhage. If the time required for resuscitation and treatment of life-threatening systemic complications exceeds six hours, infection may be established before local definitive treatment can be effected.

Immune Capacity of Patient. Local resistance depends greatly on the type of tissue injured and its blood supply and the adequacy of the systemic circulation as a whole, i.e., the presence or absence of shock. The adequacy of host resistance depends upon the integrity of the entire immune system, including the humoral globulin fractions, complement components of plasma, the activity of lymphocytes and neutrophils, and the cells of the reticuloendothelial system. Alterations of immunoglobulin, opsonin, and complement-component function have all been described in injured patients, as have suppression of chemotaxis, phagocytosis, and bactericidal capacity of neutrophils. Several humoral suppressive factors and immunosuppressive T-lymphocytes have also been identified, but the precise mechanisms and the clinical significance of these alterations of immune capacity remain undefined.

General Condition of Patient. The presence of such conditions as dehydration, shock, malnutrition, obesity, uncontrolled diabetes, and adrenal insufficiency may all lower the patient's resistance sufficiently to allow microbial invasion in a wound that would be resistant in an otherwise healthy patient. Drug therapy such as steroids, cytotoxic agents, immunosuppressive agents, and even antimicrobial agents may render the patient susceptible to infection. General exposure to radiation also lowers antimicrobial defense capacity and predisposes wounds to infectious complications.

Miscellaneous Factors. The lack of medical facilities and personnel to carry out adequate supportive care and debridement, as may exist in disaster conditions, may also increase the risk to wound infection. Drug intolerance or idiosyncrasies may limit therapy and affect the patient's response to treatment.

PROPHYLAXIS OF SURGICAL INFECTIONS

Wound and general care of the injured patient should promote prompt primary healing or timely closure of wounds and thereby minimize the opportunity for bacterial colonization, invasion, and sepsis. Since delays in wound treatment increase the likelihood of infection, initial surgical treatment should be undertaken within six hours after the injury. Primary closure is usually contraindicated (except under special circumstances) in wounds not treated within six to ten hours.

CLEANSING AND SURGICAL DEBRIDEMENT OF WOUNDS

Adequate debridement of traumatic wounds consists of meticulous removal of all dead or devitalized tissue, detached fragments of soft tissue or bone, foreign bodies and debris. In wounds of the face and hands, conservative debridement should be the rule, since both areas include essentially irreplaceable structures that are necessary for proper function and appearance. Simple shaving and cleansing of the skin, gentle irrigation of the wound with saline, conservative trimming of ragged wound edges, and removal of nonviable tissue fragments may be all that is required for debridement of such wounds.

Massive wounds of the extremities may require extensive debridement and painstaking removal of detached bone fragments, foreign bodies, and every bit of muscle and other soft tissue that is ischemic or of questionable viability. When it is obvious that an extremity is irreversibly damaged with irreparable vascular and nerve injury, amputation may be the only effective form of debridement.

IMMOBILIZATION

The traumatized part of the body should be placed at rest as much as possible. After the wound is cleansed and debrided, a bulky dressing is usually applied to place the damaged structures at rest, thereby decreasing the danger of further hemorrhage and dissemination of bacteria by muscle movement. In the case of extremity wounds, elevation may be helpful in improving the patient's comfort and minimizing or reducing local swelling. The patient should be nursed at a temperature of comfort to prevent vasoconstriction, which can further decrease local blood flow.

ADJUNCTIVE SURGICAL PROCEDURES

In the treatment of patients with specific injuries, operative procedures may be necessary to minimize contamination. A proximal colostomy in the patient with a wound of the colon will significantly decrease the bacterial flow that would otherwise pass across the site of perforation. Adequate drainage of areas such as the retroperitoneal space contaminated as a result of wounds, as well as drainage of wounds of the liver, biliary tree, and pancreas, may prevent local or disseminated infection. Early excision and skin grafting of third-degree burns of 20 percent or less of the total body surface will reduce the risk of infection. Primary excision of more extensive burn wounds is fraught with hazard and should be undertaken only by an experienced team at a treatment facility in which the necessary laboratory and nursing support is available.

PROPHYLACTIC ANTIBIOTIC THERAPY

Because all traumatic wounds are contaminated, prophylactic antibiotic therapy at the onset of treatment must be considered. In selecting the antibiotics to be used and the treatment regimen, the following general principles should be borne in mind:

1. All patients with extensive wounds should receive antibiotic treatment, preferably an agent active against gram-positive organisms and a second antibiotic active against gram-negative organisms, as a part of preoperative resuscitation. Antibiotic combinations formerly used for wound infection prophylaxis include penicillin G and streptomycin, and penicillin G and a tetracycline, neither of which is commonly used today. Recently advocated combinations include a cephalosporin and an aminoglycoside; a penicillinase-resistant penicillin and an aminoglycoside; and

when anaerobes are a consideration, clindamycin, an aminoglycoside, and a cephalosporin. Use of perioperative prophylactic antibiotics becomes more important when primary treatment has been or is likely to be delayed.

2. Antibiotic therapy may be required for the treatment of lesser wounds in patients with diabetes, extensive vascular disease, or debilitating conditions of any origin.

3. Patients with wounds involving a joint space or an open fracture should receive prophylactic antibiotic treatment.

4. Patients with penetrating wounds of the abdomen and chest in whom there is visceral injury require antibiotic therapy from the time of admission until the third to fifth day after injury, when such can be terminated if the patient's course is uneventful.

5. Animal bites and especially human bites, even when the wounds are small, require antibiotic therapy. At the present time, penicillin is the agent of choice.

6. Prophylactic antibiotic therapy should be given before initial surgery in traumatized patients so that an effective level of the antimicrobial agent will be present throughout the operation. There are no special prophylactic doses of antibiotics, and the full adult or pediatric dosage of the agent selected should be given for the duration of treatment.

7. Antibiotic prophylaxis should be continued for only three to five days after injury.

8. Patients with minor wounds of the face, not including the buccal cavity, generally do not require prophylactic antibiotic therapy.

9. Cultures should be obtained from all contaminated areas at the time of initial surgery, so that if infection develops, specific antibiotic therapy based on the organisms recovered and their antibiotic sensitivity can be employed.

10. A history of idiosyncratic or sensitivity reaction to antibiotics must be sought from each trauma patient. When the patient gives a clear history of such reactions, one should select an antibiotic that has not been used previously or to which the patient is known not to be sensitive.

11. Adequate surgical treatment is the essential component of wound management, and antimicrobial agents are only adjunctive.

TETANUS

Tetanus is caused by the anaerobic organism *Clostridium tetani* and its toxins and is characterized by local convulsive spasm of the voluntary muscles and a tendency toward episodes of respiratory arrest. It may occur as a complication in either large or small wounds, including lacerations, open fractures, burns (rare), abrasions, and even hypodermic injections. However, the fact that approximately one third of patients seen with active tetanus either have no obvious wound or have wounds considered to be insignificant emphasizes the problem of tetanus prophylaxis following unknown or minimal wounds and suggests that the disease will never be eliminated until universal active immunization has been achieved.

General Principles of Tetanus Prophylaxis

Individual Consideration of Each Patient. For each patient with a wound, the attending physician must determine what is required for adequate prophylaxis (Table 5–1).

Surgical Debridement. Regardless of the active immunization status of the patient, meticulous surgical care, including removal of all devitalized tissue and foreign bodies, should be provided immediately for all wounds. Such care is as essential for the prevention of tetanus as it is for the prevention of other types of wound infection.

Active Immunization. Tetanus toxoid is the simplest, surest, and cheapest immunologic agent available. Immunization should be started in infancy with DPT shots, sometime between 2 and 6 months of age. Two to three doses given intramuscularly 1 month apart followed by a booster at 12 months is the usual method of immunization. Another booster is administered when the child is 5 to 6 years old. Booster injections of tetanus toxoid should be given periodically, but the time schedule has not been definitely established. Basic active immunization with adsorbed toxoid requires three injections. A booster of adsorbed toxoid is indicated ten years after the third injection or ten years after an intervening wound booster.

Each patient with a wound should receive adsorbed tetanus toxoid intramuscularly at the time of injury, either as an initial immunizing dose or as a booster for previous immunization, *unless* he has received a booster or has completed his initial immunization series within the past five years. As the antigen concentration varies in different products, specific information on the volume of a single dose is provided on the label of the package.

Passive Immunization. Whether or not passive immunization with homologous (human) tetanus immune globulin should be provided must be decided individually for each patient. The characteristics of the wound, the conditions under which it was incurred, and the previous active immunization status of the patient must be considered. In those patients without previous active (toxoid) immunization, passive immunization is indicated. In the past, it was traditionally administered with equine or bovine antitoxin in a dose of 3000 to 10,000 units. Because of the danger and frequency of allergic reactions, as well as the rapid elimination of the antitoxin and the incidence of delayed serum sickness following use of equine or bovine antitoxin, passive immunization with these agents should

TABLE 5–1. PROPHYLACTIC TREATMENT OF TETANUS

Type of Wound	Patient Not Immunized or Partially Immunized	Patient Completely Immunized Time Since Last Booster Dose	
		5* TO 10 YEARS	10 YEARS +
Clean minor	Begin or complete immunization per schedule; tetanus toxoid, 0.5 ml	None	Tetanus toxoid 0.5 ml
Clean major or tetanus prone	In one arm: Human tetanus immune globulin, 250 units† In other arm: Tetanus toxoid, 0.5 ml, complete immunization per schedule†	Tetanus toxoid 0.5 ml	In one arm: Tetanus toxoid 0.5 ml† In other arm: Human tetanus immune globulin, 250 u†
Tetanus prone, delayed or incomplete debridement	In one arm: Human tetanus immune globulin 500 units† In other arm: Tetanus toxoid 0.5 ml, complete immunization per schedule thereafter†; antibiotic therapy	Tetanus toxoid 0.5 ml; antibiotic therapy	In one arm: Tetanus toxoid 0.5 ml† In other arm: Human tetanus immune globulin, 500 u†; antibiotic therapy

*No prophylactic immunization is required if patient has had a booster within the previous five years.
†Use different syringes, needles, and injection sites.
NOTE: With different preparations of toxoid, the volume of a single booster dose should be modified.

be discontinued. Instead, the safer human tetanus immune globulin (Hypertet) administered intramuscularly is recommended in the dosages noted below. It should *never* be given *intravenously* for prophylaxis. This product (Hypertet) has a half-life of protection of approximately 30 days.

Patient Record. Every wounded patient should be given a written record of the immunization provided and should be instructed to carry the record at all times and, if indicated, to complete his active immunization. For precise tetanus prophylaxis, an accurate and immediately available history of previous active immunization against tetanus is required.

Antibiotic Prophylaxis. The value of antibiotic agents in the prophylaxis of tetanus remains questionable. There is no doubt that *Clostridium tetani* is sensitive in vitro to penicillin and tetracycline, as well as other antibiotics, but there seems to be some difficulty in delivering an adequate dose of antibiotics to the susceptible bacteria before they liberate toxin. The tetanus-prone wound characteristically has a decreased blood supply and contains necrotic tissue that may prevent high antibiotic blood levels from reaching the infecting bacteria. It is recommended that antibiotic therapy not be relied upon as adequate prophylactic therapy in the place of immunization. For patients with extensive necrotic wounds, particularly those in whom debridement has been delayed or compromised, penicillin and tetracycline have often been employed as prophylaxis against other types of wound infection that may occur, as well as for prophylactic action against tetanus.

SPECIFIC MEASURES FOR PREVIOUSLY IMMUNIZED PATIENTS

When the patient has been actively immunized within the past 10 years and has a severe, neglected, or old (more than 24 hours) tetanus-prone wound, give 0.5 ml of adsorbed toxoid unless it is *certain* that a booster was received within the previous five years.

When the patient received active immunization more than 10 years previously and has not received a booster within the past 10 years:

1. To all, give 0.5 ml of adsorbed tetanus toxoid.

2. To those with wounds with an overwhelming possibility that tetanus might develop, also give 250 units of tetanus immune globulin (human), using different syringes, needles, and sites of injection.

3. To those with severe, neglected, or old wounds, give 500 units of tetanus immune globulin (human) in addition to the toxoid booster.

Antibiotic prophylaxis should also be considered for any patient with tetanus-prone wounds.

TREATMENT FOR PATIENTS NOT PREVIOUSLY IMMUNIZED

With clean minor wounds, in which tetanus is most unlikely, give 0.5 ml of adsorbed tetanus toxoid (initial immunizing dose) and complete immunization at the normally recommended intervals.

With all other wounds:

1. Give 0.5 ml of adsorbed tetanus toxoid (initial immunizing dose).

2. Give 250 units of tetanus immune globulin (human). The dose should be increased to 500 units in severe or neglected wounds.

3. Consider giving penicillin or oxytetracycline prophylactically.

4. Complete immunization at the normally scheduled intervals.

Do *not* administer heterologous antitoxin (equine) except when tetanus immune globulin (human) is not available within 24 hours and *only* if the possibility of tetanus outweighs the danger of reaction to heterologous tetanus antitoxin. Before using such antitoxin, question the patient for a history of allergy and test for sensitivity. If the patient is sensitive to heterologous antitoxin, do not use it because the danger of anaphylaxis probably outweighs the danger of tetanus; rely on penicillin or oxytetracycline. Do not attempt desensitization because it is not worthwhile. If the patient is not sensitive to equine tetanus antitoxin and if the decision is made to administer it for passive immunization, give at least 300 units.

CLOSTRIDIAL MYOSITIS (GAS GANGRENE)

TYPES OF WOUNDS WITH INCREASED RISK

Clostridial myositis is most likely to develop in wounds that have:

1. Extensive laceration or devitalization of muscle such as occurs in compound fractures and injuries from high-velocity missiles.

2. Significant impairment of the local blood supply by the injury, a tourniquet, a tight cast, a circumferential limb burn, or delayed thrombosis.

3. Gross contamination by foreign bodies.

4. Delayed treatment.

5. Inadequate treatment such as incomplete debridement or lack of immobilization.

PREVENTION

Surgery. The most effective means of preventing gas gangrene continues to be early and adequate operation. This includes wide incision, thorough debridement of all devitalized and potentially devitalized tissues, removal of contaminating dirt and all foreign bodies, and effective drainage as required. Adequate debridement is especially important in irregular deep wounds with loculations and recesses. Dead and devitalized tissue and foreign bodies must be removed at the time of initial operation. In combat wounds, in wounds for which treatment has been inordinately delayed, and in all wounds other than the face in which there has been some trauma to the soft tissues, this thorough debridement should be coupled with delayed suture of the wound. The wound should be left open for from four to seven days following the debridement, and then delayed suture should be accomplished if the wound has remained clean and shows no evidence of infection.

Antibiotics. Antibiotic therapy is of some prophylactic value when combined with proper surgical procedures. Experimental and clinical experience affirms this principle but indicates that antibiotic therapy alone cannot be relied upon to prevent clostridial myositis. Penicillin, cephalothin, clindamycin, and chloramphenicol are reported to be effective against over 80 percent of tested strains of *Clostridium perfringens,* whereas tetracycline shows effectiveness against less than 80 percent of strains.

Antitoxin. Prophylactic administration of gas gangrene antitoxin at the time of injury or shortly thereafter is not recommended. The evidence indicates that it has been of little or no practical value in prevention of clinical gas gangrene.

Hyperbaric Oxygen Therapy. Hyperbaric oxygen therapy remains unproven as a prophylactic measure in gas gangrene. Experimental evidence and limited, but favorable, clinical results suggest that hyperbaric oxygen therapy can reduce both the mortality and morbidity of established clostridial myonecrosis.

THERAPY OF ESTABLISHED INFECTIONS

GENERAL PRINCIPLES

Successful treatment of surgical infections depends largely upon the physician's realization that even the newer antibiotic agents are adjunctive to established surgical principles. Early and accurate diagnosis is of great importance in the control of surgical infections. Information should be obtained about the infecting microorganism by immediate examination of stained smears of pus and by culture of the site of infection. Biopsy at the interface of infected and uninfected tissue may be helpful in establishing the nature of infection, particularly in chronic infections of a specific nature. Daily observation of the patient and the wound is mandatory. Quantitative cultures of the margin of the wound suspected of being infected should be obtained and a biopsy of the infected wound and adjacent uninjured tissue taken for histological confirmation of microbial invasion of viable tissue, as will be present in an infected wound.

Selection of Antimicrobial Agent

Whenever possible the selection of antimicrobial agent should be made on the basis of the results of smears, cultures, and sensitivity tests and should be limited to at most two agents. In the case of life-threatening infections, treatment with a broad-spectrum agent or combination of agents should be begun, with antibiotics altered according to the results of specific sensitivity studies. Ongoing surveillance of the microbial flora of the hospital and the sensitivity patterns of the organisms causing infections in that hospital permits one, prior to obtaining culture and sensitivity test results, to initiate antibiotic therapy with those agents most likely to be effective. Treatment of serious mixed infections produced by a variety of gram-positive and gram-negative aerobic and anaerobic bacteria usually requires two antibacterial agents for treatment. Aqueous penicillin G and one of the broad-spectrum antibiotics such as a cephalosporin, an aminoglycoside, a tetracycline, or one of the newer semisynthetic penicillins may be selected. There is some laboratory evidence that antagonism may occur between two or more antibiotics. This may decrease their effectiveness and such combinations should not be employed. Clinical experience suggests that such antagonism is seldom important in vivo. Similarly, true antibiotic synergism identifiable in the laboratory has been difficult to document clinically. Repeat cultures and sensitivity tests at weekly intervals in patients with severe prolonged infections are important because of the possibility of acquired bacterial resistance or the development of secondary infections, either of which may necessitate a change in antibiotic therapy.

The majority of antibiotic agents exert only a bacteriostatic effect, which is greatest on actively growing and reproducing bacteria. Dosage of antibiotic agents must be adequate to obtain sufficient blood and extracellular fluid levels long enough to permit the natural defense mechanisms of the body to dispose of the inhibited, but often still viable, bacteria. Antibiotic therapy, when indicated, should be started as promptly as possible after injury — that is, on admission. Late treatment usually results in a limited or delayed effect with more subsequent septic complications. Local application of chemotherapeutic agents to wounds other than burns is seldom indicated. Intravenous administration of antibiotics is recommended for trauma patients so that adequate blood, fluid, and tissue concentrations will be achieved as rapidly as possible.

Surgical Intervention and Supportive Treatment

The principles of operative treatment of traumatic injuries have not been changed significantly by modern antimicrobial therapy. Antibiotic therapy should be initiated preoperatively for the indications just noted, but operation should not be delayed.

Local and general physiological derangements may be overlooked in the severely traumatized patient. They must be corrected if the full therapeutic effect of antibacterial therapy is to be obtained. Adequate replacement of fluids, electrolytes, and blood is essential in treating patients with surgical infections. General care also includes providing a comfortable ambient temperature to minimize peripheral vasoconstriction and minimize caloric demands. One must also provide sufficient calories and nitrogen to meet the increased metabolic needs of the infected trauma patient. Both the adequacy of the nutritional support regimen employed and the patient's utilization of nutrients, which can be impaired by sepsis, must be frequently monitored.

UNTOWARD REACTIONS TO ANTIBIOTIC AGENTS

The side effects of antimicrobial agents can be classified as toxicity (related to the amount of drug given), hypersensitivity reactions, idiosyncratic reactions, and superinfection. Each antibacterial agent has been shown to be capable of producing one or more of these reactions. Sensitization is a greater problem with certain antibiotics such as penicillin than with others. Certain antibiotics such as chloramphenicol and sulfonamides are capable of producing severe depression of the bone marrow, probably on the basis of idiosyncrasy. The choice of antibiotic agent is dictated by the sensitivity pattern of the offending organism, but relative safety of the individual antimicrobial agents must be considered as well. Secondary or superimposed infections usually occur by suppression of susceptible microbial strains and overgrowth of those organisms resistant to the antibiotic being administered. An example of this type of superimposed infection is the development of staphylococcal enterocolitis following antibiotic therapy. More recently the problem of Candida overgrowth in the gastrointestinal and genitourinary tracts following long-term antibiotic therapy has become more prominent, particularly in burn patients.

CLASSIFICATION OF WOUND INFECTION

Traumatic soft tissue injuries may be contaminated and infected by a variety of microorganisms, resulting in aerobic, anaerobic, gram-negative, gram-positive, or mixed infections, or even nonbacterial infections. When wound sepsis occurs, it may be classified clinically according to its pathophysiological type or bacteriologically according to its microbial etiology. Table 5–2 is a brief clinical classification of infections that may develop in traumatic wounds.

The majority of wound infections start as a cellulitis with hyperemia, edema, pain, and interference of function. Suppuration often follows as a

TABLE 5-2. CLINICAL CLASSIFICATION OF WOUND INFECTIONS

Cellulitis
Lymphangitis and lymphadenitis
Septic thrombophlebitis
Suppuration and abscess formation
Necrosis and gangrene
Bacteremia
Septicemia

result of local liquefaction of tissue and the formation of pus with the production of an abscess. Direct extension through the subcutaneous tissue and along muscle, tissue planes, or tendon sheaths is the most common route of a septic process. In severely injured patients, such as those with extensive burns or multiple trauma, hematogenous pneumonia is a frequent consequence of infection in the wound or in a previously cannulated vein. Further spread may occur by direct lymphatic, venous, and rarely by arterial routes.

ETIOLOGICAL CLASSIFICATION

Many infections are caused by a relatively small number of microbes and can be classified by clinical characteristics on the basis of causative organism.

Staphylococcal Infections. The treatment of established staphylococcal infections consists of rest, heat, elevation of the infected area, adequate surgical drainage when pus has formed, and antibiotic therapy. An infected wound should be reopened with hemostats at the point of maximum pain, swelling, or fluctuation, followed by removal of all skin sutures. The wound should be loosely packed open to keep the edges separated. The packing should be removed within 24 to 72 hours and replaced as necessary. Antibiotic therapy must begin promptly. If the organism is penicillin sensitive (a rarity today), aqueous penicillin G should be administered in doses of approximately 3 million units/24 hours. Erythromycin in doses of 200 mg every six hours orally or sodium oxacillin in oral doses of 3 to 4 gm/day are also effective against some staphylococci. Currently the majority of staphylococcal infections encountered in surgical patients are caused by penicillin-resistant organisms; one of the semisynthetic penicillins should be begun when the infection is diagnosed. Parenterally administered methicillin (4 to 6 gm/day) is a commonly used agent. If the causative organism is identified as being "methicillin-resistant," the antibiotic regimen should be altered to employ the antibiotic agent identified by sensitivity testing as being most effective against the causative organism, e.g., one of the other semisynthetic penicillins, lincomycin, a tetracycline, a cephalosporin, or even an aminoglycoside.

Streptococcal Infections. Although most frequently produced by the aerobic *Streptococcus pyogenes,* some infections are caused by the nonhemolytic *Streptococcus viridans,* anaerobic streptococci, and microaerophilic streptococci. Lesions caused by the aerobic *Streptococcus pyogenes* characteristically are invasive and show rapid early clinical progression.

The treatment of hemolytic streptococcal infections consists primarily of controlling their invasive characteristics by antibiotic therapy, rest, and warm applications, followed by surgical drainage if abscesses or cutaneous gangrene develop. Penicillin is the agent of choice in doses of approximately 3 million units/24 hours. In most instances operative treatment should be delayed until the invasive characteristics of the organism have been controlled. After operation, treatment includes rest, elevation of the part if possible, and application of warm moist compresses to the open wound.

Anaerobic Infections. Infections caused by anaerobic organisms alone are relatively infrequent, but evidence is mounting that anaerobic bacteria may contribute to the development of infections that occur after gastrointestinal tract injury. Anaerobic infections occur with highest incidence in patients with chronic debilitative diseases. In 78 to 83 percent of infections from which anaerobes are recovered, an aerobic organism is also found, most commonly *E. coli.* Many anaerobic organisms have been recovered from clinical specimens, but bacteroides is the anaerobe most frequently involved in such infections. Patients with bacteroides infection show signs of systemic toxicity and often have an inordinate leukocytosis. The wound discharge is characteristically malodorous, thin, and brackish. General supportive care must be given and antibiotic therapy should be begun (80 to 100 percent of bacteroides have been reported to be sensitive to clindamycin, chloramphenicol, or rifampin) and continued for two weeks beyond defervescence. Surgical drainage is mandatory and extensive dissection may be necessary to drain adequately the abscess cavities, which, though poorly defined, are commonly multiloculated and burrowing in character.

Gram-Negative Bacillary Infections. *Escherichia coli,* Pseudomonas, Klebsiella, and *Proteus vulgaris* are examples of organisms capable of causing wound infections in the post-traumatic period. The presence of necrotic tissue, general debility, and immunosuppression increase the likelihood of relatively nonvirulent gram-negative bacteria invading previously undamaged tissue and causing infection. A relatively long incubation period is characteristic of post-traumatic wound infections caused by these bacilli. Treatment of these gram-negative infections includes incision and drainage of abscess cavities, excision of necrotic tissue, and antibiotic therapy based on sensitivity tests. Chloramphenicol is particularly useful in many of these infections but because of the severe untoward reactions associated with its use, it generally is used in treating life-threatening infections caused by organisms resistant to all other agents. More recently, the aminoglycosides and some of the newer semisynthetic penicillins and cephalosporins have been used effectively against these gram-negative infections, particularly those caused by *Pseudomonas aeruginosa.*

Mixed or Synergistic Infections. A large and miscellaneous group of infections with a polymicrobial etiology are found in association with injuries involving the gastrointestinal, respiratory, and genitourinary tracts. The toxins and enzymes produced by the organisms responsible for such infections may cause extensive tissue necrosis, suppuration, and systemic toxicity. Examples of mixed infections include human bite infections, peritonitis, empyema, and nonclostridial cellulitis.

Human bite infections are particularly dangerous because of the potentially virulent organisms usually present in the mouth. A mixture of bacteria consisting of aerobic and anaerobic streptococci, *Bacteroides melaninogenicus,* spirochetes, or staphylococci is often found. When infections become established, radical decompression of infected areas and tissue planes by incision is necessary along with intensive antibiotic therapy and physiologically sound wound care.

Crepitant (nonclostridial) cellulitis is a mixed infection that is usually seen as a complication of wounds of the perineum, abdominal wall, buttock, hip, thorax, or neck that have been contaminated by discharges from the intestinal, genitourinary, or respiratory tracts. Proper surgical decompression of all involved areas by multiple incisions is imperative. Aqueous penicillin in doses of one million units every four to six hours is recommended along with a broad-spectrum antibiotic. Supportive therapy in this form of infection is also necessary and may be life saving.

Nonbacterial Infections. The increased magnitude of injury now treated by timely surgery and sophisticated pre- and postoperative care involving sophisticated broad-spectrum antibiotics has resulted in an increased occurrence of infections due to yeast, fungi, and viruses in critically ill patients with impaired antimicrobial defense mechanisms. Diagnosis of such infections depends upon frequent examination of wounds with impaired healing and biopsy monitoring of infected wounds for microbiological and histological examination. Specific antifungal or antiviral therapy should be begun promptly, with surgical excision of the infected tissue when indicated.

Antifungal agents include mycostatin, useful for the treatment of oral and gastrointestinal moniliasis; flucytosine, which can be administered orally for treatment of Candida, Torulopsis, and Aspergillus infections, and amphotericin B given intravenously as treatment for life-threatening systemic fungal infections. Recent enthusiastic reports on the effectiveness of miconazole indicate that it may be an effective antifungal agent.

Herpes simplex virus has been the viral agent most frequently causing infections in surgical patients. Both convalescent serum and dexamethasone have been recommended for the treatment of systemic viral infections, but their effectiveness remains unconfirmed. The effectiveness of idoxuridine, cytosine arabinoside, and adenine arabinoside for systemic herpetic infections also remains unverified by controlled trials.

CLOSTRIDIAL INFECTIONS

CLOSTRIDIAL MYOSITIS

Unfortunately, clostridial myositis is often recognized by the clinical appearance of the patient and the infected wound in more obvious, far advanced, and often irreversible states of disease. Casts, splints, or large dressings necessary for the treatment of major injuries obscure the area of the wound and make the observation and interpretation of local signs difficult. For these reasons, the dressings should be removed promptly and the wound inspected directly if there is the slightest suspicion of this infection. The most important causative microorganism is *Cl. perfringens* (Welchii). It may occur alone or in combination with other clostridia.

Clinical Manifestations. A variable interval exists between injury and the development of the lesion, sometimes a period as short as six hours, particularly in wounds associated with gross devitalization and contamination of muscle. The average incubation period is 48 hours. Pain is the earliest and most important symptom, being secondary to the rapid infiltration of the infected muscle by edema and gas.

A rapid and feeble pulse usually follows the onset of pain and is characteristically out of proportion to the elevation of the temperature. Early in the course of infection the blood pressure is normal or slightly elevated. Later it may decrease significantly, falling to shock level.

Temperature elevation in the early stages of the infection may vary considerably. Fever is not a reliable index of the severity and extent of the infectious process, but a low or subnormal temperature associated with a markedly rapid pulse may indicate a grave prognosis. The general appearance of the patient usually includes a peculiar gray pallor, weakness, and profuse sweating. The mental state is often one of apathy and indifference. Stupor, delirium, prostration, and coma are late symptoms indicative of an overwhelming infection.

Early in the course of infection the overlying skin is either white, shiny, and tense or essentially normal in appearance. A dirty-brown watery discharge with peculiar foul odor usually escapes from the wound. As the swelling increases, the overlying skin becomes dusky or bronze in appearance. In advanced cases further discoloration occurs and vesicles filled with dark-red fluid characteristically appear. Crepitation is a relatively late sign.

Laboratory and X-ray Diagnosis. Blood counts usually reveal a marked reduction in red blood cell, hematocrit, or hemoglobin levels. The leukocyte count is seldom elevated above 12,000 to 15,000. In general, no satisfactory laboratory tests exist for the early diagnosis of gas gangrene. For this reason immediate surgical exploration of any wound suspected of harboring clostridial myositis is advisable. Microscopic examination of the watery discharge usually reveals numerous red blood cells and many large gram-positive bacteria. In contrast to pyogenic infections, few pus cells are seen. *Clostridium perfringens* and other clostridia usually appear as large gram-positive bacilli with squared ends without evidence of sporulation when the exudate is prepared with Gram stain.

X-rays taken at intervals of two to four hours may aid in the diagnosis by differentiating gas in the soft tissues produced by clostridial invasion from that due to mechanical or chemical causes. If the visible gas increases in amount or linear spread along the muscle and fascial planes is evident, an earlier diagnosis of gas gangrene can be made.

Treatment. Early and adequate operation is the most effective means of treating clostridial myositis. If the diagnosis is made early, while the gangrene is relatively localized, radical decompression of the involved fascial compartments by extensive longitudinal incisions and excision of infected muscle usually arrests the process and eliminates the need for amputation. If the diagnosis is reached when the process is extensive and has caused irreversible gangrenous changes, open amputation of the guillotine type becomes necessary.

Penicillin G, cephalothin, and clindamycin, in that order, are the drugs of choice in treating this condition. The intravenous route using maximum doses is preferred, i.e., 3 million units of penicillin, every 3 hours. Chloramphenicol is also effective. Resistance of anaerobes, including the clostridial organisms, to tetracycline has relegated that agent to an inferior position for treatment of anaerobic infections. Supportive therapy, including blood transfusion, maintenance of fluid and electrolyte balance, adequate immobilization of the infected injured parts, and relief of pain, are of great value.

Effectiveness of hyperbaric oxygen therapy in treatment of clostridial myonecrosis remains unproved, but the favorable clinical experience of the Duke University group has led them to recommend its use as an adjunct to adequate surgical therapy. In cases of severe toxemia with septic shock, intravenous steroids should be considered. All secondary operations designed to facilitate healing or restore function of the wounded extremity should be postponed until the infection has been brought under complete control.

The use of polyvalent gas gangrene antitoxin remains controversial. Fifty thousand units of the antitoxin given intravenously at once and every 4 to 6 hours up to a total dosage of 250,000 units seems to have been helpful in some cases in controlling the severe toxemia of gas gangrene. Many surgeons, however, continue to doubt the efficacy of gas gangrene antitoxin.

CLOSTRIDIAL CELLULITIS

Clostridial cellulitis is a septic crepitant process involving the epifascial, retroperitoneal, or other connective tissues. Its incubation period is usually three to four days and its onset is ordinarily more gradual than gas gangrene. Systemic effects are usually less than with clostridial myositis. However, clostridial cellulitis is not a condition to be regarded lightly. The spread of infection in the tissue spaces may be rapid and extensive, necessitating prompt radical surgical drainage.

Prevention of clostridial myositis and clostridial cellulitis depends primarily on thorough and complete initial debridement of wounds. Dead and devitalized tissue and foreign bodies must be removed at the time of initial surgery. All wounds in which there has been severe trauma to the soft tissue and wounds from high-velocity missiles should be thoroughly debrided, packed open, and frequently inspected. Delayed suturing can be done four to seven days later if the wound has remained clean. The use of gas gangrene antitoxin has not proved to be of value in the prophylaxis of these infections.

Treatment.   The debridement of the wound involved with anaerobic cellulitis is the most important step in the management of these patients. All devitalized tissue must be excised. When the infection follows fascial planes extending from the traumatized area of the wound, long incisions must be made to open these areas and excise the necrotic fascia. Following debridement the wounds may be gently cleansed with a surgical soap and water before a dressing is applied. Intensive systemic antibiotic and supportive therapy similar to that listed for clostridial myositis should also be used for this serious infection.

TETANUS

Established tetanus is a clinical emergency. Its treatment consists primarily of supportive and symptomatic measures to prevent the complications (usually respiratory) that cause death.

Serotherapy.   Considerable controversy has arisen over the effectiveness of serotherapy in the treatment of established tetanus. Protective antibody levels can be obtained with the injection of tetanus antitoxin, but whether or not these protective levels are of benefit to a patient who has fixation of tetanus toxin in the central nervous system remains debatable. However, there are experimental data indicating that tetanus antitoxin can inactivate circulating toxin and toxin as it is liberated from the wound. Accordingly, intramuscular human tetanus immune globulin has been recommended in a dosage of 3,000 to 6,000 units, which will establish protective serum levels persisting for up to 14 weeks after injection. Other authorities recommend the immediate intravenous administration of 10,000 units of human tetanus immune globulin.

Surgical Excision of Wound.   If a primary wound is present it should be surgically excised or extensively debrided with removal of all foreign material and necrotic tissue. Injection of the area with antisera one hour prior to surgical incision is recommended.

Sedation and Muscle Relaxant Drugs.   Sodium pentothal has been a drug of choice for general sedation of the patient with tetanus to control convulsive seizures. It has been administered in dilute solution (0.5 to 1.0 gm/1000 ml) in a continuous slow intravenous drip. The dosage is adjusted to produce sleep, from which the patient can be aroused by moderate external stimuli to obey commands. Should a convulsive seizure occur, a 2.5 percent solution of pentothal is injected intravenously immediately. A syringe with this more concentrated pentothal solution should be connected by a stopcock to the continuous intravenous drip tubing.

A constant intravenous infusion of diazepam (Valium) 10 to 20 mg/kg of body weight per 24 hours may be adequate to control seizure and muscle spasms. To control severe tetanic contractions curare, succinyl choline, or methocarbamol may be used with mechanical ventilation necessary for those patients receiving the muscle relaxants.

Tracheal Intubation. Early tracheal intubation employing a cuffed endotracheal tube may be of benefit in treating severe cases. An endotracheal tube provides a constant open route for suctioning and prevents aspiration. Alternatively, tracheostomy decreases the anatomical dead space and provides a route for long-term access to the lower tracheobronchial tree.

Mechanical Respirators. The use of a mechanical ventilator may be helpful for ensuring adequate ventilation in the presence of heavy sedation. Adequate humidification of the inspired air should be provided to prevent crust formation and drying of the tracheobronchial mucosa.

Constant Nursing Attendants. A special nurse or physician should be at the patient's bedside at all times. This is extremely important so that convulsive seizures and episodes of respiratory arrest can be immediately recognized and treated immediately.

External Stimuli. The patient should be kept in a darkened, quiet room, and all forms of stimulation should be kept to a minimum. Loud sounds or sudden stimulation of any type may excite seizures and cause respiratory arrest.

Adequate Fluid, Electrolyte, and Calorie Intake. Fluids should be administered in sufficient volume to prevent dehydration and maintain electrolyte balance yet avoid fluid overload. Adequate nutrition, preferably by an enteral route, should be provided. If an endotracheal or tracheostomy tube is in place, simultaneous placement of a nasogastric tube may compress the intervening esophageal and tracheal walls with resulting necrosis and fistula formation. Obviously, the smallest caliber feeding tube should be used in such patients. Intravenous hyperalimentation may be necessary to achieve calorie balance in patients requiring extended care.

Chemotherapy. Antibiotics do not affect tetanus toxoid that is already present in the circulation or bound to tissues. However, invasive wound infection or complicating pneumonia may require specific antibiotic therapy as determined by sensitivity tests on the organisms identified in culture samples.

Steroid Therapy. Although not used routinely, steroid therapy has been employed in a few severe cases of tetanus in which the prolonged course of the disease seemed to threaten adrenal exhaustion. The effectiveness of such treatment is unproved.

Hyperbaric Oxygen. Since hyperbaric oxygen has no apparent effect upon tetanus toxins already present in the patient's tissue, its use appears to have no influence on the course of clinically established tetanus.

Hygiene and Positioning. Prolonged coma, obtundation, disturbed muscle tone, and therapeutic considerations such as prolonged mechanical ventilation require that the skin be kept clean and dry and the patient frequently turned to prevent formation of decubitus ulcers. Special care should also be taken to prevent the development of fecal impaction, urinary retention, and atelectasis. Carefully planned and reliably executed physical therapy should be carried out to prevent development of limb contractures.

Chapter

6

Burns and Other Thermal Injuries

Heat, cold, chemicals, and electricity — alone or in combination — produce injuries that share many of the same pathophysiological mechanisms but often require differing forms of treatment. The consequences of massive intravascular fluid loss and of extensive tissue destruction dominate the early care of patients with such injuries. Since patients are seen at varying intervals after injury or may be transferred from the primary receiving facility with only partially complete treatment, the initial phase of care is considered to include the first 48 hours postburn and may be of longer duration.

THERMAL INJURIES

Thermal injury to the skin disrupts capillary integrity, allowing loss of large volumes of plasma-like fluid into the extravascular tissues. Most of the immediate problems affecting the acutely burned patient, including hypovolemia, airway obstruction, and extremity ischemia, arise from the massive tissue sequestration of fluid.

First Aid

At the scene of the accident, the burning process should be stopped by extinguishing flames, or removing the patient from an electric contact or from further exposure to a chemical agent. Thereafter, the burned patient is managed like any victim of trauma, and care of associated injuries usually takes precedence over treatment of the burn wound (except in the case of those patients with chemical burns). Because running allows spread of the flames to the upper parts of the body and face, the patient should be placed flat on the ground and the fire extinguished by water or blankets, or by slowly rolling the patient over. When used for a brief period immediately following injury, application of running water or a towel wet with cold water may be soothing and may limit the extent of injury. Such treatment

84

should be terminated when tissue temperature returns to body temperature, particularly in patients with large burns, who can develop systemic hypothermia. Thereafter, the patient should be wrapped in clean sheets and blankets to maintain body temperature and transported to a treatment facility. The burn wound requires no specific attention at this time.

Carbon monoxide poisoning is common following thermal injury and may cause headache, dizziness, and confusion. If a burned patient exhibits any central nervous system symptoms, some degree of carbon monoxide poisoning should be presumed to be present. It is prudent to treat all burned patients at the scene of the accident with humidified 100 percent oxygen to accelerate the dissociation of any carbon monoxide from oxygen. Inhalation injury usually produces no immediate problems following burn injury. However, if airway obstruction appears to be imminent or if other injuries render the airway unstable, an endotracheal tube should be inserted, especially if the patient is unconscious.

The condition of burned patients with no associated injuries is usually stable immediately following injury, and the patient can be safely transported to a hospital for definitive care. (Excessive speed and disregard of traffic signals by the driver of the transporting ambulance are seldom necessary.) The patient should not be given oral fluids or food, and if the trip to the hospital is expected to exceed 30 to 45 minutes, an intravenous catheter should be inserted for fluid administration.

HISTORY

Most patients with even large burns are alert immediately following injury, and a careful medical history can be obtained while the physical examination and initial treatment are being carried out. The patient's family can often provide additional information regarding events surrounding the injury. Certain details are important in relation to resuscitation therapy, potential complications, and ultimate mortality. Those treating the patient should know the preburn weight and the exact time of injury, since resuscitation fluid estimates for the first 24 postburn hours are calculated on the basis of extent of burn and body weight.

Damage to the respiratory tract occurs more commonly when the patient is burned in a closed space or by steam than by flash burns in an open area. A decreased level of consciousness at the time of injury explains the deep and extensive burns often present in the patient who is acutely intoxicated, postictal, or unconscious at the time of burning. Pre-existing diseases, such as diabetes, chronic alcoholism, chronic lung disease, and congestive heart failure, must be identified, because they predispose to future complications and are associated with an increased mortality. Chronically administered medications such as digitalis, anticonvulsants, insulin, and replacement hormones must be continued during hospitalization. Known allergies proscribe use of the involved medication.

Physical Examination

All clothing, jewelry, and dentures are removed. Associated injuries are searched for, and their treatment may take precedence over that of the burn. Estimation of the severity of the thermal injury is necessary both for planning initial care and for predicting future morbidity and mortality.

Initially, the extent of burn can be quickly estimated in an adult by using the Rule of Nines, in which various anatomical regions represent 9 percent of the total body surface or a multiple thereof. Thus, the head represents 9 percent of the total body surface area, each upper extremity 9 percent, the anterior trunk 18 percent, the posterior trunk 18 percent, and each lower extremity 18 percent. The perineum represents 1 percent of the body surface. In children, the head accounts for a larger proportion of the body surface, and the lower extremities contribute proportionately less. The use of a surface area chart (Fig. 6–1) allows a more detailed estimate of burn extent, and the area of burn should be recorded while the patient is undergoing initial wound debridement.

Although the depth of the burn is less important than the extent of burn in initial triage decisions and immediate care, it significantly influences the decision on need for in-hospital care, the incidence of burn wound infection, and the risk of death, and determines the need for skin grafting and functional results (Table 6–1). A *first-degree burn*, such as that produced from excessive sun exposure, involves only the most superficial layers of the skin and is of little physiological importance. The involved skin is slightly erythematous and painful and exhibits no blisters. Such burns are not included in the estimate of burn size. The *second-degree burn* extends deeper into but not through the skin and is often called a partial-thickness burn. Such burns are most commonly caused by flash ignitions or spill scalds. The appearance of a second-degree burn varies with the depth of the injury. A superficial second-degree burn is moist and pink to bright red in adults, and is covered with a serous exudate. These burns are often exquisitely painful and are sensitive to touch and air movement. They usually heal within three weeks. Deep second-degree burns are less sensitive (but not anesthetic), appear darker or pale and colorless, and are less pliable. Such burns heal slowly, often with hypertrophic scarring, and are susceptible to conversion to full-thickness injuries during episodes of infection or poor perfusion.

A *third-degree burn* destroys the entire depth of the skin and may extend into the underlying subcutaneous tissue. An injury involving the underlying muscle is sometimes called a "fourth-degree burn." Third-degree burns are frequently caused by immersion scalds, flames, chemicals, and electricity. Since all dermal elements are destroyed, full-thickness burns require grafting for closure. Such burns are dry and have an unyielding leathery texture. These burns may be black and charred, yellow-brown or translucent in appearance, and thrombosed veins are often visible beneath the surface. Since the cutaneous nerve endings have been destroyed, third-degree burns are anesthetic. Lesser intensities of heat cause deeper burns in children, and the characteristics of burn depth in adults do not necessarily apply to burns in children. A red moist burn, especially if caused by a scald, is more often a full-thickness injury in a child. When the severity of burns in both children and adults is estimated, more often than not the extent is overestimated, while the depth is underestimated.

RESUSCITATION

A secure cannula should be inserted into a large-caliber accessible vein in the upper extremity or into a central vein. The cannula is preferably

BURN ESTIMATE AND DIAGRAM
AGE vs. AREA

Area	Birth 1 yr.	1–4 yr.	5–9 yr.	10–14 yr.	15 yr.	Adult	2°	3°	Total	Donor Areas
Head	19	17	13	11	9	7				
Neck	2	2	2	2	2	2				
Ant. Trunk	13	13	13	13	13	13				
Post. Trunk	13	13	13	13	13	13				
R. Buttock	2½	2½	2½	2½	2½	2½				
L. Buttock	2½	2½	2½	2½	2½	2½				
Genitalia	1	1	1	1	1	1				
R.U. Arm	4	4	4	4	4	4				
L.U. Arm	4	4	4	4	4	4				
R.L. Arm	3	3	3	3	3	3				
L.L. Arm	3	3	3	3	3	3				
R. Hand	2½	2½	2½	2½	2½	2½				
L. Hand	2½	2½	2½	2½	2½	2½				
R. Thigh	5½	6½	8	8½	9	9½				
L. Thigh	5½	6½	8	8½	9	9½				
R. Leg	5	5	5½	6	6½	7				
L. Leg	5	5	5½	6	6½	7				
R. Foot	3½	3½	3½	3½	3½	3½				
L. Foot	3½	3½	3½	3½	3½	3½				

TOTAL

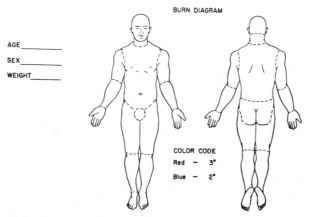

BURN DIAGRAM

AGE_____

SEX_____

WEIGHT_____

COLOR CODE

Red — 3°

Blue — 2°

Figure 6–1. Surface area chart used to "map" extent of burn. Note change with age of the proportion of total body surface represented by the head and lower extremities.

TABLE 6–1. CLINICAL CLASSIFICATION OF BURN DEPTH

| | First-degree | Second-degree (Partial Thickness) | | Third-degree (Full Thickness) |
		SUPERFICIAL	DEEP	
Color	Bright red	Red and mottled	Dark red or pale yellow to off-white	Very dark red in children; pearly white, charred; translucent and parchment-like. Bronzed – strong acid injury; dissolution of skin with exposed deep tissues – strong alkali injury
Surface	Dry with focal exfoliation	Blisters with copious exudate	Denuded surface with minimal exudate	Dry and leathery with thrombosed dermal and subdermal vessels visible. Smooth and silky – strong acid injury; liquefaction necrosis – strong alkali injury
Sensation	Painful	Painful	Diminished pinprick sensation; intact dermal sensation	Anesthetic except for deep pressure sensation in subdermal tissues
Time for healing	3–6 days	10–21 days	More than 3 weeks	Grafting always required
Cause	Sun or minor flash injury	Flash injury; spill scalds	Scalds of longer duration; flash of high intensity; brief exposure to flame	Flame burns; strong chemicals; contact with hot objects; electricity; prolonged scalds

inserted through unburned skin, but when this is not feasible, reliability of venous access is more important than violation of the burn wound. Fluid administration through a needle inserted into a peripheral vein is unreliable, since tissue edema and movement during transportation may dislodge the needle. Most physicians treating acutely ill patients are skilled in the techniques of percutaneous cannulation, and cutdowns are rarely necessary.

The burn injury produces a defect in the capillary barrier with loss of intravascular electrolytes, proteins, and water across the damaged vessels. The net effect is an ongoing plasma volume deficit, which is the central feature of burn shock. The goal of fluid resuscitation is to replace and maintain effective plasma volume during the period of capillary leakage, and resuscitation should commence as soon after thermal injury as possible, before the patient has incurred a large plasma volume deficit. Lactated Ringer's solution approximates the ideal balanced electrolyte solution and is used in most resuscitation regimens. Because of both the large volumes required for resuscitation and the relative glucose intolerance of acutely injured individuals, resuscitation fluid should not contain glucose. The adult fluid dosage of lactated Ringer's solution should be estimated as 2 ml/kg body weight/percent body surface burned, utilizing the *full* extent of the burn for calculation (Table 6–2). Because of a higher ratio of body surface area to mass, children require relatively more fluid, and their resuscitation needs should be estimated as 3 ml/kg body weight/percent body surface burned. Approximately one half of the calculated dosage will be required during the first eight hours following injury, and the remainder over the subsequent 16 postburn hours. Additional electrolyte-free fluid need not be given during the first 24 postburn hours. No colloid-containing fluids need be administered during the first

TABLE 6–2. **BURN PATIENT FLUID RESUSCITATION**

First 24 hours postburn
1. Adult: Lactated Ringer's solution, 2 ml/kg body weight/% burn
2. Child: Lactated Ringer's solution, 3 ml/kg body weight/% burn
    a. Calculate fluid dose on basis of total extent of burn
    b. Plan upon administering one-half of calculated dose during the first 8 hours postburn
    c. Adjust infusion rate to obtain hourly urinary output of:
        a. 30–50 ml in adult
        b. 1 ml/kg body weight in children weighing less than 30 kg

Second 24 hours postburn
1. Colloid-containing fluid (e.g., fresh-frozen plasma, albumin diluted to physiologic concentration in saline):
    a. 0.3 ml/kg body weight/% burn for patients with burns of 30–50%
    b. 0.4 ml/kg body weight/% burn for patients with burns of 50–70%
    c. 0.5 ml/kg body weight/% burn for patients with burns of more than 70%
2. Electrolyte-free water to meet metabolic needs and maintain urinary output

postburn day, since intravascular colloid continues to be lost across the damaged capillary surface. Although 10 to 15 percent of the red blood cell mass is initially lost by direct trauma and by continued hemolysis, burned patients are usually polycythemic during the first 48 postburn hours because of the proportionately greater loss of plasma volume. Blood is therefore not given unless pre-existing anemia or concurrent hemorrhage intervenes. Later, as plasma volume is restored, red cells are given in quantities sufficient to maintain the hematocrit over 30 percent.

This formula for fluid resuscitation of burned patients is only an *estimate*, and the volume actually administered to any patient is adjusted according to his physiological response to injury and therapy. Adequacy of resuscitation is determined by scheduled repeated observation of a number of clinical indices of organ function by both the physician and the nursing personnel.

The patient's general condition and vital signs should be assessed at least hourly. Disturbances of mentation, such as confusion and agitation, are uncommon in the adequately resuscitated patient and suggest hypovolemia and the need for increased fluid. Tachypnea and anxiety are more often caused by hypoxia and respond to oxygen administration. Pulse rate in an adult should be less than 120 beats per minute. Blood pressure obtained by a cuff sphygmomanometer is unreliable because of massive tissue edema and peripheral vasoconstriction. A Doppler ultrasonic flow probe used in conjunction with an occlusive cuff alleviates many of these difficulties but may still give erroneously low blood pressure measurements, and other indices of tissue perfusion must be relied upon.

Urinary output is the most reliable and conveniently obtained indication of adequate tissue perfusion. A urethral catheter should be inserted immediately following admission to the treatment facility and connected to a closed drainage system. After a urinalysis is obtained, the initial urine obtained should be discarded and measurement of hourly outputs begun. For adults and for children over 30 kg body weight, 30 to 50 ml/hour is an acceptable rate of urine production and indicates adequate fluid replacement. For children weighing less than 30 kg, the rate of fluid infusion should be adjusted to obtain an hourly urinary output of 1 ml/kg body weight. Urinary outputs in excess of these guidelines result in over-resuscitation, cause increased tissue edema, and predispose to pulmonary complications later in the first postburn week. Over-resuscitation occurs most often when burn formulae have been blindly followed and the infusion rate not adjusted according to the patient's physiological response. Conversely, oliguria is nearly always due to insufficient fluid administration, and diuretics are rarely indicated.

Higher urinary volumes may be necessary in several specific instances: extensive electrical injury, crush injury, deep thermal injury with muscle necrosis, and white phosphorus burns inappropriately treated with concentrated solutions of copper sulfate (greater than 1 percent copper sulfate). If hemochromogens appear in the urine, urinary output is increased to 75 to

100 ml/hour by the infusion of additional fluids and, if necessary, by an osmotic diuretic. Mannitol, 12.5 gm, is added to each liter of lactated Ringer's solution until the hemochromogens disappear from the urine. When diuretics have been given, however, urinary output is no longer a reliable indicator of fluid resuscitation adequacy.

Although rarely needed, monitoring of central venous pressure or pulmonary capillary wedge pressure may be indicated during the resuscitation of high-risk patients. Such patients include the elderly, those with significant pre-existing cardiopulmonary disease, those requiring greater than expected fluid volumes, and patients in whom resuscitation has been inordinately delayed. The central venous pressure rarely exceeds 5 cm of water during the period of resuscitation, and higher levels are often associated with cardiopulmonary disease. Because of high respiratory rates and increased pulmonary vascular resistance, the flow-directed pulmonary artery catheter more accurately reflects the acutely burned patient's intravascular volume than does a central venous catheter. Mechanical ventilatory support must be temporarily stopped to obtain accurate readings of the pulmonary capillary wedge pressure.

Laboratory studies are of ancillary value only and are more useful after the first postburn day. The hematocrit should return to normal by 48 to 72 hours, and serum electrolytes and BUN generally remain normal during all stages of resuscitation if the patient is properly managed. The arterial pH may be decreased soon after injury, particularly if a long delay has intervened prior to resuscitation. The metabolic acidosis arises from poor tissue perfusion and generally ameliorates with adequate fluid administration. If significant acidosis persists after restoration of vital signs and urinary output, intravenous sodium bicarbonate is indicated.

The patient should be weighed directly on admission and at least daily thereafter. A weight gain of 15 to 20 percent of initial body weight occurs during the initial resuscitation. During the second 24 postburn hours (and subsequent days), fluid therapy is directed toward replacing urinary and evaporative fluid losses at a rate that allows a slow, controlled loss of the weight gained during the first postinjury day. The patient usually begins to diurese on the second postburn day in response to osmotically active tissue breakdown products and to early mobilization of tissue edema fluid. Cutaneous thermal injury destroys the water vapor barrier of the skin, and large quantities of water are lost by evaporation. This loss is proportional to burn size and can be estimated according to the formula: evaporative water loss (ml/hr) = (25 + percent body surface burned) × total body surface area in square meters. This formula estimates the lower limit of evaporative loss, which increases with high environmental temperatures and air flow and may exceed nine liters per day. The adequacy of hydration should be monitored by daily determination of body weight, serum osmolality, and serum sodium concentration. Hypernatremia should be treated by judicious administration of increased amounts of electrolyte-free water.

With completion of resuscitation at the end of the first postburn day, total body sodium is increased by as much as 2500 to 3000 mEq. The large urinary and evaporative losses contain little sodium, so that normal body tonicity must be regulated by the administration of electrolyte-free water. Sodium-containing fluids only add to the sodium excess already present and further increase edema formation, especially in the elderly. A useful guide to fluid replacement after the first postburn day is to administer dextrose in water at a rate predicted to replace evaporative loss plus an allowance for an adequate urine output. The actual rate is then adjusted to allow a daily weight loss of 2 to 3 percent of body weight, so that the patient has returned to his preinjury weight by postburn day 10. Urinary output is not replaced volumetrically, even if diuresis is massive. Hyponatremia almost always arises from excessive administration of electrolyte-free water and not from a deficit in total body sodium. Hyponatremia in children not uncommonly precipitates convulsions, which occur during the first two postburn days in 80 percent of episodes.

After the first postburn day, capillary integrity is restored, and plasma protein deficits can be rectified by administration of colloid-containing solutions. Colloid equivalent to 0.3 to 0.5 ml plasma/kg body weight/percent burn is administered on the second postburn day to restore plasma volume. Thereafter, plasma proteins are most effectively maintained by adequate nutrition. Potassium supplements are not necessary during the first 24 to 48 postburn hours and are dangerous if given in the presence of massive tissue destruction, acidosis, or hemolysis. If hyperkalemia develops at this time, the patient should be placed on a cardiac monitor and treated by intravenous administration of 30 to 40 units of regular insulin added to 1 liter of 10 percent glucose solution and, in acidotic patients, 150 to 300 mEq of sodium bicarbonate. Administration of an ion exchange resin (Kayexalate) is also given in a dosage of 20 to 30 gm every 6 hours orally or 100 gm per rectum as a retention enema. Dialysis may be necessary in refractory cases. Massive renal losses of potassium begin after the second postburn day and may exceed 600 mEq per day. The serum potassium level should be monitored and losses replaced by addition of potassium to the intravenous fluids in the amount needed to maintain the serum concentration at or slightly above 3.5 mEq/L.

INHALATION INJURY

Respiratory difficulties accompanying thermal injury are caused by obstruction of the upper airway, impairment of ventilatory exchange, and, later, development of infection of the lower airway and lung. Facial and neck burns, especially those around the lips and nose, should alert the physician to the possibility of respiratory tract injury. An unyielding third-degree burn encircling the thorax can cause impairment of ventilatory exchange, which is relieved by chest escharotomy. Hoarseness, stridor, audible airflow turbulence, and the production of carbonaceous sputum indicate potentially severe inhalation injury. Diagnostic procedures should be carried out to define the extent of injury. Tracheostomy is no longer performed routinely in burned patients. When a stable airway is required, an endotracheal tube is preferred. Indications for tracheal intubation include (1) acute upper airway obstruction, or impending obstruction, (2) edema of laryngeal structures, (3) inability to prevent aspiration or to handle copious secretions (bronchorrhea) induced by inhalation injury, and (4) severe lower airway inhalation injury with acute respiratory failure.

The pharynx is visualized directly, and the vocal cords and supraglottic structures are examined by mirror laryngoscopy. Erythema, edema, and mucosal blebs confirm the presence of serious upper airway injury. Further instrumentation of the upper respiratory tract can precipitate complete obstruction and is avoided. Upper airway edema is maximal during the first 48 hours following injury and then decreases. If significant swelling is present but obstruction is not imminent, the patient can be treated every two to four hours for a total of 24 to 36 hours with aerosolized racemic epinephrine (0.5 ml of a 2.25 percent solution diluted to a volume of 2 ml with saline). Fluid administration is kept to the minimum consistent with good organ perfusion. The patient is placed in a semirecumbent position and treated with humidified air or oxygen as indicated, and, except for very careful insertion of a nasogastric tube, no manipulation or mechanical irritation of the swollen supraglottic structures is permitted. If the patient with known upper airway injury is treated in this fashion, he must be continuously and carefully observed by experienced personnel who can immediately recognize and treat progressive airway obstruction.

If obstruction appears imminent or if a patient with inhalation injury is going to be transported under conditions that preclude continuous evaluation of the airway, a nasotracheal tube should be inserted after application of a topical vasoconstrictor and anesthetic to the nasopharynx. The nasotracheal tube can be passed over a flexible fiberoptic bronchoscope, which not only allows negotiation of injured air passages under direct vision but also permits safe insertion in patients with suspected or proven neck injuries. Except for severe facial or neck injuries, tracheotomy is rarely indicated as an emergency. Following tracheal intubation, humidified air or oxygen is administered by a T-shaped connector or a ventilator, depending on the functional status of the lungs. Sterile technique is always used during routine care of the tube and during tracheobronchial toilet. Tissue edema begins to recede 48 hours after injury, and, in the absence of other respiratory disease, extubation is usually possible by the fifth postburn day.

Except for steam inhalation, thermal injury to the lower tracheobronchial tree and lung parenchyma is rare. Rather, the noxious products of incomplete combustion and smoke are either inhaled or forced down the airway by the overpressure of an explosion, and cause a chemical tracheobronchitis or bronchiolitis. If the injury to the tracheobronchial tree is severe, unrelenting bronchospasm and profuse bronchorrhea may develop within hours and proceed to irreversible respiratory failure. More commonly, inhalation injury becomes apparent only after the third post-burn day, when mobilization of sequestered tissue fluid begins. The chest roentgenogram and arterial blood gases are often normal for several days following injury and do not predict the presence of inhalation injury.

Flexible fiberoptic bronchoscopy provides accurate information about acute infraglottic inhalation disease even in the absence of upper airway injury. After topical anesthesia, the examination is easily performed at the bedside; general anesthesia is both unnecessary and extremely hazardous in acutely burned individuals. Edema, erythema, focal hemorrhage, ulceration, and deposition of particulate carbonaceous material in the tracheobronchial mucosa indicate lower airway injury. Congestion and focal hemorrhage will not be seen in inadequately resuscitated patients who will exhibit a pale mucosa, and this false-negative finding is avoided by performing bronchoscopy only after resuscitation has restored tissue blood flow. False-positive results are occasionally encountered in patients with chronic bronchitis and a long smoking history. The accuracy of diagnosis of inhalation injury can be enhanced by use of the ^{133}Xenon ventilation/perfusion lung scan and various tests of pulmonary function, but facilities for performing such tests may not be available during the early care period.

Patients with inhalation injury are treated symptomatically according to the severity of disease (Table 6–3). Encouragement to cough, frequent repositioning, incentive spirometry, and administration of humidified oxygen as indicated by arterial blood gases are effective general measures. Chest percussion and the use of routine intermittent positive pressure breathing have not been found useful and may produce complications (rib fracture, wound injury, pneumothorax, and gastric distention). Bronchodilators, administered either intravenously or by nebulizer, effectively treat bronchospasm. Profuse bronchorrhea or purulent secretions are removed by nasotracheal aspiration or through a rigid ventilating bronchoscope. The small orifice of the standard diagnostic fiberoptic bronchoscope limits

TABLE 6–3. TREATMENT OF INHALATION INJURY

1. Administer warm humidified oxygen
2. Encourage coughing
3. Incentive spirometry
4. Endotracheal toilet — obtain culture of secretions
   a. Catheter suction
   b. Bronchoscopy
5. Bronchodilators
6. Endotracheal intubation
   a. Acute obstruction
   b. Need for prolonged access to lower airways
7. Mechanical ventilation
8. Steroid administration (for intractable bronchospasm)
9. Antibiotic administration (for specific indication)

its use for such a purpose. The arterial carbon dioxide tensions of burned patients usually vary between 30 and 35 torr, and increasing levels above this range often herald respiratory failure hours before hypoxia develops or pneumonia is evident on chest roentgenogram. Once respiratory insufficiency develops, an endotracheal tube should be placed and ventilation supported by mechanical means. The need for positive end expiratory pressure (PEEP) is determined by the $AaDO_2$ as calculated from measurements of arterial blood gases. The amount of PEEP that can be safely utilized depends on the response of the arterial blood gases and cardiac output to such therapy.

Prophylactic steroids are ineffective in preventing the complications of inhalation injury and may accentuate small airway obstruction and infection. Prophylactic systemic and aerosolized antibiotics offer no protection from later pulmonary infection and promote the rapid emergence of drug-resistant organisms. Bronchopneumonia is the most common sequel of inhalation injury, and antimicrobial therapy is determined by the sensitivity patterns of the organisms recovered from endobronchial cultures. In addition to regular physical examinations, the respiratory status of thermally injured patients is monitored by daily chest roentgenograms, arterial blood gases, and sputum cultures.

Peripheral Circulation

Following thermal injury and subsequent resuscitation, fluid accumulates in the interstitial spaces, and tissue pressure increases. Skin damaged by a full-thickness injury is unyielding and will not stretch as tissue volume increases. If such a burn involves the circumference of an extremity, increasing tissue pressure will impede arterial blood flow. The clinical indications of impaired circulation to an extremity with a circumferential third-degree burn include cyanosis of the distal unburned skin, delayed capillary refilling, paresthesias, deep pain, and in late stages, paralysis of the extremity. Skin surface sensory changes are less meaningful because of skin damage by the burn. Swelling and coolness to touch of distal unburned skin is a reflection of the generalized vasoconstriction following thermal injury and does not require surgical therapy. Burn wound edema makes palpation of distal extremity pulses difficult. The Doppler ultrasonic flowmeter gives a more accurate assessment of peripheral blood flow, and its use averts unnecessary surgical procedures. The distal palmar arch pulses of the upper extremities and the posterior tibial pulses of the lower extremities should be examined, but only after intravascular volume and systemic blood flow have been restored.

All burned extremities should be elevated to a level higher than the heart by suspending the involved extremities in slings attached to intravenous fluid poles. The slings can be fashioned from lengths of stockinette or thick burn pads and custom-fitting orthoplast splints that partially encircle

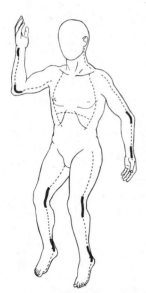

Figure 6–2. Outline drawing showing preferred sites for escharotomy incisions. Heavy lines across joints emphasize importance of incising eschar present over joints.

the arm and extend above the elbow. Active exercises are carried out for five minutes every hour during the first 48 hours postburn. After this time, edema fluid begins to mobilize as the patient begins to diurese, and tissue pressure returns to normal.

If prophylactic measures fail, escharotomy is indicated to prevent necrosis of the ischemic tissue. The escharotomy incision is placed through insensate third-degree burn and the superficial fascia. Once totally transected, the edges of the eschar will spontaneously separate, exposing the underlying subcutaneous fat, which should not be further incised. No anesthesia is needed for this procedure, which can be carried out in the intensive care ward. When escharotomy is properly performed, blood loss associated with it is minimal. To avoid laceration of tendons and nerve trunks, all extremity incisions are placed in the midmedial or midlateral lines, or both, of the limb (Fig. 6–2). The location of these lines is best identified when the hand is fully supinated into the anatomical position. If the hand is left pronated, the incision may inadvertently be carried directly across the antecubital space and may endanger the underlying structures. The incision should begin at the proximal margin of the constricting eschar, extend distally across all involved joints, where the nerves and vessels are most tightly constricted, and terminate at the distal margin of circumferential eschar. An unincised constricting band proximal to an otherwise completed escharotomy, especially around a joint, will act as a tourniquet and prevent restoration of blood flow. If escharotomy through a deep burn fails to re-establish peripheral circulation, fasciotomy is indicated. Following placement of escharotomy incisions, the resulting wounds are covered with topical antimicrobial agents.

Some evidence suggests that digital escharotomies preserve function of severely burned fingers. Such incisions are placed along the lateral aspect of the thumb and along either the lateral or medial aspect of the other fingers. The incisions should be just slightly posterior to the midlateral or midmedial lines of the digit to avoid the neurovascular bundles. The volar attachments of Cleland's ligaments should be divided in the course of incising the eschar. A circumferential third-degree burn of the thorax may occasionally impair respiratory exchange and require that a chest wall escharotomy be performed. Thoracic wall escharotomy incisions are placed along the anterior axillary lines, beginning at the tip of the clavicle and extending to the lower costal margin. If the third-degree burn extends onto the abdominal wall, the two incisions are connected along the lower costal margin.

ADDITIONAL IMMEDIATE CONSIDERATIONS

Ileus. Ileus frequently occurs early postinjury in patients who sustain burns larger than 25 percent of the body surface. All patients with extensive burns should have a nasogastric tube inserted, the stomach emptied of gastric secretions, and oral intake precluded. Motility usually returns after the second postburn day, and oral intake can then be resumed. Immediately following thermal injury, antacids are begun as prophylaxis against Curling's ulcer. Antacid (30 ml each hour) is injected into the nasogastric tube and, if needed, is supplemented to maintain the gastric pH above 5. When the nasogastric tube is removed, the same quantity of antacid is given orally. The administration of cimetidine also appears to be effective in prevention of the clinical complications of Curling's ulcer. Cimetidine can be given parenterally (400 mg every 4 hours) even in the presence of ileus. When gastrointestinal motility returns, administration is continued orally at a dosage of 300 mg every 6 hours.

Antibiotics and Tetanus Prophylaxis. Group A beta streptococcal cellulitis in the early postburn period is now uncommon, and prophylactic penicillin is not administered because its use hastens the emergence of antibiotic-resistant gram-negative organisms. The narrow border of erythema surrounding the edges of the burn wound after the first several postburn days is usually not infectious in origin but is caused by an inflammatory reaction to tissue breakdown products. Streptococcal infection is indicated by enlargement of this erythematous border in conjunction with systemic signs of sepsis. The administration of penicillin at this time is followed by rapid resolution of the infection. Tetanus prophylaxis is based on the prior immunization status of the patient as described in Chapter 5.

Analgesia. While a second-degree burn can be exquisitely painful, a third-degree burn is insensate and causes surprisingly little discomfort.

During resuscitation, small doses of morphine (3 to 5 mg for an adult) or meperidine (30 to 50 mg) are judiciously administered intravenously at intervals determined by the patient's physical condition and response. In order to ensure effectiveness, all analgesics are given only by intravenous injection. The repeated subcutaneous or intramuscular injection of analgesics during the early postburn period of hypovolemia and poor tissue perfusion will be ineffective for pain relief and can result in profound respiratory depression and hypotension when blood volume has been restored, tissue perfusion improves, and the multiple doses are simultaneously absorbed. Narcotic overdosage is treated by intravenous injection of the specific antagonist, naloxone. If sedation is needed for a patient being maintained by a mechanical ventilator, morphine is adequate. In the rare situation in which muscle relaxants are necessary, depolarizing blocking agents such as pancuronium bromide are utilized in preference to succinylcholine, which can cause fatal hyperkalemia in traumatized patients.

WOUND CARE

When admission procedures are completed and the patient's condition stabilized, the burn wound is gently debrided by personnel wearing gowns, masks, and gloves. This is a convenient time to estimate the extent of the burn. Unless associated injuries warrant operative intervention, the initial wound debridement is not of sufficient magnitude to warrant general anesthesia, which may precipitate shock and cardiopulmonary arrest if resuscitation is incomplete and significant hypovolemia exists. The patient is placed in the Hubbard tank, the loose nonviable skin is removed, and the body hair is shaved from the burned areas. The surgeon should avoid vigorous mechanical debridement, which will further damage the injured tissue. The burn wound is then gently bathed with an antibacterial detergent, covered with a topical antimicrobial agent, and left open. Mafenide acetate (Sulfamylon) and silver sulfadiazine (Silvadene) creams are the most commonly used topical chemotherapeutic agents. Silver sulfadiazine is especially popular because it causes little pain, is easily applied, and can be conveniently covered with occlusive dressings during patient transfer. Once each day, the topical cream is washed off and the burn wound inspected by the patient's physician. Because of its ability to penetrate the eschar, mafenide acetate cream is the agent of choice for neglected burns, for very deep thermal or electrical burns, and for burns infected with anaerobic or gram-negative organisms. The use of various iodine preparations has been associated with hypernatremia, hyperosmolality, and systemic absorption of iodides. In addition, the effectiveness of the iodine-containing topical agents remains unconfirmed.

Patients with facial burns are placed with their heads slightly elevated (above the level of the heart) until resuscitation is complete; thereafter, they should be placed in the Fowler's position to facilitate edema resorption. The eyes of any patient with facial burns should be examined immediately upon admission; any globe or corneal injury is noted and, if necessary, treated. As facial edema forms, the lids swell and protect the globe and cornea. When the lid edema resolves, lid retraction may occur and expose the cornea. The exposed cornea should then be protected by hourly instillation of artificial tears or periodic application of ophthalmic ointments.

Burned hands must be elevated and active motion carried out for five minutes every hour to reduce edema formation and the need for escharotomy. Occlusive dressings that obscure signs of impaired blood supply to the hand should be avoided during the resuscitation period. Following resuscitation, a progressive program of active motion of burned joints is continued under the supervision of a physical therapist to minimize dysfunction and prevent subsequent deformity. Patients with perineal burns do not require colostomy to divert the fecal stream. Regular bowel function keeps the anus dilated and prevents anal stricture formation. If the glans penis is burned, a urethral catheter should be left in place until the burn heals (severe burns of the labia are treated in a similar fashion). However, if the penile corpora are extensively burned, a suprapubic cystostomy should be performed. Burned perineal tissue should be allowed to demarcate, and early excision of such burn wounds is not indicated. All adjacent viable skin should be saved for future coverage of perineal structures. Exposed testicles are salvageable unless the tunica is ruptured and the testicular contents extruded, in which case orchiectomy is indicated.

DECISION ON TREATMENT SETTING

Although some triage has occurred by virtue of the patient's being brought to a treatment facility, the physician must now decide whether to treat the patient as an outpatient, to admit him directly to the hospital, or to transfer him to a specialized burn treatment facility. The major determinant of patient disposition is the severity of the burn injury, as indicated in Table 6–4. Minor burns are cleansed with soap and water and allowed to dry. Blisters or bullae less than 2 cm in diameter may be left intact or simply drained, but larger bullae, which commonly rupture and become infected, should be debrided. The use of dressings is optional and depends upon the location of the burn and the patient's desires. If dressings are used, they should be changed every three days and the wound inspected. If healing is progressing satisfactorily, a dressing is reapplied; but if infection develops, the patient should be admitted to the hospital and the wound treated with a topical chemotherapeutic agent.

TABLE 6–4. TRIAGE CRITERIA

I. Minor burn injury: Can be treated on outpatient basis and admitted for grafting of small full-thickness burns.
   A. Second-degree burns
      1. Less than 15% total body surface in adult
      2. Less than 10% total body surface in child
   B. Third-degree burns: Less than 2% of total body surface

II. Moderate uncomplicated burn injury: Can be treated at a general hospital by personnel with experience in burn care or at a specialized burn treatment facility.
   A. Second-degree burns
      1. 15–25% of total body surface in adult
      2. 10–20% of total body surface in child
   B. Third-degree burns: 2–10% of total body surface

III. Major burn injury: Best treated at burn unit or burn center
   A. Second-degree burns
      1. More than 25% of total body surface in adult
      2. More than 20% of total body surface in child
   B. Third-degree burns: More than 10% of total body surface
   C. Patients with lesser burns but with complicating features:
      1. Significant burns of hands, feet, face, or perineum
      2. Inhalation injury
      3. Significant fractures or other mechanical trauma
      4. Significant pre-existing disease, e.g., diabetes
      5. Either extreme of age; less than 5 or more than 60

PATIENT TRANSFER

Once the decision has been made to transfer the burned patient to an appropriate treatment facility, the referring medical staff should contact directly the surgeon who will be responsible for continuing that patient's care to ensure that the patient is properly prepared. The patient should be transferred as soon as his physical condition has stabilized, since movement of the patient becomes progressively more dangerous as delayed complications begin to emerge. Resuscitation can be in progress during transfer, but the patient's vital signs and urinary output should verify that he is sufficiently stable to be transferred. Escharotomies, if needed, should be carried out before transfer. To prevent aspiration pneumonia, a nasogastric tube is inserted and secured with umbilical tape tied around the head. The intravenous catheter is covered with a secure dressing, and the urethral catheter is taped to the abdominal wall. A chest roentgenogram is obtained to confirm the absence of intrathoracic disease. If a central venous cannula has been inserted or if the patient has sustained a blast injury, the roentgenogram should be examined carefully for evidence of a pneumothorax, which is best seen on a film exposed during expiration. A pneumothorax of *any* size is treated by tube thoracostomy before transfer. Because the high noise intensity in most ambulances and aircraft prevents adequate physical examination, an endotracheal tube should be inserted prior to evacuation in any patient with signs of respiratory embarrassment.

The wound can be covered with a topical antimicrobial agent and wrapped with thick layers of gauze or can be merely covered with bulky but not constricting dressings. Blankets are used to maintain body temperature but should be removed if the patient becomes hyperthermic during transfer. If the patient is evacuated by air, humidified oxygen is given to counter the effects of the lowered atmospheric pressure and humidity in the aircraft cabin. Low-hanging ceilings and decreased ambient pressure necessitate administration of intravenous solutions from plastic bags placed in pressure devices. The patient should be accompanied by experienced burn care personnel with proper equipment (such as Doppler flow meters, extra intravenous fluids, chest tubes) available en route. With this preparation, nearly all burned patients can be safely transported during the early postburn period. However, if the following conditions are present, transportation should not be attempted: (1) pneumonia, (2) congestive heart failure unresponsive to treatment, (3) ventricular arrhythmias, (4) hyperpyrexia exceeding 39.4° C, or (5) recent gastrointestinal bleeding. The cause of the hyperpyrexia must be found and treated. If the patient bleeds massively during transportation, no blood bank or operating room facilities will be available.

CHEMICAL INJURIES

Because chemical agents continue to produce damage as long as they are in contact with tissues, chemical injuries demand immediate local treatment. The principal goal of treatment is removal of the offending agent by immediate lavage with copious amounts of water. Any dry alkali powders should be brushed off clothing and exposed body parts prior to lavage. While irrigation is in progress, all clothing, including gloves and shoes, is removed to aid in eliminating the chemical agent and to permit performance of a thorough physical examination. During this process, the various members of the treatment team must avoid injuring themselves by avoiding contact with any residual agent. A search for specific neutralizing agents wastes valuable time, and use of such materials may produce further injury as a result of the heat generated by an exothermic neutralization reaction. While strong acids can usually be removed by water irrigation in a relatively short period of time (approximately 30 to 60 minutes), strong alkalis often remain in injured tissues after many hours of irrigation and can be completely removed only by subsequent surgical debridement. Premature cessation of irrigation of alkali-injured tissue is often followed by further destruction, especially of periorbital and ocular tissues.

Once the offending agent has been successfully removed, the extent of injury is determined, and treatment is instituted using the guidelines

TABLE 6-5. PITFALLS IN TREATMENT OF CHEMICAL BURNS

1. Delayed or inadequate water lavage
2. Failure to remove clothing soaked with offending chemical
3. "Normal well-tanned" appearance of injured skin misinterpreted, causing underestimation of extent of burn
4. Delayed or inadequate eye irrigation
5. Failure to diagnose inhalation injury due to gaseous agent
6. Treatment of phosphorus burns with dilute 0.5–1.0% copper sulfate solution as a soak or a more concentrated solution as a wash

established for thermal injuries. The most common error in the management of chemical injuries is underestimation of the extent of injury (Table 6-5). Skin that is damaged by chemical agents often appears early to be soft and bronzed, and such areas can be mistakenly judged to be "suntanned" or to be superficially injured, when in fact deep, full-thickness necrosis has occurred. Unremoved clothing may not only hide injured tissue but also maintain contact of body parts with large quantities of chemical agents. Chemical injuries affecting a large portion of the body surface require fluid resuscitation, using the same guidelines as for thermal injuries.

Wounds containing white phosphorus require a different initial approach. White phosphorus ignites at temperatures over 34° C, and tissue damage following contact arises from heat-induced coagulation necrosis. White phosphorus injuries commonly result from munition explosions with subsequent impaction of particles in exposed tissues, and further tissue destruction may occur if the embedded phosphorus particles ignite as the particles are removed. Patients with white phosphorus burns are most safely and expeditiously treated by either submerging the affected body parts in water or normal saline or by wrapping the involved part in water-soaked dressings for transportation to a surgical facility where any embedded particles and surrounding necrotic tissue can be debrided. Identification of impacted particles can be facilitated by use of an ultraviolet lamp in the darkened surgical theater. The extracted phosphorus particles are kept covered with water to avoid ignition on contact with air, and all operating theater personnel must be made aware of the danger of such an occurrence. Washing with a 1 percent copper sulfate solution impedes oxidation by forming an easily identified blue-gray cupric phosphide coating on exposed particles and can be used in the initial care of white phosphorus burns. However, its inappropriate application as a soak or in concentrations greater than 1 percent may cause hemolysis and renal failure, and the use of copper sulfate offers little advantage over water or saline.

Wounds caused by metallic sodium or magnesium should not be irrigated, since water reacts violently with these agents and potentiates tissue loss. Embedded particles of these compounds are removed and placed in methanol, and all necrotic tissue is then debrided.

Phenolic compounds are partially removed by the mechanical effects of water irrigation, but since such agents are not water soluble, the wound subsequently should be flushed with an appropriate solvent (glycerol, polyethylene glycol, or propylene glycol). Burns caused by hydrofluoric acid should be lavaged with large quantities of water. However, continued deep pain indicates further tissue injury, and such wounds should be explored and debrided. Although advocated in the past, local injection of calcium gluconate in and around the wound offers no proven benefit. Recently the injection of calcium gluconate into the artery serving the involved part has been recommended as a means to limit both symptoms and tissue destruction.

Chemical injuries of the eyes demand immediate treatment that must be initiated before the ophthalmologist is available. As with other chemical injuries, copious irrigation with water or physiological saline is vital. A topical anesthetic may be needed to counteract the intense blepharospasm that may prevent sufficient exposure for examination and irrigation. Cycloplegic and miotic agents are instilled to ameliorate the effects of iritis. With alkali-induced ocular injuries, the necessary prolonged irrigation can be facilitated by a scleral contact lens with an irrigating side arm. Neutralizing agents and topical steroids are contraindicated. Areas of necrotic tissue may require excision and coverage with conjunctival flaps.

ELECTRICAL INJURIES

Electricity produces damage by causing heat-induced coagulation necrosis, and treatment of such injuries in many ways resembles that of conventional thermal injury. Because superficial tissues lose heat faster than deeper tissues, a misleadingly small surface wound often conceals extensive deep damage and may lead to inadequate wound care and fluid management.

At the scene of injury, the patient should be carefully removed from any continued contact with the electrical source. If respirations and pulse are undetectable, cardiopulmonary resuscitation is instituted. Cardiac arrhythmias are often present, and all electrically injured patients should be continuously monitored by electrocardiographic means until cardiac stability has been established. Ventricular arrhythmias are usually treated by intravenous administration of lidocaine (50 to 150 mg as a bolus over a 1- to 2-minute period, followed by a constant infusion of 1 to 4 mg per minute). A cannula is secured in a vein of adequate caliber. An indwelling urethral catheter is placed. A balanced electrolyte solution (usually lactated Ringer's solution) is administered to effect a urinary output of 30 to 50 ml per hour. If hemochromogens appear in the urine, signifying muscle or massive red cell destruction, fluid management is altered as described previously.

Other injuries are commonly associated with electrical injuries, and a thorough physical examination should be carried out. Vertebral fractures may occur as a consequence of tetanic contraction of the paravertebral muscles, and fractures of the skull and long bones are found in patients who have fallen from a height after electrical contact. Even if asymptomatic, the electrically injured patient should be transported in a cervical collar and appropriate roentgenograms of the spine obtained after admission to a treatment facility. After splinting for transportation, fractures of a burned extremity are treated definitively by skeletal traction and never with a cast or internal fixation.

The surface burn, which may be quite large if the patient's clothing ignited, is covered with a topical antimicrobial agent. The absence of pulses and stony hardness of muscle compartments, whether directly beneath the surface burn or in a remote location, indicate subfascial injury and dictate surgical exploration. Fasciotomy, not escharotomy, and inspection of all underlying structures are mandatory for assessment of tissue viability. Because heat dissipates more readily from superficial than from deep muscles, the exploration must be carried down to bone, even in the absence of superficial damage. Necrotic tissue is excised to prevent subsequent infection and electrolyte abnormalities (usually hyperkalemia). Since nonviable tissue may initially appear healthy, the wounds are thereafter inspected daily, and further debridement is carried out as needed. All explored wounds are packed open and closed at a later date, after a bed of granulation tissue has developed. Ancillary diagnostic procedures, such as arteriography and radionuclide scanning of the muscle, serve mainly to confirm what is evident on physical examination and surgical exploration, but may be useful in determining extent of deep tissue injury in the presence of equivocal findings.

A number of complications are specifically associated with electrical injuries (Table 6–6). In addition to direct destruction of nerves with accompanying neurological defects, delayed effects may appear. This emphasizes the need to admit all patients with high-voltage electric injury to a hospital, where a thorough neurological examination should be performed daily with recording of all positive findings. Days to weeks later, a syndrome resembling polyneuritis may affect peripheral nerves at sites remote from the injury, producing a predominantly motor dysfunction. Similarly, delayed spinal cord disorders may present as hemiplegia, quadriplegia, or an ascending paralysis resembling the Guillain-Barré syndrome. Because the large volume of the trunk allows dissipation of electric energy, visceral injuries are rare; nevertheless, daily abdominal examination will detect the few injuries that do occur. Cataracts not uncommonly form as a consequence of electrical injury, particularly that of the head and neck, and may appear years later. Consequently, an early baseline examination of the eyes should be recorded in all patients with high-voltage electric injury, with follow-up examinations carried out at six-month intervals.

TABLE 6-6. SPECIAL DIAGNOSTIC AND TREATMENT CONSIDERATIONS FOR PATIENTS WITH HIGH VOLTAGE ELECTRIC INJURY

Complication	Cause	Evaluation	Treatment or Prevention
Early death	Cardiopulmonary arrest	Physical examination	Cardiopulmonary resuscitation
Oliguria	Underestimation of fluid needs based on small surface injury	Hourly urinary output	Increase fluid administration rate
Acute renal failure	Hemochromogens in small volume of urine	Examination of urine	Increase fluid administration plus use of osmotic diuretic
Hyperkalemia	Muscle destruction	EKG and serum electrolyte measurements	Insulin, glucose, calcium, bicarbonate infusion; ion exchange resins; dialysis
Deep tissue necrosis	Direct effect of current	Palpation, arteriography, radionuclide scanning	Surgical exploration, debridement, and amputation as indicated after condition is stabilized
Neurological deficits A. Peripheral nerves B. Long tracts of spinal cord	Direct or delayed effect of current	Serial neurological examinations; EMG testing	Symptomatic with physiotherapy to maintain function
Cataract formation	Delayed effect of current	Serial eye examinations	Lens extraction
Cholelithiasis	Unknown	Physical examination and roentgenographic studies of biliary tract	Cholecystectomy

Electric injuries of the mouth are especially common in children who chew on electrical cords. The oral commissures usually are burned severely, and the labial artery not infrequently bleeds massively as the eschar begins to separate. Such patients should be admitted for observation but require no early surgical intervention, since these burns characteristically result in considerably less tissue destruction than estimated immediately after injury.

Persons struck by lightning frequently sustain cardiopulmonary arrest and pronounced central nervous system deficits. However, with the use of cardiopulmonary resuscitation and other appropriate care for all lightning injury patients, the majority survive and recover complete neurological function. The attendant burn is usually superficial and heals rapidly.

COLD INJURIES

Exposure to cold temperatures can produce a spectrum of physiological derangements, varying from direct tissue damage (frostbite, immersion foot, trench foot, and chilblain) to severe total body hypothermia. Such injuries are now seen with increasing frequency as the popularity of winter sports rises and as the elderly population increases.

FROSTBITE

Frostbite results from the actual freezing of tissue and produces damage by tissue ice crystallization, cellular dehydration, and microvascular occlusion. The skin and subcutaneous tissues of exposed body parts, especially the hands, feet, nose, and ears, are most often affected, and the severity of injury is enhanced by such factors as wet clothing, air movement (chill factor), peripheral vascular disease, and decreased level of consciousness. The severity of frostbite varies with the degree and duration of exposure to low temperatures. *First-degree frostbite* causes superficial edema and hyperemia of the skin without necrosis. *Second-degree frostbite* induces hyperemia and blister formation, with partial-thickness necrosis of the skin. *Third-degree frostbite* results in necrosis of the entire skin thickness and may also involve underlying subcutaneous tissue. *Fourth-degree frostbite* results in necrosis of the skin and all deeper structures, including bone, and terminates in gangrene of the extremity.

The tissue reaction after thawing provides a useful guide to the true extent of permanent damage. With more superficial injuries, the affected body parts demonstrate a rapid return of blood flow through both the surface capillary beds and the deeper arteriovenous shunts. The involved extremity becomes bright red and warm, rapidly swells, and soon develops massive vesicles filled with straw-colored fluid. Healing is rapid and is usually complete within two weeks. In contrast, blood flow remains depressed following thawing of a severely frozen body part. The skin is cool, deep red to purple, and later may form small blisters containing hemorrhagic fluid. Although sensation and distal muscle function are often absent, distal movement is usually possible, since tendons are resistant to cold injury and the proximal muscles are intact. Such severely injured tissue will eventually mummify and demarcate. Most cases of frostbite lie between these two extremes, and accurate assessment of tissue viability may be impossible until demarcation is complete, a process that may require many weeks. The eventual extent of tissue loss commonly is much less than initial observations would indicate.

The single most effective means of tissue salvage is rapid rewarming of the affected part in a circulating water bath at 42° C. Slow rewarming is less effective, and the use of dry heat, such as from a fire, is dangerous, since the injured part lacks sufficient sensation to prevent a burn injury from occurring. Thawing in cold water or rubbing with ice potentiates tissue loss and should be avoided. No alcohol should be given to the patient. Body temperature should be maintained, the affected part elevated, and mechanical trauma minimized by foot cradles, cotton between digits, and absolute bed rest. Blisters should be left intact, and the injured tissue is gently cleansed daily. Unless infection supervenes (wet gangrene), surgical debridement has no place in the early treatment of frostbite; escharotomy and fasciotomy rarely improve tissue salvage. Tetanus prophylaxis is based on the patient's prior immunization status and on the circumstances of injury. Antibiotics are utilized only if an open wound was present prior to freezing or if infection subsequently develops. Frostbite involving large portions of the body may, as thawing occurs, produce large blood volume deficits, in which case fluid resuscitation is required. The beneficial effects on tissue salvage of sympathectomy (either by nerve trunk section or by pharmacological agents), low molecular weight dextran, heparin, and corticosteroids remain unproved.

NONFREEZING COLD INJURY

Nonfreezing cold injury is more common than frostbite and occurs in more temperate conditions. The common etiological features of trench foot and immersion foot are dependency and immobility of the lower extremity in a wet environment. Trench foot develops in a few days at temperatures near freezing. Immersion foot evolves over a longer period of time at more moderate temperatures. Treatment consists of rapid rewarming and the meticulous local care described previously for frostbite. The vesicles, which form after rewarming, coalesce into a superficial eschar, which subsequently sloughs. Deep injury is uncommon, and the involved extremities most often heal spontaneously. Pernio, or chilblain, occurs after chronic exposure to dry, cold temperatures just above freezing, with subsequent formation of small, superficial ulcers on exposed body parts. These lesions heal spontaneously with cessation of exposure.

Hypothermia

Severe total body hypothermia (body temperature below 34° C) is associated with a variety of signs and symptoms that depend on how fast body temperature has fallen. Signs following immersion in cold water include low body temperature, coldness of the patient's skin to touch, and shivering. Hypothermia of slower onset, as is particularly common in elderly or intoxicated persons, frequently elicits no shivering and is often overlooked because most clinically available thermometers do not record below 34° C. Nearly all patients demonstrate a decreased level of consciousness, and vital signs, although variable, tend to be depressed. Because of intense vasoconstriction, a Doppler ultrasonic flowmeter is useful for detecting pulsatile blood flow.

Any wet clothes are removed, following which the hypothermic patient should be rewarmed expeditiously with careful monitoring and support of vital signs. If hypothermia is of moderate severity (body temperature 30° to 34° C) and the patient is shivering, he can usually be passively rewarmed by wrapping in warm blankets and administering warm fluids.

If body temperature is lower or shivering is absent, if body temperature fails to rise with passive rewarming methods, or if cardiopulmonary arrest has occurred, the patient must be actively rewarmed. This is best accomplished by prompt immersion into a circulating water bath at 42° C. To avoid the potential problem of rewarming collapse, some authors advocate internal rewarming by peritoneal dialysis, cardiopulmonary bypass, or mediastinal lavage, but such invasive procedures have not produced superior results. Intravascular volume deficits, especially common when hypothermia is slow in onset, must be carefully replaced. Electrolyte abnormalities (hypokalemia is most common) are corrected as indicated by laboratory studies. Cardiac arrhythmias are usually supraventricular in origin and disappear with restoration of normal body temperature; ventricular irritability, which occurs infrequently, is treated by intravenous administration of lidocaine, as previously described. When body temperature has returned toward normal, associated injuries and pre-existing diseases (e.g., frostbite, drug overdose, diabetes mellitus) should be identified and treated. Recovery from hypothermia is related to underlying disease, and as such, mortality exceeds 80 percent in the elderly but is only 10 percent in previously healthy young patients.

REFERENCES

1. Pruitt BA Jr: The Burn Patient: I. Initial Care. *In* Current Problems in Surgery, Vol. XVI, No. 4, April 1979.
2. Pruitt BA Jr: The Burn Patient: II. Later Care and Complications of Thermal Injury. *In* Current Problems in Surgery, Vol. XVI, No. 5, May 1979.
3. Pruitt BA Jr: Advances in fluid therapy and the early care of the burn patient. World J Surg 2:139, 1978.
4. Curreri PW, Asch MJ, Pruitt BA Jr: The treatment of chemical burns: Specialized diagnostic, therapeutic and prognostic considerations. J Trauma 10:634, 1970.
5. Baxter CR: Present concepts in the management of major electrical injury. Surg Clin North Am 50:1401, 1970.
6. Strandness DE Jr, Sumner DS: Hemodynamics for Surgeons. *In* Cold Injury. New York, Grune & Stratton, pp. 582–620, 1975.

7

Anesthesia

In caring for the injured patient, a major objective of the anesthesiologist is to allow necessary surgery to take place as quickly as possible. Nevertheless, the principles of good anesthetic management in the perioperative period must be observed. Indeed, the degree of attention to these principles may often determine whether the patient survives.

PREOPERATIVE MANAGEMENT

HISTORY

The comprehensiveness of the history will depend upon the urgency of the situation and the state of consciousness of the patient. At the very minimum, however, the anesthesiologist should determine the time and nature of the injury, time and nature of last food intake, medications the patient takes, previous illnesses (including chronic alcoholism), specific allergies, and untoward events associated with previous anesthetics administered to the patient or close relatives.

Of particular concern is a history of temperature elevation (malignant hyperpyrexia), prolonged apnea (abnormal pseudocholinesterase), jaundice or other evidence of hepatic disturbance, delayed emergence from general anesthesia, and cardiovascular catastrophies (severe dysrhythmias, heart failure, cardiac arrest).

If time permits, it is desirable to obtain information concerning previous or present illnesses. Conditions that are likely to influence the choice and course of anesthesia include asthma, chronic obstructive pulmonary disease, recent myocardial infarct (three to six months), chronic renal disease, hepatic disease, central nervous system disorders (myasthenia gravis, myotonia congenita and dystrophica), endocrine disease (diabetes, adrenal dysfunction, hyperthyroidism) and hematological disease (sickle cell disease or trait).

PHYSICAL EXAMINATION

A complete physical examination is desirable, but even an abbreviated examination can yield valuable information to the anesthesiologist.

Airway. Even a cursory examination of the airway will forewarn the anesthesiologist of anatomical abnormalities or injuries to the upper airway that may make intubation difficult or impossible. If respiratory obstruction is present, it should be relieved immediately. Ordinarily, one should be able to insert an oral or nasal endotracheal tube quickly and easily, but if endotracheal intubation is not possible, tracheostomy should be performed without delay. An endotracheal tube should also be inserted when the patient is unconscious or semiconscious in order to protect the airway from aspiration of foreign materials and to provide adequate ventilation to the patient. Further, it should be noted that when a patient is unconscious as a result of a basilar skull fracture, it is possible inadvertently to insert a nasotracheal tube (or a nasogastric tube) into the cranial vault. Extreme caution must be used to avoid this.

When intubating a patient with suspected injury of the cervical spine, it is essential that the head not be manipulated, lest quadriplegia or even death ensue. Our approach to this problem is to have the head and neck stabilized in a fixed position while the patient is intubated in the awake state with the aid of a fiberoptic laryngoscope or bronchoscope.

Patients with maxillofacial injuries present a different problem. One must be careful to avoid dislodging loose teeth or bone fragments. Additionally, it is essential to examine the oropharynx for foreign material that may be aspirated. These patients should be intubated in the awake state under direct vision. Loose teeth, bone fragments, and blood present in the oropharynx should be scrupulously removed. When there is actual damage to the tracheobronchial tree, it may be necessary to use a double-lumen endotracheal tube (Robertshaw, Carlens) to isolate the injured segment. In severe laryngeal injury or transection of the trachea, tracheostomy is unavoidable.

Following intubation, one may need to use positive pressure to ventilate a patient whose respiration is either depressed or absent. If a pneumothorax is present as a result of rib fractures or other chest trauma, the positive pressure may produce a tension pneumothorax. It is essential, therefore, that the physician be alert to the possibility of pneumothorax and if such is present provide chest drainage prior to the initiation of positive pressure respiration.

Circulation. Except under desperate circumstances, surgery should not commence until the circulatory signs show evidence of reasonable recovery of circulatory hemodynamics (see Chapter 2). At least two large cannulae (14 to 16 gauge) should be in place before induction of anesthesia when massive blood loss has occurred or is anticipated. There is a tendency for many physicians, especially in emergency facilities, to overutilize subclavian puncture. Unless the physician is experienced with performing that technique, the incidence of pneumothorax may be quite high. In most emergency situations, peripheral veins are available for venipuncture. In those instances in which they are not, or when central venous pressure monitoring is deemed necessary, cannulation of either the external or internal jugular vein is a safe alternative to subclavian puncture and is preferred by a number of physicians.

Premedication. All patients who have suffered injury should be presumed to have a full stomach. The regurgitation and aspiration into the lung of highly acid stomach contents (pH less than 3.0) will frequently result in severe pulmonary injury (Mendelson's syndrome).[1] Many anesthesiologists advocate the use of oral antacids preoperatively to raise the pH of the stomach contents. In addition, the administration of cimetidine 300 mg intravenously will inhibit the secretion of further acid.

Other medication administered in the preoperative period will depend upon the physical and emotional status of the patient. If the patient is apprehensive, tranquilizers such as diazepam or hydroxyzine are useful. Diazepam should be administered intravenously (2.5 to 5.0 mg), since it is poorly absorbed by the intramuscular route. Conversely, hydroxyzine may be administered intramuscularly in a dose of 25 to 50 mg for the average adult patient.

Narcotics should be reserved for those patients who are in pain. When indicated, it is best to administer small doses of short-acting narcotics such as fentanyl intravenously. This method of administration allows titration of sufficient narcotic to relieve pain without undue depression of the respiratory and central nervous systems. An anticholinergic agent is useful to dry secretions. Atropine, scopolamine, and glycopyrrolate are satisfactory, but the latter seems to have some advantages over the others. Glycopyrrolate does not produce central nervous system effects, causes less tachycardia, and may decrease acidity of gastric contents.

INTRAOPERATIVE MANAGEMENT

SELECTION OF ANESTHETIC TECHNIQUE

The selection of an anesthetic technique for a patient will be determined by the capability and experience of the person who administers the anesthetic, the site(s) of surgery, and the physical status of the patient. Ordinarily, a patient whose circulatory system is unstable will not tolerate spinal or epidural anesthesia that is sufficiently high to block the sympathetic nervous system. These patients are managed better under general anesthesia. Conversely, spinal anesthesia that is limited to a lower extremity or the perineal area may be useful on occasion. If the site of surgery is limited to an extremity or a circumscribed area on the head or trunk, local infiltration or regional nerve block is a valuable technique.

GENERAL ANESTHESIA

Since the injured patient who requires emergency surgery is at risk from aspiration of gastric contents, it is essential to protect the airway. Ideally, the patient should be *intubated in the awake state*. Local anesthesia of the vocal cords or trachea will depress the glottic and cough reflexes and therefore should be avoided. Careful explanation of the procedure to the patient is essential to success of the technique.

For patients who are intoxicated or otherwise uncooperative, and in instances when a rise in intracranial or intraocular pressure must be avoided, a *rapid sequence technique* of induction and intubation should be used. This technique involves:

1. Preoxygenation for 2 to 5 minutes before induction of anesthesia
2. Slight head-up position
3. Induction with a standard dose of ultra short-acting barbiturate (3 to 4 mg/kg) and a relaxant (curare 3 mg followed by succinylcholine 1.5-2 mg/kg *or* pancuronium 0.15-0.2 mg/kg)
4. Obstruction of the esophagus by pressure on the cricoid cartilage (Selick's maneuver)
5. Intubation with inflation of the balloon as quickly as possible.

If the patient's circulatory system is stable, inhalation agents or intravenous agents may be used to maintain anesthesia. For patients who have sustained severe injury, massive hemorrhage, or both, a narcotic-and-relaxant technique is usually preferable to inhalation agents, since with it myocardial depression can be avoided.

REGIONAL ANESTHESIA

Anyone who uses a local anesthetic drug to produce anesthesia must be thoroughly familiar with the pharmacological properties of that drug. At the very least, one must know the maximum safe dose of the drug and use the lowest effective concentration. One must prevent rapid absorption of the drug by avoiding direct intravascular injection and by adding epinephrine to the injectate, except when specifically contraindicated. One must also be able to recognize and treat untoward reactions.

The drug most commonly used for infiltration local anesthesia is lidocaine. The maximum safe dose is approximately 6 to 7 mg/kg with 1:200,000 epinephrine and 4 to 5 mg/kg without epinephrine. A concentration of 0.5 percent lidocaine is sufficient to produce anesthesia for the repair of superficial wounds, and it should be mixed with 1:200,000 epinephrine except when the injection is made in the immediate vicinity of end arteries (fingers, toes, etc.).

Toxicity secondary to local anesthetics is almost always the result of a high blood level of the local anesthetic agent. Allergy to local anesthetics is extremely rare (less than 0.5 percent). A high blood level may result from an excessive dose of drug, rapid absorption, delayed biotransformation, or a combination of these. Prevention of local anesthetic reactions by adherence to the aforementioned principles is a primary objective.

If toxicity should occur, however, the physician must be able to recognize the signs and symptoms and initiate treatment before severe permanent injury to the central nervous system or the cardiovascular system or both ensues. The early signs of toxicity are dizziness, tinnitus, and decrease in blood pressure. The ECG findings include a slight prolongation of the P-R interval and widening of the QRS complex. Severe toxicity is characterized by muscle tremors and twitching that may progress to convulsions, apnea, and severe depression of blood pressure and pulse rate. The ECG reveals marked prolongation of the P-R interval and widening of the QRS complex. Treatment includes ventilating the patient with 100 percent oxygen, endotracheal intubation, use of vasoactive drugs such as ephedrine or metaraminol to combat cardiac depression, and control of convulsions with a small dose of diazepam (2.5 to 5 mg) or an ultra short-acting barbiturate such as thiopental (50 to 75 mg).

For operations on the extremities, intravenous regional anesthesia or nerve blocks are extremely valuable techniques, for these avoid the problem of aspiration of gastric contents and do not ordinarily depress the respiratory, circulatory, or central nervous systems.

INTRAVENOUS REGIONAL ANESTHESIA

The major advantages of intravenous regional anesthesia are its simplicity and reliability — yet in this simplicity lies its greatest danger. It is not a technique to be used everywhere by anyone. It should be used only where adequate equipment is available for monitoring and resuscitation, and only by a physician skilled in the management of untoward reactions to local anesthetic agents. Intravenous regional anesthesia is particularly applicable to emergency surgery on the extremities because sedation is not required ordinarily; it is highly reliable and it has a rapid onset and short recovery period. The only absolute contraindications to its use are allergy to local anesthetic drugs (a rare occurrence), and those conditions that preclude the use of a tourniquet.

Upper Extremity. A double tourniquet is placed on the upper arm. After exsanguination of the extremity with an Esmarch bandage or by gravity drainage when the injury precludes the use of an Esmarch bandage, the proximal tourniquet is inflated to 250 torr. In the average adult patient, 50 ml of 0.5 percent lidocaine without epinephrine is then injected intravenously. After ten minutes, the distal tourniquet is inflated, and the proximal tourniquet is deflated to avoid tourniquet pain.

Lower Extremity. The technique is essentially the same as for the upper extremity, except that a larger volume of solution is injected. A 0.25

percent solution is prepared by diluting 75 ml of 0.5 percent lidocaine with 75 ml of normal saline. After exsanguination of the extremity and inflation of the proximal tourniquet to 350-400 torr, 150 ml of the 0.25 percent solution is injected. Again, after ten minutes, the distal tourniquet is inflated and the proximal tourniquet is deflated. Because the thigh is so much larger than the upper arm, wider tourniquets are used on the lower extremity.

At the completion of the surgical procedure, the tourniquet may be deflated completely if a period of 40 minutes has elapsed since injection. For shorter procedures, one should use a *cycled deflation technique*. This technique consists of deflation for five seconds followed by reinflation for one minute. This procedure is repeated two to three times. *Under no circumstances should the tourniquet be released prior to 15 minutes after injection.*

Possible complications of intravenous regional anesthesia include local anesthetic toxicity secondary to inadvertent release of the tourniquet, incomplete anesthesia and unsatisfactory operating conditions because of inadequate exsanguination, and nerve damage because the tourniquet pressure is either too high or too prolonged. Inadvertent release of the tourniquet is a technical error that is best avoided by a careful check of the equipment before use. Equally careful attention should be given to adequate exsanguination of the extremity by using both gravity drainage and an Esmarch bandage. After inflation of the tourniquet and removal of the Esmarch bandage, one should feel for a distal pulse to be sure that the tourniquet pressure is sufficiently high to have completely obliterated the pulse. Excessive tourniquet pressure on the other hand may cause nerve damage and the pressure delivered by the inflating mechanism should be checked for accuracy against an ordinary mercury manometer. Furthermore, a tourniquet should not remain inflated for longer than two hours under any circumstances. If the surgical procedure takes longer than two hours, the anesthesia can be extended by utilizing a continuous technique,[2] or by converting to a general anesthetic. In either event, the tourniquet can be deflated for a period of five minutes and then reinflated for an additional 60 to 90 minutes.

In summary, intravenous regional anesthesia is a technically simple technique of anesthesia for surgery of any extent on the distal portions of the upper or lower extremities. The technique is safe and reliable, provided that one pays careful attention to detail and avoids technical errors.

NERVE BLOCKS (UPPER EXTREMITY)

Unlike intravenous regional anesthesia, brachial plexus block requires considerable technical skill and requires more time. The technique, however, is more versatile because the use of a tourniquet is not required.

Consequently, procedures of longer duration can be performed without interruption under brachial plexus block than can be performed under intravenous regional anesthesia. Various approaches to block of the brachial plexus may be used, depending upon the site of surgery and the nature of the injury to the patient. The popular techniques available include axillary block, interscalene block, and subclavian perivascular block. A combined cervical and brachial plexus block via the interscalene approach allows surgery on the shoulder as well as the upper extremity. Techniques for performing these blocks are described by Winnie and others.[3-6] The blocks are also described in standard textbooks on regional anesthesia.[7, 8] The axillary approach to the brachial plexus is the safest of the three because there is no danger of pneumothorax, a distinct possibility with any of the supraclavicular approaches.

AXILLARY NERVE BLOCK (TECHNIQUE)

The patient lies supine with the arm abducted. The axillary artery is palpated and a 4 to 5 cm needle is inserted in a slightly cephalad direction just lateral to the artery. Correct placement of the needle is determined by marked pulsation of the needle. A peripheral nerve stimulator may be used to ensure correct placement. Paresthesiae are not sought using this technique because of possible nerve damage. If a paresthesia is encountered, however, the needle should be withdrawn slightly before injection of the drug. Ordinarily, 35 to 40 ml of a 1 percent solution of lidocaine or 0.5 percent bupivacaine is sufficient to provide adequate anesthesia. The application of digital pressure just distal to the site of injection will help to drive the solution cephalad so that anesthesia of the musculocutaneous nerve will be obtained. This nerve leaves the lateral cord of the brachial plexus high in the axilla, and therefore is frequently missed. Performing the block as far cephalad in the axilla as possible will also help to ensure adequate block of the musculocutaneous nerve. The lateral antebrachial cutaneous branch of the musculocutaneous nerve provides sensory anesthesia to the entire lateral side of the forearm. Consequently, failure to anesthetize this nerve may render the entire block ineffective.

Since one needs to use a large volume of local anesthetic solution, it is essential to use the lowest effective concentration; e.g., 1 percent lidocaine or 0.5 percent bupivacaine. This precaution is all the more essential because vascular absorption from the axilla is quite rapid. The addition of epinephrine 1:200,000 to the local anesthetic agent will help to slow absorption and reduce the peak blood level attained.

NERVE BLOCKS (LOWER EXTREMITY)

Surgery on the lower limb may be performed by combined sciatic and femoral nerve block[9] or lumbar plexus anesthesia.[10] These blocks require more technical skill than upper extremity blocks. Consequently, they are ordinarily used only by anesthesiologists experienced in regional anesthesia. Others usually prefer intravenous regional anesthesia or low spinal anesthesia.

NERVE BLOCKS (FACE)

There are three nerve blocks that can be performed in the face region that are both simple and safe: supraorbital nerve block, infraorbital nerve block, and mental nerve block. Labat's techniques for performing these blocks are presented in the following paragraphs.

Supraorbital Block

Operations on the forehead may be performed by block of the supraorbital and supratrochlear nerves. These nerves are blocked by first palpating the supraorbital foramen located on the upper border of the orbit 2.5 cm from the midline and then injecting 1 to 2 ml of a local anesthetic at this point and also 1 cm medially.

Infraorbital Nerve Block

This nerve, a continuation of the maxillary nerve, exits through the infraorbital foramen located on the lower border of the orbit 2.5 cm from the midline. Operations of the lower lid, the side of the nose, and the upper lip may be performed when this nerve is blocked. The needle is inserted at a point 2.5 cm lateral to the ala nasae. It is directed cephalad at an angle of 45 degrees toward the infraorbital foramen. This foramen can be palpated approximately 1 cm below the midpoint of the lower border of the orbit. Injection of 2 to 3 ml of anesthetic solution at this point will produce an effective block.

Mental Nerve Block

Operations on the mucous membrane and skin of the lower lip can be performed under mental nerve block. This nerve is blocked as it exits from the mental foramen. This foramen is located 2.5 cm from the midline and midway between the margins of the mandible. It passes downward, forward, and inward. A line is drawn perpendicular to the lower margin of the jaw 2.5 cm from the midline. This line is then bisected. A wheal is raised 1.5 cm from the midpoint along a line bisecting the upper outer quadrant.

The needle is directed along this plane at an angle of 45 degrees with the skin until bone is contacted and then maneuvered until it enters the foramen. At this point, 1 cc of solution is injected.

MONITORS

Regardless of whether general or regional anesthesia is selected, it is essential that all injured patients be monitored carefully. Routine monitoring for all patients should include monitoring of blood pressure, temperature, and ECG. If the patient has sustained a major injury, has had considerable blood loss, or is in poor physical condition generally, it is desirable to insert a central venous pressure or Swan-Ganz catheter and an indwelling arterial catheter. If there is a possibility of intracranial injury, the state of consciousness of the patient should be monitored both preoperatively and postoperatively. A convenient method for monitoring the state of consciousness is the Glasgow scoring method[12] (see Fig. 12–1). This system assigns numerical values to three parameters: eye movement, motor response, and verbal ability. A decrease in score indicates that the patient may be developing an intracranial hematoma (see Chapter 12).

POSTOPERATIVE MONITORING

Careful monitoring of the patient should continue into the postoperative period. Since vomiting and aspiration can occur on emergence as well as induction, the endotracheal tube should not be removed until the patient is completely awake. If the patient has undergone major intracranial, intra-abdominal, or intrathoracic surgery, it is prudent to leave the endotracheal tube in place and maintain the patient on a ventilator for 24 hours or longer.

Narcotic drugs should be used judiciously to control pain in the postoperative period. Intercostal block with a long-acting agent such as bupivacaine 0.5 percent with 1:200,000 epinephrine will provide good pain relief for intrathoracic and some upper abdominal surgery and decrease the requirement for narcotic drugs. Both the inability to breathe deeply because of pain, and respiratory depression from narcotic drugs can lead to atelectasis and pneumonia. Inspiratory maneuvers should be strongly encouraged as early as possible in the postoperative period, and the importance of this should be stressed to the patient preoperatively if possible. If the patient experiences difficulty in clearing his airway of mucus postoperatively, chest physiotherapy is useful. In recalcitrant atelectasis, bronchoscopy may be vital, especially in the obtunded patient and in the patient who has sustained thoracic trauma.

REFERENCES

1. Mendelson CL: Aspiration of stomach contents into the lungs during obstetrical anesthesia. Am J Obstet Gynecol 52:191, 1946.
2. Brown EM: Continuous intravenous regional anesthesia. Acta Anaesth Scand Suppl XXXVI, 1969, pp 39–45.
3. Winnie AP: Interscalene brachial plexus block. Anesth Analg 49:455, 1970.
4. Winnie AP, Collins VY: The subclavian perivascular technic of brachial plexus. Anesth Analg 25:353, 1964.
5. DeJong RH: Axillary block of the brachial plexus. Anesthesiology 22:215, 1961.
6. Eriksson E, Skarby HG: A simplified method of axillary block. Nord Med 68:1325, 1962.
7. Bonica JJ: The Management of Pain. Philadelphia, Lea and Febiger, 1953.
8. Moore DC: Regional Block, 9th ed. Springfield, Illinois, Charles C Thomas, 1971.
9. Gjessing J, Harley N: Sciatic and femoral nerve block with mepivacaine for surgery on the lower limb. Anaesthesia 24:213, 1969.
10. Winnie AP, Ramamurthy S, Durrani Z: The inguinal perivascular technic of lumbar plexus anesthesia. The "3 in 1 block." Anesth Analg 52:989, 1973.
11. Adriani J: Labat's Regional Anesthesia, 3rd ed. Philadelphia, WB Saunders Company, 1967.
12. Jennett B, Bond MR: Assessment of outcome after severe brain damage. Lancet 1:1031, 1976.

Chapter

8

Chest

Thoracic injuries are the primary cause of death in up to 25 percent of traffic fatalities and are a contributing factor in a further 50 percent. In addition, penetrating thoracic trauma continues to be a common lesion in major urban hospitals throughout North America. Clinical events may progress with great rapidity in these patients, and it is likely that more avoidable deaths occur in patients with this group of injuries than any other. Prompt recognition and immediate action at the scene of the accident, during the transport of the patient, and in the emergency department may be life-saving.

INITIAL ASSESSMENT

The importance of immediate establishment of an adequate airway and the maintenance of effective ventilation cannot be overemphasized. The upper airway may be obstructed by blood, gastric contents, teeth, or foreign material, requiring only oral and nasopharyngeal suctioning for removal. In the unconscious patient, the tongue can frequently obstruct the airway, in which case the problem is easily solved by pulling the tongue or jaw forward or inserting an oropharyngeal airway. Endotracheal intubation is the most effective method of securing and maintaining a patent airway in the injured patient. Hyperventilation with 100 percent oxygen using a mask and a muscle relaxant such as succinylcholine (0.5 to 1.0 mg/kg) may occasionally be required to intubate the hypoxic restless patient. If the patient is ventilating but inadequately, "blind" nasotracheal intubation is often accomplished more easily than orotracheal intubation and is more comfortable for the patient. The use of a fiberoptic bronchoscope may be helpful in accomplishing intubation under direct vision in the presence of multiple facial bone fractures, cervical spine injuries, laryngeal fractures, or cervical tracheal injuries.

Emergency cricothyroidotomy should be performed if endotracheal intubation cannot be accomplished readily in the obstructed or nonventilating patient. Once an endotracheal or cricothyroidotomy tube is in place, aspiration of blood or gastric contents can be prevented, continuous tracheobronchial toilet is easily carried out, and controlled ventilation is possible. After the obstructed airway and all other life-threatening situations have been controlled, a careful initial examination of the disrobed patient can take place.

Evaluation of the adequacy of ventilation should be a primary concern. The rate, depth, and difficulty of respiration should be quickly assessed. Restlessness and combativeness should be considered to be due to hypoxemia or hypotension until proved otherwise. Simple inspection of lip and skin may provide evidence of hypoxemia. However, cyanosis may not develop until late, if at all, in patients with low hemoglobin levels. The size, location (exit and entrance), and nature of chest wounds should be noted. All penetrating wounds should be considered as sucking chest wounds and a watertight dressing applied. Paradoxical movement of the chest wall may be obvious on inspection, but obesity, chest wall hemorrhage, and subcutaneous emphysema may mask a major flail segment. Local crepitus and the palpation of mobile rib or sternal segments also suggest a flail segment. No examination of the chest is complete without a careful assessment of the abdomen (Chapter 10), including peritoneal lavage when indicated.

Examination of the neck will determine the position of the trachea, which may be deviated away from the side of a tension pneumothorax. Jugular venous distention suggests pericardial tamponade or increased intrathoracic pressure. Subcutaneous emphysema should alert the examiner to potential pulmonary, tracheal, or esophageal disruption. Severe crushing trauma to the thorax may produce the syndrome of "traumatic asphyxia" characterized by subconjunctival hemorrhages, petechiae or reddish discoloration of the skin of the face, neck, and shoulders, and varying neurological deficits.

Percussion and auscultation of the chest are useful in detecting the hyper-resonance of a tension pneumothorax or the dullness associated with a significant hemothorax. Hamman's sign, a "crunching" sound during systole over the mid and left anterior chest wall, is present in 50 percent of patients with a pneumomediastinum. The initial stable condition of a chest trauma victim may be deceiving and repeated careful examinations are essential.

A history of the mechanism of trauma from the patient or a witness of the accident is also invaluable. Knowledge of the caliber, velocity, and trajectory of the wounding missile may be helpful in the assessment of penetrating thoracic trauma. Previous medical history including current medication, allergies, and pre-existing cardiopulmonary status should be documented.

DIAGNOSTIC STUDIES

The single most important diagnostic study is the upright posterior-anterior (PA) chest film. Nevertheless, it must be stressed that in certain circumstances, active treatment such as chest tube insertion for tension pneumothorax must be initiated without a chest x-ray being available. The PA chest film will help quantitate a hemothorax or pneumothorax and may confirm mediastinal or subcutaneous emphysema. The integrity of the diaphragm and the presence of intrathoracic viscera can be assessed by chest x-ray. Serial chest x-rays are invaluable in following pulmonary contusion and assessing the adequacy of chest tube drainage.

Traumatic rupture of the aorta is suggested by a number of chest roentgenographic signs, including widening of the mediastinum, an apical cap, haziness or obliteration of the aortic knob, deviation of the trachea or esophagus to the right, depression of the left main stem bronchus, obliteration of the usual clear space between the aorta and the left pulmonary artery, and fracture of the first or second ribs. With any of these changes, serious consideration should be given to arteriography, which should demonstrate the ascending aorta, the arch vessels, and the descending thoracic and abdominal aortas in more than one plane.

An accurate hemodynamic assessment as obtained by CVP, Swan-Ganz PA catheter, arterial blood pressure, and hourly urine outputs is useful in assessing the quality of tissue perfusion. Arterial blood gases provide the best evaluation of the adequacy of ventilation. The need for repeated blood gas studies can be met by the insertion of a radial artery cannula.

The fiberoptic bronchoscope is invaluable as a diagnostic aid in assessing the integrity of the tracheobronchial tree and is useful therapeutically in removing bronchial plugs and the increased tracheobronchial secretions associated with chest trauma.

MANAGEMENT OF COMPROMISED VENTILATION

The most common causes of impaired ventilation following injury are:

1. Airway obstruction
2. Loss of normal negative intrapleural pressure and occupation of pleural space by air (pneumothorax) or blood (hemothorax)
3. Pulmonary contusion
4. Disruption or instability of chest wall or diaphragm.

PNEUMOTHORAX

Traumatic pneumothorax (Fig. 8–1) may be classified as simple or closed, open or communicating ("sucking chest wound"), or tension. A pneumothorax is often quantitated as the percentage of the volume of the hemithorax occupied by extrapulmonary air. Progressive accumulation of air in the pleural space may result in a tension pneumothorax with positive

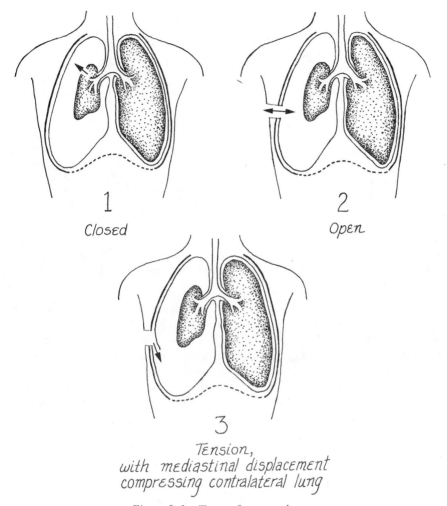

1

Closed

2

Open

3

*Tension,
with mediastinal displacement
compressing contralateral lung*

Figure 8–1. Types of pneumothorax.

intrapleural pressure and a resulting shift of the mediastinum and compression of superior and inferior venae cavae, reducing venous return, and cardiac output. The clinical findings depend upon the size of the pneumothorax and consist of tachypnea, dyspnea, chest wall pain, hyperresonance, and decreased breath sounds over the involved hemithorax. The diagnosis is readily confirmed by chest x-ray.

Tube thoracostomy via the second or third intercostal space in the midclavicular line or preferably high in the midaxillary line using a No. 24 or No. 28 Argyle chest tube is the accepted treatment for a pneumothorax. The chest wall or axilla is prepped with an antiseptic and draped. The skin, subcutaneous tissues, and pleura are infiltrated with 2 percent lidocaine. A

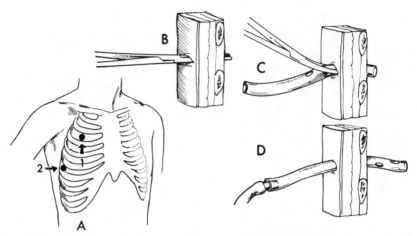

Figure 8–2. Hemostat technique for tube thoracostomy for closed drainage of the chest. *A*, sites for insertion: upper-anterior for air, lower-lateral for fluid. *B, C, D*, steps in introduction of the tube. (Modified after Netter. CIBA Clinical Symposia, 1971.)

1 to 2 cm incision is made 2 to 3 cm below the selected interspace and deepened through subcutaneous tissue and pectoralis muscle using blunt dissection with a Kelly hemostat. The intercostal muscle is penetrated with the hemostat, which is kept on the superior margin of the rib to avoid the intercostal vessels. A chest tube is then placed in the tip of the hemostat and pushed into the pleural space, directed upward, and fixed carefully with a skin suture (Fig. 8–2). The tube is attached to an underwater drainage system and 10 to 20 cm H_2O suction. If a water-seal is not available, a Heimlich valve or simple flutter valve is used (Fig. 8–3). The presence of a

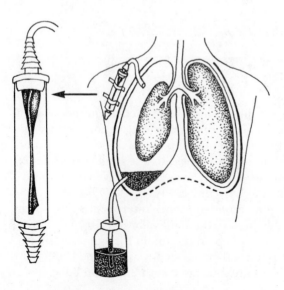

Figure 8–3. The upper anterior chest tube is attached to a Heimlich one-way valve useful in transport of a patient with a pneumothorax. The lower chest tube provides dependent drainage for a hemothorax and is attached to a conventional underwater drainage system.

large air leak with failure of the lung to expand or the development of increasing subcutaneous emphysema suggests a major pulmonary laceration or rupture of the trachea or a bronchus, which should be evaluated with emergency bronchoscopy. Pneumomediastinum in association with pneumothorax raises the question of a perforated esophagus requiring endoscopic or contrast studies of the esophagus.

Every penetrating injury should be considered as an open or communicating pneumothorax. A large chest wall opening subjects the lung to atmospheric pressure, and effective ventilation is impossible. The wound should be covered immediately with a watertight dressing and at least one chest tube should be inserted remote from the chest wall wound. With large chest wall defects, endotracheal intubation and positive pressure ventilation may be needed to provide effective ventilation during transfer to the operating room. Thorough debridement of the chest wall and management of the pulmonary or cardiac injuries are carried out as needed in such patients before closure of the chest wall defect. In some instances local muscle or myocutaneous flaps may be required.

Hemothorax

Blood in the pleural space may originate from lung, chest wall, heart, great vessels, or from injured intra-abdominal viscera associated with a ruptured diaphragm. The clinical findings will depend upon the magnitude of blood loss and may be a combination of hypovolemic shock and hypoxemia. Dyspnea, decreased air entry, and dullness to percussion over the involved hemithorax herald a significant hemothorax. Hemothorax demonstrable on chest x-ray means that at least 200 to 300 ml of blood have accumulated. A small hemothorax requires no specific therapy and will resorb spontaneously. A moderate-sized hemothorax (500 to 1000 ml) is best managed with a large-bore chest tube (32F or 36F) inserted in the fifth or sixth intercostal space in the midaxillary line. Initial drainage of approximately 1500 ml or drainage greater than 200 to 300 ml/hr for three to four hours is an indicator for early thoracotomy. Measurement of hourly chest tube drainage and serial chest x-rays are essential for accurate measurement of continued intrathoracic bleeding.

Pulmonary Contusion and Chest Wall Instability

A simple rib fracture is the most common chest injury. Rib fractures may be multiple and may also include costochondral separations that are not visible on the chest x-ray. Multiple rib fractures or a combination of rib fractures, costochondral separations, and a sternal fracture may lead to an

TABLE 8-1. PRINCIPLES OF MANAGEMENT OF SEVERE
LUNG CONTUSION

1. Restrict IV fluid
2. Lasix 40 mg on admission and daily for 3 days post-trauma (selectively)
3. Methylprednisolone 500 mg IV stat and q6h for 72 hours (controversial)
4. Salt-poor albumin 25 mg daily
5. Blood losses replaced with plasma or whole blood
6. Vigorous tracheobronchial toilet
7. Morphine and intercostal blocks for control of chest wall pain
8. Supplemental nasal O_2 to maintain PO_2 above 80 mm Hg
9. Mechanical ventilation via endotracheal tube if PO_2 below 60 mm Hg on room air

unstable segment of chest wall, or a "flail chest." This results in the paradoxical indrawing of the involved chest wall segment with inspiration. Decreased vital capacity, increased airway resistance, and decreased functional capacity are associated with this lesion. The mechanical instability of the chest wall may be treated initially by compression of the chest wall by sand bags.

A major flail segment that results in hypoxemia as judged by an arterial PO_2 below 60 on room air is initially best treated with "internal pneumatic stabilization" with endotracheal intubation and positive pressure ventilation using a volume-cycled respirator. Long-term endotracheal intubation may require the use of tracheostomy, especially if there is evidence of vocal cord damage, if the secretions are difficult to manage, or if the patient does not tolerate the endotracheal tube well.

Recently it has been pointed out that a flail chest is usually associated with pulmonary contusion. Pulmonary contusion, defined as damage to lung parenchyma resulting in edema and hemorrhage without accompanying laceration, is most commonly associated with blunt trauma but also occurs with penetrating injuries, especially those due to high-velocity missiles. The interstitial and intra-alveolar hemorrhage and edema lead to airway collapse, increase in pulmonary vascular resistance, reduced lung compliance, ventilation-perfusion imbalance, and systemic hypoxemia. There is experimental and clinical evidence that pulmonary contusion is aggravated by rapid administration of large quantities of crystalloids. Amelioration by steroids is still debatable.

In the light of these changes, vigorous treatment of the associated pulmonary contusion is a fundamental factor in the management of flail chest (Table 8–1). Many patients with flail chest can be treated successfully with careful attention to fluid balance and the maintenance of efficient tracheobronchial toilet, coughing, and deep breathing. However, individuals with other severe injuries and those not responding adequately to this therapy should be provided with ventilatory assistance promptly. The use of long-term positive pressure ventilation in the face of multiple rib fractures will occasionally require the insertion of chest tubes bilaterally in order to prevent tension pneumothorax if the ventilatory pressure exceeds 50 to 60 cm of water.

DIAPHRAGMATIC RUPTURE

Diaphragmatic rupture is rare, but if not recognized and treated quickly, it can intensify any respiratory insufficiency following chest trauma. It is usually associated with blunt trauma to the lower chest and abdomen. The rupture can occur at any point of the diaphragm, but 95 percent involve the left hemidiaphragm. The natural pleural-peritoneal pressure gradient of 5 to 10 cm of water favors the movement of abdominal viscera into the thorax. A maximal inspiratory effort may raise this gradient to 50 to 100 cm of water. The major early physiological consequence is the space-occupying effect of abdominal viscera in the thorax. The diagnosis is suspected on clinical grounds by a decreased air entry and presence of any x-ray abnormality of the diaphragm or lower lung fields. X-ray evidence of a nasogastric tube curling back up into the chest or barium studies showing bowel in the chest may be confirmatory.

Immediate insertion of a nasogastric tube for decompression of the stomach is essential. Endotracheal intubation and positive pressure ventilation may be required for stabilization of the patient to allow transfer for surgical repair of the diaphragm. The high incidence of associated intra-abdominal injuries mandates an abdominal approach to the repair. Serious concomitant intrathoracic injuries are uncommon but are best dealt with by a separate thoracotomy rather than a combined thoraco-abdominal approach.

MANAGEMENT OF THE WIDENED MEDIASTINUM

Widening of the mediastinum on a chest x-ray following blunt chest trauma must immediately suggest a traumatic rupture of the aorta. The dramatic increase in the incidence of traumatic rupture of the aorta over the last three decades closely parallels the increase in high-speed motor vehicle accidents. This lesion is frequently overlooked due to severe associated injuries. The clinical features are summarized in Table 8–2. Unfortunately, the roentgenograms taken on critically injured patients are often misleading. A-P films taken at short distances with poor inspiration and the patient lying flat tend to make the mediastinum appear wider than it really is.

TABLE 8–2. TRAUMATIC AORTIC DISRUPTION

History:	High-speed horizontal or vertical deceleration injury
Clinical:	Retro-sternal or interscapular pain, upper limb hypertension
Radiological:	Widened superior mediastinum, depression of left main stem bronchus, deviation of esophagus, left hemothorax, fracture of sternum or first rib, apical cap, haziness of aortic knob

A high index of suspicion should prompt immediate complete aortography to localize damage that may be present virtually anywhere in the aorta but that is just distal to the left subclavian artery in 95 percent of cases. Of the trauma patients having aortography because of a widened mediastinum, about 30 to 50 percent will have a ruptured thoracic aorta.

A high incidence of early death (30 percent in six hours and 60 percent in 48 hours) caused by completion of the tear of the aorta in those who reach the hospital alive demands early surgical intervention. Repair of the rupture has often been performed in conjunction with systemic heparinization and left heart cardiopulmonary bypass. The heparinization, however, may increase bleeding from any major head or abdominal injuries, which are present in at least 60 percent of these patients. As a consequence, an ascending-to-descending aortic shunt has been used as an alternative. It has generally proved effective and does minimize bleeding from associated injuries. Most recently, clamping and direct suturing of the aortic tear without a graft, using Arfonad to control proximal aortic hypertension, has been receiving increasing favorable attention in carefully selected cases. The frequency of the most dreaded postoperative complication, paraplegia, is increased with prolonged shock with aortic clamping without a bypass or shunt for more than 20 minutes.

INDICATIONS FOR URGENT THORACOTOMY

The indications for urgent thoracotomy are summarized in Table 8–3. The most frequent indication is a penetrating wound of the heart, which is discussed in Chapter 9. Suspicion of cardiac tamponade or evidence of massive intrathoracic bleeding is a strong indication for an immediate thoracotomy as an integral part of resuscitation. Cardiac arrest caused by a thoracic or abdominal injury is an indication for immediate thoracotomy with open cardiac massage, compression or clamping of the descending thoracic aorta, and control of any intrathoracic bleeding. The thoracotomy may be done in the emergency department if it contains full operating room facilities. Otherwise, it is best done in the operating room. The key to success is the immediate recognition of the need for a thoracotomy.

TABLE 8–3. **INDICATIONS FOR URGENT THORACOTOMY**

1. Hemopericardium with cardiac tamponade
2. Penetrating cardiac injury with cardiac arrest
3. Massive hemothorax or continued chest tube drainage
4. Rupture of aorta or major branch
5. Rupture of tracheobronchial tree
6. Rupture of diaphragm
7. Rupture of esophagus
8. Sucking chest wall injury

COMBINED THORACOABDOMINAL WOUNDS

It is important to remember that vital abdominal viscera are protected by the lower portions of the thorax. Penetrating wounds of the chest below the fourth intercostal space anteriorly frequently involve the abdominal cavity. Wounds of entrance and exit must be carefully assessed and should be covered with a radiopaque marker just before any x-rays are done. Significant intra-abdominal pathology may be indicated by the findings of peritoneal irritation, abdominal distention, or roentgenographic demonstration of free air under the diaphragm. Diagnostic peritoneal lavage has been useful in the diagnosis of associated intra-abdominal injuries but cannot be totally relied upon, especially in the early hours after injury. Recovery of peritoneal dialysis fluid through a previously placed chest tube is obvious evidence of a diaphragmatic injury.

As a general principle, injuries to the diaphragm and intra-abdominal contents are best dealt with through a separate midline abdominal incision; evidence of serious intrathoracic bleeding or pathology is best dealt with by a separate thoracotomy rather than by a combined thoracoabdominal incision. Wounds of the right hemithorax frequently involve the liver and are best managed according to the principles outlined in Chapter 10. A complete repair of the diaphragm and separate infradiaphragmatic drainage of liver wounds will help minimize the incidence of bile leakage into the pleural cavity and empyema.

MANAGEMENT OF TRAUMATIC ASPHYXIA

No specific therapy is required for this clinical syndrome in which sudden high intravascular pressures produce a severe reddish or red-blue discoloration of the skin in the upper portions of the body. The extravasation of red blood cells into the interstitial tissue frequently also produces cerebral and pulmonary changes. Therapeutic efforts should be directed toward associated injuries such as hemopneumothorax, cardiac contusion, great vessel injuries, and ruptured diaphragm. Steroids have been advocated for associated cerebral edema. Neurological manifestations, including unconsciousness, are usually transient. The ultimate outcome is related to severity of associated injuries.

ESOPHAGEAL INJURY

The esophagus may be injured by penetrating wounds of the mediastinum, particularly at the thoracic inlet. However, esophageal injuries are most frequently caused by an esophagoscope at the time of endoscopy. Spontaneous rupture of the esophagus may also occur following vigorous vomiting. Esophageal injury must always be ruled out in any penetrating mediastinal wound, particularly in the presence of a pneumomediastinum. Severe substernal pain, leukocytosis, and fever following endoscopic examination of the esophagus or forceful vomiting suggest a perforation of the esophagus. Subcutaneous emphysema in the neck under such circumstances is almost diagnostic. There is frequently an associated pleural effusion, and if the parietal pleura has been disrupted, there may be a hemopneumothorax.

The diagnosis of an esophageal injury may be confirmed by having the patient swallow a small amount of methylene blue and discovering the dye in fluid recovered by thoracocentesis or in chest tube drainage. Water-soluble contrast media may also demonstrate a perforation but not infrequently fail to reveal a subsequently proven laceration. A carefully performed dilute barium examination under fluoroscopy is more accurate.

The treatment of esophageal perforation or laceration is early thoracotomy with opening of the mediastinal pleura, two-layer closure of the perforation, and coverage of the repair with a gastric, intercostal muscle, pleural, or pericardial flap. Systemic antibiotics and effective drainage of the pleural space with large chest tubes are an integral part of the management.

CORROSIVE ESOPHAGITIS

Esophageal burns may follow the ingestion of acid or alkaline, solid or liquid caustic agents. Children between 2 and 4 years of age are the most frequent accidental victims. Adults are usually involved following accidental ingestion or a suicide attempt.

The key to successful management of corrosive burns to the esophagus is the early identification of the etiological agent and accurate assessment of the depth and extent of injury. The ingestion of lye is frequently associated with severe laryngeal and pharyngeal injury. Antidotes are ineffective unless given instantly. Gastric lavage is contraindicated because of the risk of perforating the esophagus or inducing vomiting with exacerbation of the original injury.

Hoarseness, stridor, and dyspnea suggest laryngeal involvement. Substernal or interscapular and abdominal pain suggest a mediastinal or peritoneal injury. All patients should be admitted and observed for evidence of airway compromise. Esophagoscopy as soon as the patient's condition is stable is indicated to assess accurately the extent and depth of injury. Because of the risk of perforation, the esophagoscopist should stop as soon as evidence of a circumferential burn is demonstrated. Wide-spectrum prophylactic antibiotics should be administered in full dosage. Steroids (such as dexamethasone 4 to 6 mg every 6 hours) are usually also given, but their efficacy has recently been questioned.

Minor superficial burns will heal without sequelae, but a deeper burn may progress to a corrosive stricture requiring long-term dilatation. Swallowing of a lead shot on a heavy silk suture as soon as a circular injury is found may be useful in deep mucosal injuries. This will allow relatively safe dilatation of the esophagus in the chronic stage of this injury.

REFERENCES

1. Kirsh M, Sloan H: Blunt Chest Trauma: General Principles of Management. Boston, Little, Brown & Co., 1977.
2. Mulder DS, Wallace DH, Woolhouse FM: The use of the fiberoptic bronchoscope to facilitate endotracheal intubation following head and neck trauma. J Trauma 15:638, 1975.
3. Graham JM, Mattox KL, Beall AC: Penetrating trauma of the lung. J Trauma 19:665, 1979.
4. Trinkle JK, Richardson JD, Franz JD, et al: Management of flail chest without mechanical ventilation. Ann Thorac Surg 19:355, 1975.
5. Hood RM: Traumatic diaphragmatic hernia. Ann Thorac Surg 12:311, 1971.
6. Kouchoukas NT, Lell WA, Kays RB, Samuelson PN: Hemodynamic effects of aortic clamping and decompression with a temporary shunt for resection of descending aorta. Surgery 85:25, 1979.

9

Cardiac Injuries

Improved emergency communication and transportation systems have brought to hospitals an increased number of patients with cardiac injuries who previously would have died at the scene of the accident or in the ambulance. The penetrating cardiac wounds usually produce striking signs and symptoms, whereas the cardiac damage due to blunt trauma, which is much more common, is more subtle and easily missed.

PENETRATING WOUNDS

ETIOLOGY

The great majority of penetrating wounds of the heart are stab or gunshot wounds. Stab wounds of the heart usually involve only one chamber, seldom cause damage to intracardiac structures, and usually have an obvious track. However, gunshot wounds are much more likely to cause through-and-through and intracardiac injuries. In addition, the track of a bullet is unpredictable and much more likely to damage other organs. As a consequence, the morbidity and mortality from gunshot wounds are much greater than for stab wounds.

PATHOPHYSIOLOGY

The main hemodynamic problems caused by penetrating cardiac wounds are hemorrhage and pericardial tamponade. The bleeding may rapidly progress to hypovolemic shock or death. The tamponade results in impaired diastolic filling of the heart; however, it also limits the amount of bleeding from the myocardial wound and may thereby be life-saving, at least temporarily. Damage to the proximal portion of a major coronary artery is uncommon, but it may result in arrhythmias or infarction with resultant cardiogenic shock.

If the pericardial and myocardial wounds are small, which is the usual situation in patients who arrive alive at a hospital, the main problem is tamponade. These patients will usually improve rapidly, at least temporarily, with pericardiocentesis. If the myocardial wound is large and the pericardial wound small, the patient develops tamponade rapidly and is usually in severe shock when first seen. If the pericardial wound is large, the patient generally rapidly exsanguinates.

DIAGNOSIS

Clinical

All patients in shock with a penetrating wound of the chest between the midclavicular line on the right and midaxillary line on the left should be considered to have a cardiac injury until proved otherwise.

Virtually all patients with a penetrating wound of the heart will have some tamponade, with varying degrees of hypovolemia. If the only problem is tamponade, the neck veins will usually be distended to some degree, the blood pressure (particularly the pulse pressure) will tend to be low, and occasionally the heart tones are faint or muffled. This combination of signs, often referred to as Beck's triad, can be very deceptive and many false positives and false negatives occur. If the patient has a tamponade but is hypovolemic, the neck veins will not be distended until or unless the blood volume is adequately restored. Conversely, chest injuries can cause the patient to breathe abnormally or strain, raising the central venous pressure (CVP) and distending the neck veins in the absence of tamponade. Even with a large tamponade, the heart tones are usually clear, and this is the least reliable sign in Beck's triad.

A paradoxical pulse, characterized by a drop in systolic blood pressure of more than 15 mm Hg during normal inspiration, should also suggest tamponade. Agitation, lack of cooperation, and air hunger are often present but may occur with any chest injury causing hypoxemia or shock.

Pericardiocentesis

All patients in shock with a possible cardiac injury should have pericardiocentesis. This is primarily a diagnostic procedure, but removal of as little as 5 to 10 cc of blood from the pericardium may cause a dramatic improvement in cardiac output and blood pressure.

Technique. The main approaches for pericardiocentesis are precordial and paraxiphoid. With the precordial approach, a 16- or 18-gauge needle is inserted into the fifth intercostal space 2 to 3 cm lateral to the sternal border, so as to avoid the internal mammary vessels that lie 0.5 to

1.0 cm from the sternum. The use of this precordial approach is more direct but more apt to result in false negatives or false positives and with it the midportion of the anterior descending coronary artery can easily be lacerated.

Use of the paraxiphoid approach is much safer. An 18-gauge spinal (10 cm) needle should be used. The skin is punctured with a knife blade 2 cm below the costal border adjacent to the xiphoid. If a metal needle is used, the pericardiocentesis should be done with constant electrocardiographic monitoring, if such monitoring will not result in delay of the pericardiocentesis. The ECG monitoring is best done by attaching the V-lead from the ECG to the metal needle with an insulated wire with alligator clips at both ends.

The needle is passed upward and backward at an angle of 45 degrees for 4 or 5 cm until the point seems to enter a cavity. Most physicians direct the needle toward the left shoulder; however, directing the needle toward the right shoulder is less likely to result in penetration of a cardiac chamber. One aspirates frequently as the needle is advanced and, if no blood is obtained, a stylet is inserted or 0.5 to 1.0 cc of saline is injected to be certain that the needle is not plugged. The needle is then carefully passed farther until blood is obtained, cardiac pulsations are felt, or the ECG shows inversion of the QRS.

Most of the blood in the pericardial cavity is clotted and consequently one can usually remove only 2 to 3 cc at a time and in a rather erratic fashion. Easy removal of larger quantities of blood usually indicates that the blood is being aspirated from a cardiac chamber. If a plastic catheter or needle is used for the pericardiocentesis, it should be left in place for continuous drainage of the intrapericardial blood until the cardiac wound is surgically repaired.

About 25 percent of patients with acute tamponade will have a negative pericardiocentesis; therefore, failure to aspirate blood does not rule out tamponade.

X-ray

X-ray studies may delay urgent operation and are of little assistance in diagnosing a cardiac lesion except in the infrequent case with intrapericardial air. Significant enlargement of the heart shadow by an acute tamponade is unusual. Furthermore, lack of change in the size of the cardiac silhouette on serial chest films does not exclude the diagnosis of cardiac injury.

The main reason for obtaining x-rays is to rule out other injuries, particularly hemopneumothorax. However, if a large hemothorax or pneumothorax is suspected and the patient's condition is unstable, the chest tube(s) should be inserted without obtaining x-ray confirmation. Furthermore, if the involved chest cavity is to be opened almost immediately, delaying the procedure to insert the chest tube(s) is unwise.

ECG and Echocardiography

ECG changes are usually nonspecific. ST-T wave changes may indicate pericardial irritation or may merely reflect associated ischemia or hypoxia. Echocardiography, although potentially very helpful in diagnosing the presence of pericardial fluid, is usually not immediately available and there are occasional false positives and false negatives.

TREATMENT

Fluid Replacement

It is essential that patients with penetrating wounds of the chest have two or three large intravenous cannulae placed, with at least one cannula in a leg vein in case the superior vena cava or one of its major branches is injured. An adequate or preferably an increased blood volume helps to maintain cardiac output until the tamponade can be relieved.

Cardiorrhaphy

It-is now generally believed that all patients with suspected injury to the heart should have an emergency thoracotomy to assess accurately the injuries, to relieve the tamponade completely, and to repair any injuries found. An immediate thoracotomy is particularly important if the patient has persistent shock and when his condition is deteriorating.

After an endotracheal tube has been inserted, the chest is opened either through an anterior thoracotomy or midsternotomy. The transpleural approach through a long incision in the fifth left anterior intercostal space is usually preferred because it is quicker and does not require a sternal knife or saw. If additional exposure is found necessary, the adjacent cartilages may be divided at the sternum. In some cases it may be necessary to divide the sternum transversely so that the incision may be extended into the right thorax. Some surgeons prefer a sternal-splitting approach, particularly if need for cardiopulmonary bypass is suspected.

If an anterior thoracotomy incision is used, the internal mammary vessels must be ligated. The pericardium is incised parallel to the phrenic nerve and opened widely. All the blood is rapidly removed and the wound in the heart is located. Bleeding from the heart is controlled by pressure over the wound with a finger. Repair of the myocardial injury is done best with interrupted, pledgetted horizontal mattress sutures using 2–0 nonabsorbable material swedged onto a long slender curved needle. The pericardium is either approximated with a few widely spaced interrupted sutures or it is left open to prevent recurrent tamponade. The only potential problem with a wide-open pericardium is possible adhesion to the sternum or lung. Herniation is only a problem if a portion of the heart, usually the apex, becomes entrapped in a partial pericardial closure.

Open Cardiac Massage

If the cardiac arrest occurs before transport to the operating room, an endotracheal tube should be inserted and emergency left anterolateral thoracotomy performed in the emergency department to provide open cardiac massage. Closed massage is ineffective in these patients. The bleeding site can usually be controlled with a fingertip while the massage is being performed. In some instances, bleeding from a cardiac wound can be controlled nicely by inserting a Foley catheter through the myocardial opening and pulling the inflated balloon up against the wound opening. In addition, clamping or compressing the descending thoracic aorta increases almost threefold the blood flow to the heart and brain. One must, however, be careful not to cause left ventricular distention or central hypertension. Alternate massage of the heart and ascending aorta may further improve coronary blood flow.

Standard open CPR techniques must be used if the heart is in standstill (asystole) or has only weak ventricular fibrillation. Administration of sodium bicarbonate (1 mEq/kg) or adrenalin (3 to 5 ml of 1:10,000, intracardiac, intravenously or even intratracheally) may help achieve a coarse fibrillation, which is easier to defibrillate with internal paddles (40 watt-sec is usually adequate).

Coronary Artery Injuries

Suture-ligation of the cut ends is the treatment of choice for lacerations of small or distal coronary vessels. Suture ligation may also be applied to injuries of the proximal coronary arteries if there is no evidence of cardiovascular impairment; however, such patients must be observed closely. If arrhythmias, dysfunction, or an infarct develops, saphenous vein–coronary artery bypass should be performed. Standby cardiopulmonary bypass equipment is generally essential for such surgery to be performed properly.

Intracardiac Injuries

If heart failure is not present at the time of injury, valvular or septal repairs are best performed electively with cardiopulmonary bypass at a later date after full cardiac catheterization.

BLUNT TRAUMA

Cardiac damage due to blunt trauma is being recognized with increased frequency. Cardiac injury is now considered the most common unsuspected visceral injury responsible for death in fatally injured accident victims.

MECHANISMS OF INJURY

The mechanisms involved in cardiac damage from blunt trauma include acceleration and deceleration, compression, and injury caused by a sudden increase in intrathoracic or intra-abdominal pressure. The damage is more extensive if the trauma occurs during the isovolemic phases of the cardiac cycle.

The spectrum of cardiac injuries that may result from blunt trauma include myocardial contusion, pericardial effusion, septal defects, and rupture of valvular structures or cardiac chambers.

MYOCARDIAL CONTUSION

Incidence

Myocardial contusion occurs much more frequently than is generally recognized. In carefully monitored patients admitted to hospitals with severe blunt chest trauma, the incidence is probably at least 20 to 25 percent and has been reported to be as high as 76 percent.

Pathology

The pathological changes usually consist of subendocardial hemorrhage, which is the apex of a much larger cone of myocardial damage. This damage can include focal myocardial edema, interstitial hemorrhage, myofibrillar degeneration, and focal myocytolysis. Shock, hypovolemia, and excessive catecholamine release may greatly aggravate these changes.

The boundaries of damage are usually sharply demarcated in contrast to the hemorrhage often associated with myocardial infarction.

In some instances there is full-thickness damage that may closely resemble an infarction. This type of injury is most apt to occur if there is concomitant coronary vascular occlusion caused by arterial spasm, intimal tears producing a flap, or by compression from adjacent hemorrhage and edema. In some instances transient hypotension may cause complete occlusion of a previously severely diseased vessel.

Usually there is complete clinical recovery with minimal residual scarring following a myocardial contusion. However, in some cases, softening and fibrotic replacement of the contused myocardium are followed by thinning of the scar, which leads to dilatation and aneurysm formation.

Diagnosis

Cardiac contusions are among the most frequently missed or delayed diagnoses in injured patients admitted to the hospital. The reasons for delay in diagnosis are often related to (1) attention directed toward other severe injuries, (2) lack of evidence of thoracic injury, or (3) lack of evidence of cardiac injury on initial examination.

Clinical. In some instances a tachycardia that is completely out of proportion to the degree of trauma or blood loss may be the first tipoff to the diagnosis. Aside from evidence of significant chest wall injury, the only other physical signs helpful in establishing the diagnosis are the presence of a friction rub or abnormality in heart sounds.

ECG. The diagnosis of myocardial contusion is made primarily by ECG. It is crucial that myocardial contusion be suspected in all patients with significant blunt injury to the chest (particularly by steering wheel) and that serial ECG's be obtained for at least 48 hours in all such cases.

ST-T wave abnormalities present on admission or developing after 24 to 48 hours and persisting for several days can usually be accepted as evidence of myocardial contusion. The development of a bundle branch block or an arrhythmia should also alert the physician to the possibility that the myocardium has been contused. Persistent electrocardiographic changes or the development of significant Q waves suggest more than simple contusion and are probably indicative of extensive myocardial scarring with possible formation of a ventricular aneurysm.

High-frequency electrocardiograph (HF-ECG) employing a cathode ray tube and an expanded time scale may be particularly helpful. HF-ECG has demonstrated notching and slurring in the QRS complex that were not apparent on the conventional ECG. Such changes have been seen as early as three minutes after trauma and have persisted for weeks after the conventional ECG reverted to normal.

Enzymes. SGOT, LDH, and CPK levels are usually elevated in patients with severe blunt chest trauma because of injuries of liver, lung, bone, brain, and skeletal muscle. Consequently, they are of little value in diagnosing cardiac injuries. CPK myocardial isoenzymes should be theoretically more specific, but in most patients with blunt chest trauma all fractions have been elevated even without other evidence of myocardial contusion.

Other Studies. Technetium scanning has been suggested as a possible diagnostic technique for identifying cardiac contusion, but it is apt to be positive only with large lesions. Low cardiac output as measured by impedance cardiography may provide the most sensitive test for cardiac contusion. However, such changes are nonspecific, and this technique may be difficult to apply in some patients with thoracic injury.

Cardiac catheterization and coronary angiography are useful for outlining the extent of myocardial injury and coronary artery disease in patients who suffer definite myocardial infarction with cardiospecific enzyme and ECG changes. They should be undertaken in patients in whom cardiac symptoms persist after the injury and in those suspected of having coincident coronary artery or other cardiac disease.

Treatment

If a myocardial contusion is suspected, the patient should be treated as if he had an acute myocardial infarction. Particular attention must be directed to prevention and treatment of complications, especially arrhythmias and congestive heart failure. Continuous cardioscopic monitoring is important in this regard. The avoidance of fluid overload in management of patients with cardiac contusion cannot be overemphasized.

Anticoagulants should be avoided in patients with cardiac contusion because most patients have other significant injuries that may be complicated by anticoagulants. Furthermore, the effects of anticoagulation upon the cardiac injury are uncertain, and these agents may be particularly risky in patients with cardiac contusions accompanied by hemopericardium.

PERICARDIAL EFFUSIONS OR TAMPONADE

Pericardial injury should be suspected with severe blunt trauma to the chest, particularly if there is electrocardiographic or other evidence of myocardial damage. Hemopericardium can lead to tamponade within minutes or as late as a week or more after the injury. Retained pericardial blood can also cause late constrictive pericarditis.

Pericardial lacerations usually occur across the base of the heart near the junction of the visceral and parietal pericardium. Cardiac herniation caused by pericardial rupture is rare but should be suspected if shock or severe heart failure is present and the patient has blood in the pericardium with an unusual ECG or chest x-ray. If cardiac tamponade is suspected, pericardiocentesis should be performed. If the diagnosis of tamponade is established or a herniation is suspected, thoracotomy should be performed via a left anterior thoracotomy or median sternotomy incision.

SEPTAL DEFECTS

Septal defects after blunt chest trauma are rare but should be looked for carefully, particularly if there is any evidence of myocardial damage. The interventricular septum near the apex is particularly susceptible to perforation. Diagnosis may be difficult because rupture of chordae tendineae or papillary muscles or both cause mitral or tricuspid insufficiency. This insufficiency may closely mimic a septal perforation.

The murmurs of traumatic ventricular septal defect rarely appear soon after injury and are usually detected only several days or weeks later. In most cases abnormal electrocardiographic findings (especially supraventricular arrhythmias, conduction disturbances, or QRS abnormalities) may be the first signs of significant cardiac injury. The triad of chest trauma, systolic murmur, and an infarct pattern on the electrocardiogram should suggest the diagnosis of interventricular septal defect.

Although small traumatic defects may close spontaneously, surgical closure — preferably six to eight weeks after the trauma — is the treatment of choice. The presence of congestive heart failure may require earlier operation.

Isolated atrial septal defects due to blunt trauma are extremely rare and most of these patients die rapidly unless surgical repair can be performed immediately.

VALVE INJURIES

Rupture of the aortic valve is the most common valvular lesion in older patients who survive nonpenetrating cardiac injury. Blunt trauma rarely may also lacerate the papillary muscles or chordae tendineae of the mitral valve. The prognosis for rupture of the mitral papillary muscle is grave and death usually occurs within a few days after the injury. The tricuspid valve is rarely involved in blunt trauma and does not usually cause a severe hemodynamic problem.

The identification of heart murmurs after severe blunt trauma to the chest in any patient without a history of heart disease should alert the physician to the possibility that the patient's aortic valve has been damaged. The diagnosis of traumatic aortic valvular insufficiency is usually made when a loud, musical, high-pitched diastolic murmur is heard in a dyspneic trauma patient who has chest pain and previously had no murmur. As the lesion worsens, the diastolic pressure decreases. Peripheral signs of aortic insufficiency, such as visible capillary pulse, Corrigan's pulse, pistol shot sounds over the brachial and femoral vessels, and Duroziez's murmur (biphasic arterial bruit) also may become evident. Echocardiography may occasionally be diagnostic, but cardiac catheterization is essential prior to surgical therapy. The avulsion type of valve injury most frequently seen after blunt chest trauma makes leaflet repair difficult and tenuous; consequently, replacement is the recommended procedure.

CHAMBER RUPTURE

Rupture of a cardiac chamber is the most common injury noted in autopsy examinations of patients after blunt cardiac trauma. Most of these patients die rapidly from exsanguination or tamponade. Shock not responding properly to fluid replacement or transfusions or both may represent cardiac tamponade from a ruptured cardiac chamber. A positive pericardiocentesis in an individual with persistent shock after blunt trauma is an indication for immediate surgery, preferably with cardiopulmonary bypass support. This usually provides the only chance for survival from a heart chamber rupture.

FOLLOW-UP

It is important that patients with proven or suspected cardiac injury be closely observed, not only throughout their hospital stay but also later, for initially undiagnosed injuries or complications. One must look particularly for post-traumatic pericarditis, ventricular septal defect, valvular defects, ventricular aneurysm, and aortic, pulmonary, or coronary fistulas or chamber communication. When such problems are found and it appears that the defect endangers the patient's life, cardiac catheterization should be performed as soon as possible, followed by surgical repair. However, if the patient tolerates the lesion well, cardiac catheterization and subsequent repair should be performed electively six to eight weeks later.

RECOMMENDED READINGS

1. Demuth WE, Baue AE, Odom JA: Contusions of the heart. J Trauma 7:443–455, 1967.
2. Parmley LF, Manion WC, Mattingly TW: Nonpenetrating traumatic injury of the heart. Circulation 18:371–396, 1958.
3. Szentpetery S, Lower RR: Changing concepts in the treatment of penetrating cardiac injuries. J Trauma 17:457–461, 1977.
4. Wilson RF, Steiger Z, Thoms N, Arbulu A: Cardiac injuries. In Walt AJ, Wilson RF (eds.): Management of Trauma: Practice and Pitfalls. Philadelphia, Lea and Febiger, 1975, pp. 323–335.
5. Wilson RF, Murray C, Antonenko D: Nonpenetrating thoracic injuries. Surg Clin N Am 57:17–36, 1977.

10

Abdomen

Damage to the abdominal viscera may be caused by penetrating trauma (most commonly by stabs or gunshots) or blunt trauma (automobile accidents or direct blows). The type and size of the missile or the severity of impact is usually reflected in the degree of visceral damage, but so many individual variations occur that clinical speculation is dangerous. The clinical picture, especially in blunt trauma, may not reflect the serious and even potentially lethal nature of the visceral damage for hours or days. Small wounds may hide large problems; large wounds may sometimes pose only small problems. Consequently, skepticism and alertness are vital.

Most surgeons believe that gunshot wounds that may have traversed the peritoneal cavity require laparotomy because over 97 percent of these will have caused some degree of visceral damage. In contrast, stab wounds are universally now treated much more selectively.

Certain principles form the keystones of accurate diagnosis:

1. In cases in which internal injury is in doubt, repeated frequent examination is essential to early diagnosis.

2. Concomitant injuries, especially of the chest, may take precedence in treatment over the abdominal injury.

3. Patients with a head injury are especially difficult to assess and shock should never be attributed to cerebral damage; peritoneal lavage has great value in these patients.

4. Certain constellations of injuries are commonly associated, e.g., fractures of the ribs on the right side with ruptures of the liver; fractures of the ribs on the left side with splenic injury; pelvic fractures and bladder rupture; fractures of lumbar pedicles and intestinal transection in seat belt injuries.

5. The diaphragm extends to the fourth intercostal space, and injuries that may on superficial examination appear to be limited to the thorax may in fact have a diaphragmatic and abdominal component.

6. The pathway of intra-abdominal missiles cannot necessarily be predicted from the sites of the entrance and exit wounds because these vary with the position of the patient at the moment of injury and with possible deflections of the missile.

7. In penetrating wounds, the patient's back and anal region must be as carefully examined as the flanks and ventral surface.

8. Seat belts may cause complete transection of the intestine with only minimal clinical signs early on; the roentgenographic demonstration of free peritoneal air may be greatly delayed in injuries of the small intestine.

9. Signs of ecchymosis of the abdominal wall due to a seat belt should always raise serious suspicion of underlying visceral damage.

10. Hematuria mandates the need for an intravenous pyelogram (IVP), but serious renal or ureteral injury may occasionally be present in the absence of hematuria. Consequently, a case can be made for routine IVP in all severe abdominal trauma.

11. The presence of a pelvic fracture with its concomitant blood loss and retroperitoneal hematoma makes intra-abdominal visceral injury much more difficult to assess.

12. The administration of narcotics should be avoided until a definitive decision has been made about the need for operation, because narcotics may obscure clinical signs.

PLAN OF MANAGEMENT

Most deaths from abdominal injury are caused by early hemorrhage or later peritonitis. As soon as the patient arrives in the emergency department, his clinical state should be rapidly assessed and special attention given to ensuring adequate ventilation and avoidance of aspiration. If the patient is in stable condition, a full history is obtained and a systematic physical examination, including a rectal examination, is conducted. Special note is made of any possible recent ingestion or aspiration of food, alcohol, or drugs. Any degree of respiratory distress is given immediate priority. The possibility of airway obstruction, a pneumothorax or hemothorax, or a ruptured diaphragm should be considered. The presence of shoulder-tip pain reflecting subphrenic irritation is always significant. The fact that about 75 percent of patients with blunt injury to the abdomen have concomitant injury to the head, chest, or extremities must be kept in mind throughout. Similarly, any penetrating injury below the fourth intercostal space may well have affected an intra-abdominal organ.

When the patient shows evidence of impending or established shock, the process of assessment is accelerated. Oxygenation is provided, one or more intravenous cannulae are inserted into veins of an extremity (by antecubital cutdown or by direct puncture of the subclavian or internal jugular veins), and blood is sent to be typed and crossmatched. Hypovolemia is corrected if possible by a balanced salt solution. The patient is stripped and thoroughly examined, back and front. Evidence of tire marks, fractures, flail chest, subcutaneous emphysema, rupture of abdominal muscles, localized tenderness or rigidity, and blood in the rectum (on digital examination) and stomach (via nasogastric tube) is sought. Auscultation of the abdomen may be helpful, although the presence of bowel sounds at this stage does not preclude the possibility of serious abdominal injury. Vital signs are monitored and a Foley catheter is inserted to follow the quantity of urine produced and the presence of blood or sugar in the urine. The abdominal girth is measured to serve as objective evidence for any subsequent increase. When it is thought that an intra-abdominal injury may be present, prophylactic intravenous antibiotics effective against aerobic and anaerobic organisms are given immediately, pending a final decision about the need for operation. If aspiration is feared or severe stress is threatened, intravenous cimetidine is advocated by some to reduce gastric acid prophylactically.

If the patient's condition is stable, roentgenograms may be obtained. Special attention should be given to (1) the contour of the diaphragm on both sides, (2) the presence of free air under the diaphragm, (3) the position of the stomach bubble, (4) the possibility of trapped retroperitoneal air (especially to the right of the upper lumbar vertebrae; this is usually indicative of a retroduodenal rupture), (5) obliteration of the psoas shadow, (6) fracture of the lumbar pedicles.

If hematuria is noted or if a wound suggests the possibility of renal damage, an infusion IVP should be obtained. In selected cases, a retrograde cystogram may be necessary too, because an IVP should not be relied upon to assess the integrity of the bladder or lower ureter. Thorough mapping of the urinary system is of vital importance in all blunt injuries with hematuria, especially when a pelvic fracture is present.

Angiography has a limited place in the immediate care of these patients and will seldom assist in the determination of the need for emergency laparotomy. Nevertheless, angiography may be extremely valuable under certain circumstances: (1) In the presence of a nonfunctioning kidney on IVP, preliminary renal arteriography will outline the state of the renal arteries. (2) Arteriography is a highly desirable preliminary to abdominal exploration whenever a bruit is present. (3) In the presence of pelvic fractures associated with marked hemorrhage, angiography may demonstrate the bleeding point and provide a base for the embolization of the lesion, thus reducing blood loss. This may serve as definitive treatment. (4) Occasionally, arteriography may expose an unexpected source of bleeding or an area of visceral damage such as a bleeding spleen or a ruptured diaphragm. (5) As the surgical approach to splenic injury has become more conservative, arteriography has been used as a technique of defining, following, and, through embolization, treating selected splenic damage.

PLACE AND TECHNIQUE OF PERITONEAL LAVAGE

Peritoneal tap and subsequently peritoneal lavage (PL) have permitted a much more rational approach to the management of abdominal trauma.

When the peritoneal cavity contains a great deal of blood, a tap in one or more quadrants may give an immediate diagnosis. In more subtle circumstances, however, peritoneal lavage is required. Peritoneal lavage has its greatest value in the assessment of the patient with head injury, paraplegia, hypotension without obvious evidence of blood loss externally or into the thoracic cavity or a fracture site, and in patients with an increasing but relatively asymptomatic abdominal distention. PL does not take precedence over clinical judgment. In a sense, PL serves strongly to reinforce a clinical view that leans toward avoiding laparotomy.

Peritoneal lavage is accurate in about 97 percent of cases, with false positives associated mainly with pelvic fractures and technical errors. False negatives are most often associated with retroperitoneal injuries such as pancreatic or duodenal lacerations, tears of the small intestine, and ruptures of the diaphragm.

It is important that there be agreement about what constitutes a positive reading, and there has recently been some controversy on this definition. Given meticulous performance of the technique, however, most surgeons are agreed on indications for laparotomy: (1) about 75,000 RBC's/ml lavage fluid, (2) the presence of more than 500 WBC's/ml (remembering that it often requires three or four hours for this reaction to develop), and (3) the presence of bile or intestinal contents. An elevated amylase level in the lavage fluid is so seldom present that many no longer consider this a necessary measurement.

The "open" technique of PL whereby the point of insertion of the catheter through the peritoneum is directly visualized has become the most widely accepted technique, especially in the relatively obese patient. The insertion of a catheter over a guide wire is currently being explored.

After the bladder has been emptied, local anesthesia is injected through the midline of the abdomen down to the peritoneum. A small skin incision is made a short distance below the umbilicus or through the inferior rim of the umbilicus and a peritoneal dialysis catheter is carefully inserted. If aspiration reveals no gross blood or abnormal contents, about 1000 ml of lactated Ringer's solution (300 to 500 ml in children) is infused into the peritoneal cavity. When feasible, the patient is gently moved from side to side to ensure thorough irrigation of the peritoneal cavity. The bottle is then lowered to create a siphon effect and the returning fluid is carefully observed. A useful, rapid, and practical method of assessing whether or not the quantity of blood in the aspirate is significant is a failure to be able to read newsprint through the returning fluid.

It should be noted that insertion of the cannula may be hazardous in patients who have had previous intra-abdominal operations that have created adhesions. Also, in patients with a fractured pelvis, the catheter is better inserted above the umbilicus to avoid the possibility of a false-positive reading because of any associated extraperitoneal hematoma. Intra-abdominal visceral injuries occur in about 25 percent of patients with severe pelvic fractures and may be much more difficult to diagnose on clinical grounds because of the referred pain of the fracture and associated ileus. A clear PL is valuable as a negative indicator; a positive bloody lavage is much more confusing because it may reflect only the extraperitoneal hematoma.

INDICATIONS FOR OPERATION

Previously, laparotomy was advocated for all gunshot wounds of the abdomen and the great majority of stab wounds, but this idea has been modified in recent years. Exploration is still generally performed in gunshot wounds in which the possibility exists that the missile has penetrated the peritoneal cavity or passed very close to it. In contrast, careful and continuous clinical observation of selected stab wounds has obviated the need for laparotomy in many patients.

Modern surgical policies are designed to avoid unnecessary laparotomy but also to ensure that operative treatment of significant wounds is not unduly delayed. It is important to remember that about 15 percent of patients with positive clinical findings suggestive of visceral damage turn out to have negative findings at laparotomy. In contrast, about 30 percent of patients with negative or minimal clinical findings have positive findings at operation. Against this background, some surgeons prefer to explore abdominal stab wounds under local anesthesia and to discharge the patient from the hospital if the peritoneum is intact and no other lesions are present. When the peritoneum is not intact, peritoneal lavage is performed; if the PL is negative, the patient is admitted to the hospital and observed for 24 hours. On the other hand, if the peritoneal lavage is positive, the patient is taken to the operating room for exploration. In patients with multiple stab wounds in whom it is not practical to explore each of these individually, peritoneal lavage is relied upon to reinforce clinical decisions. Many surgeons routinely prefer to do a peritoneal lavage and to use the results as the index for operation rather than local wound exploration.

In our zeal to avoid unnecessary operations, however, it is important to remember that precedence is given to the time-honored indications for exploratory celiotomy in abdominal injuries. These include (1) evidence of continuing blood loss that cannot be clearly attributed to an extra-abdominal source, (2) increasing tenderness or rigidity or distention of the abdomen, (3) evidence of developing peritonitis, (4) the presence of free air on a roentgenogram, (5) an enlarging intra-abdominal mass, or (6) the demonstration of positive peritoneal lavage. In centers in which surgeons do not see many cases of abdominal injury and in which there are fewer trained observers in the hospital, a judiciously conducted laparotomy becomes more justifiable than reliance on watchful waiting.

OPERATIVE TREATMENT

When no urgency is present as measured in terms of hours, correction of any diabetes and abnormalities of acid-base and volume is carried out.

The induction of anesthesia is always a time of special hazard because of the dangers of aspiration and a sudden fall in blood pressure caused by vasodilatation. Steps to minimize these dangers should be taken.

A midline incision, especially in gunshot wounds in which the extent of damage is less predictable, remains the most useful incision in trauma, being relatively bloodless, rapidly made, generous of access to all areas, and easily enlarged. If necessary, this incision may be extended proximally to splitting of the sternum and so facilitate control of the supradiaphragmatic inferior vena cava or exposure of associated cardiac wounds. The midline incision also lends itself to easy extension into either side of the chest when there is pulmonary damage.

The presence of an abdominal tamponade, especially in a patient responding poorly to intravenous fluids, is a grave prognostic sign. When the peritoneal cavity is opened and the tamponade released, the danger of sudden collapse from fresh hemorrhage is a common hazard. Consequently, preparation should always be made ahead of time for immediate compression of the subdiaphragmatic abdominal aorta digitally, by sponge sticks, by aortic compressor, or by vascular clamp; alternatively, a preliminary left thoracotomy with supradiaphragmatic occlusion of the aorta by an arterial clamp may be preferred.

Control of hemorrhage is the primary objective, definitively or by temporary direct compression. In massive hemorrhage, the spleen, liver, aorta, and inferior vena cava are the most likely sources and manual compression over large sponges is the most effective initial approach. With maximal control achieved, rapid exploration follows. The bowel is systematically inspected. All holes are temporarily occluded with appropriate clamps to avoid further spillage. Single holes in vessels or hollow organs are viewed with great suspicion — an exit wound must be assiduously searched for. In the bowel, the mesenteric or omental areas may easily hide the perforation. If necessary, hematomas should be freely opened in the course of the search. Attention is paid to the retroperitoneal areas, and hematomas around the great vessels are opened after proximal and distal control has been assured. (See Chapter 11 for a discussion of perirenal hematomas.) In the pelvis, however, when pelvic fractures are present, hemorrhage may be extremely difficult to control if the tamponading pressure is released, and conservatism is preferable when there is no sign of expansion of the hematoma or associated visceral injury.

SPLEEN

The spleen is the intra-abdominal organ most frequently injured by blunt trauma and is often accompanied by rib fractures on the left. Penetrating injuries of the lower left thorax should also arouse suspicion of splenic or other visceral injury. This may be confirmed by peritoneal lavage. The clinical features of splenic injury include signs of blood loss, abdominal pain in the left upper quadrant, and pain in the left shoulder. The white blood cell count is often markedly elevated (20,000 to 30,000 per mm³). Roentgenographic findings include an increased density in the left upper quadrant, obliteration of the left renal and psoas shadows, and an elevated left hemidiaphragm. Displacement of the stomach bubble and downward displacement of the colon are sometimes seen.

Slow or delayed hemorrhage with a subcapsular hematoma may be difficult to diagnose. Angiography or isotopic scintiscanning may be invaluable in these circumstances, especially in the poor-risk patient in whom the added effects of an unnecessary laparotomy may tip the balance adversely.

Splenectomy is now known to increase susceptibility to overwhelming sepsis, especially in children under the age of 4, less so in those between 4 and 16 years, and least in adults. Concern over the increased vulnerability of the splenectomized patient to lethal septicemia by encapsulated organisms primarily makes it important to attempt to preserve the injured spleen whenever possible.

In children, in whom most splenic injuries follow blunt trauma and in whom the splenic lesion is commonly isolated, confirmation by ultrasonography, isotopes, or angiography may be followed by close nonoperative observation in the hospital, preferably in an intensive care unit. In older patients and in patients with multiple injuries, the spleen may be salvaged at least in part in about 50 percent of cases. Unless approximately 30 percent of the spleen can be preserved, efforts at conservation are not justified because immunological protection will not be provided. When the prolonged operating time and blood loss incurred in attempted repair of the spleen outweigh the potential hazard of any subsequent septicemia, splenectomy should be performed. This is particularly important to consider in aged patients, in patients who have been in deep shock, and in patients with multiple injuries or marked spillage of intestinal content.

It is technically important first to mobilize the spleen freely when attempting splenic repair. Repair may often be effected by simple catgut suture of the segmental blood supply, reinforced by Avitene, Gelfoam, and possibly omentum. Partial resection of a segment of the spleen with meticulous oversewing of the cut edge may be necessary in larger injuries. Ligation of the splenic artery and embolization are seldom called for. Most surgeons do not drain the splenic area unless there has been bacterial contamination or concomitant pancreatic damage.

Pneumovax should be administered to all patients who undergo splenectomy, with a booster dose being given approximately every three years. Infants and children should be given daily oral penicillin; compliance is important but difficult to achieve. The parents of children and all adults should be specifically warned about the early and fulminant manifestations of postsplenectomy sepsis, advised to have penicillin close at hand, and informed that they should consult their doctor immediately if any symptoms indicative of this type of infection should appear. Note should be made in the patient's chart that this has been done.

LIVER

Injuries to the liver are often associated with blunt trauma to the right side of the abdomen and lower thorax. Injuries of sufficient force to lacerate the liver are associated with injuries to other organs in about 90 percent of cases.

Hemostasis is the main problem in hepatic injuries. Small wounds that are not bleeding at laparotomy with the patient normotensive may or may not be sutured prophylactically. Drains are not necessary in these isolated injuries. Hemorrhage associated with large lacerations requires suture control with large chromic catgut on atraumatic needles, preferably by precise ligation of the bleeding area whenever possible. In some cases, however, horizontal mattress sutures encompassing substantial amounts of liver substance may be unavoidable. This includes attempted approximation of bleeding missile tracks deep in the substance of the liver that cannot be approached otherwise and in which it is hoped that compression will induce hemostasis. Most surgeons prefer to drain the perihepatic area with carefully placed sump or Penrose drains or both types.

In the presence of extensive hepatic bleeding, temporary compression of the area between and against gauze packs may be helpful in defining the extent of the problem and permitting blood transfusions to stabilize the patient's condition. When bleeding continues despite this manual compression, it is highly likely that the bleeding is originating from the inferior vena cava or the hepatic veins. Partial and temporary hemostatic control may be enhanced by manual compression of the portal triad temporarily. As soon as possible, selective occlusion of the appropriate hepatic artery should be obtained. Total hepatic blood flow should not be interrupted for more than 15 minutes at a time.

Most hepatic bleeding can be controlled by local measures. When these fail, ligation of the hepatic artery may produce dramatic hemostasis without subsequent liver failure if postoperative precautions to combat hypovolemia, hypoxia, and infection are taken. The hepatic artery should be ligated as close to the liver as possible. If both lobes are involved, it may be necessary to ligate the common hepatic artery. If possible, ligation of the hepatic artery proper should be avoided. Hepatic artery ligation should not be done until reasonable local attempts at hemostasis have failed; this technique cannot be done with assured impunity because it is sometimes followed by sepsis or re-bleeding.

When hepatic artery ligation fails, partial or complete resection of the injured lobe may be unavoidable. It should be recognized that the associated mortality in these circumstances remains very high.

In desperate circumstances in which both lobes of the liver are cracked or disrupted or in which hepatic artery ligation is unsuccessful and resection not feasible, firm temporary packing of the area with gauze for five to six days may be life-saving. This technique is particularly valuable in hospitals that are not equipped for major hepatic surgery. Such patients, after stabilization, can be transferred to a center where more definitive treatment can be accomplished. In point of fact, bleeding will have stopped in most of these patients when the packs are removed. These patients should be given heavy doses of broad-spectrum antibiotics for coverage.

In any case of hepatic bleeding that wells up from the depths and does not respond to the previously outlined methods, the possibility of a torn inferior vena cava or hepatic vein must be seriously considered. In these injuries, it will be necessary to stent the inferior vena cava by a cannula inserted through the right atrium or through the abdominal inferior vena cava to provide a conduit for the return of blood to the heart so that the vascular injury may be repaired under direct vision. Mortality remains high with this technique and sometimes diligent tamponading and packing may pay unexpected dividends.

In cases of torrential hemorrhage, the use of the Cell-Saver returning the patient's own blood from the peritoneal cavity to the general circulation may be life-saving. While contamination by microorganisms is not to be desired, autotransfusion of contaminated blood has been given without obvious untoward effects.

With hepatic bleeding controlled, consideration should be given to the avoidance of possible future complications. T-tube decompression of the common bile duct should be used only if the extrahepatic biliary tree is injured and not for purposes of decompressing the liver. Hemobilia following hepatic injury is uncommon. When it occurs, it is most likely to originate from a missile track or crack deep in the liver substance, appearing within a few weeks or months after injury. Bleeding is at first intermittent and is almost always associated with some degree of intra-hepatic infection. The patient may be jaundiced and present with either hematemesis or melena. Diagnosis is easily made by hepatic angiography and the primary treatment of most cases today is by embolization of the lesion with Gelfoam, muscle, or other occluding substances. Patients with treated hepatic injury should be warned of the remote possibility of this delayed event.

PORTAL VEIN

When the bleeding is seen to be coming from the portal vein, the surgeon is faced with a limited number of options. When possible, portal venorrhaphy is ideal. If the wound is tangential, repair may be relatively simple but in a number of cases end-to-end anastomosis may be necessary and in some this may entail considerable mobilization of organs in the area, especially the pancreas. As the technical problems may be immense, portal vein ligation presents an alternative and is certainly preferable to porta-caval shunt. Contrary to what used to be believed, ligation of the portal vein in humans does not necessarily result in the death of the patient.

PANCREAS

The clinical symptoms of pancreatic trauma may be deceptively mild for many hours or even days or weeks, especially when the posterior peritoneum has remained intact and has contained both the retroperitoneal hematoma and the contents of any ruptured ductules. Severe injuries are characterized by the classical signs of shock and peritonitis, which usually occur in conjunction with damage to adjacent organs.

The interpretation of the serum amylase level in pancreatic trauma is potentially deceptive. About 20 percent of patients with a transected pancreas have normal serum amylase levels at the time of operation. Conversely, hyperamylasemia is present in patients with abdominal trauma who have no pancreatic injury, the amylase originating from nonpancreatic sources as proved on isoamylase studies. Consequently, hyperamylasemia per se is not an indication for laparotomy. On the other hand, a rising serum amylase level is significant, especially in association with abdominal pain, because the biochemical change may reflect a leaking duct or a developing pseudocyst. Accurate preoperative diagnosis of these complications may be enhanced by the use of ultrasonography and CT scanning. While preoperative endoscopic retrograde pancreatography or later intraoperative transduodenal pancreatography has been advocated, few surgeons attempt these diagnostic maneuvers in the acute situation.

About one third of pancreatic injuries are caused by blunt trauma and about two thirds by penetrating trauma. Injury to surrounding vessels is the most common cause of morbidity and death. Patients who are in shock, which is almost invariably due to hemorrhage, have a mortality rate of about 40 percent. Associated colonic injuries are the second commonest threat to life because sepsis frequently intervenes later.

The head of the pancreas is injured in about 40 percent of pancreatic injuries and in half of these, the duodenum is also involved. In order of descending frequency, concomitant injuries of the liver, spleen, stomach, colon, small intestine, and kidney occur and are reflected in the clinical picture.

Isolated injuries of the pancreas are uncommon, occurring in only about 5 percent of patients with pancreatic injuries.

The main objectives of surgical treatment are to obtain hemostasis, conservatively debride any destroyed pancreas, and promote drainage. Any retroperitoneal hematoma overlying the pancreas should be very carefully explored after the greater omentum has been detached from the transverse colon. The body and the tail can be thoroughly explored through the lesser sac; the head of the pancreas is best evaluated by reflecting the right colon and mobilizing the retroperitoneal duodenum. Hemostasis in the pancreatic substance should be obtained by suture ligation using nonabsorbable sutures.

Simple wounds — stabs and small-caliber low-velocity missile wounds — are treated by suture repair and sump drainage for as long as substantial drainage occurs. Attempts at primary pancreatic duct reconstruction have been notoriously unsuccessful. When the main pancreatic duct has been transected, resection of the body and tail is the treatment of choice, usually with splenectomy; the transected end of the pancreas may or may not be drained into a Roux-en-Y jejunal loop.

Severe injuries to the head of the pancreas, when accompanied by injuries to the duodenum and biliary tree, may require pancreatoduodenectomy, but considerable evaluation of the situation is necessary before embarking on this extensive procedure. In the majority of cases, wide and efficient drainage of the area and acceptance of a subsequent (usually transient) fistula is preferable. When this latter procedure is decided upon, the institution of early total parenteral nutrition is a fundamental feature. In addition, closure of the pylorus and diversion of the gastric contents via a gastroenterostomy may be added selectively.

STOMACH

In most injuries of the stomach, blood is present in the nasogastric aspirate. All defects are managed by a two-layer closure. It is important to look for and repair wounds of the posterior gastric wall. Wounds of the cardiac end of the stomach seldom require a thoracoabdominal incision because they can usually be well exposed for suture by division of the triangular ligament of the left lobe of the liver.

DUODENUM AND SMALL INTESTINE

Injuries of the duodenum usually result from gunshot, stab, or crushing wounds. These wounds are frequently associated with injury to the pancreas, bile ducts, and inferior vena cava. Early diagnosis and attention to concomitant injuries are essential to a satisfactory outcome. In blunt duodenal trauma, especially when the patient is intoxicated, clinical signs may not be clinically apparent for as long as 12 to 18 hours. Nevertheless, abdominal roentgenograms during this time may show retroperitoneal air, and a Gastrografin swallow may demonstrate perforation of the duodenum. Retroperitoneal hematoma and bile staining in the area of the duodenum make it mandatory to mobilize the duodenum extensively for adequate exposure of its posterior surface and adjacent structures.

Small clean wounds of the duodenum may be treated with simple closure and drainage accompanied by nasogastric suction (Fig. 10–1). Severe wounds in the first portion of the duodenum may be treated by a Billroth II distal gastrectomy. Severe wounds in the second and third portions of the duodenum with concomitant pancreatic injury present the surgeon with an extremely difficult problem of management — primary

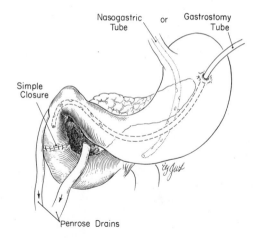

Figure 10-1. Repair of duodenal rupture with slight to moderate injury of the adjacent pancreas.

closure is frequently followed by fistula formation. If the associated pancreatic injury is not severe but the duodenal laceration is quite extensive, the following options are available: (1) The laceration may be closed and the area well drained. (2) A gastroenterostomy with a decompressive duodenostomy may be added to the repair. (3) A recently introduced alternative is closure of the pylorus by staples (the pylorus will reopen spontaneously), repair of the duodenum, establishment of a gastrojejunostomy (the addition of vagotomy in the patient without an ulcer diathesis is seldom needed), and drainage of the duodenopancreatic region. In any case, where the area of duodenal repair appears less than perfect, the suture line may be buttressed by an onlay graft of jejunum where a loop is tacked around the injured area (Fig. 10-2) or, in special

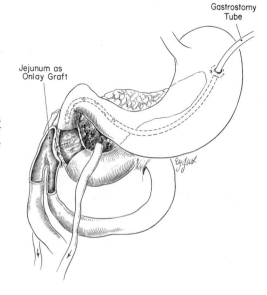

Figure 10-2. In more severe injuries of the duodenum, an onlay graft of jejunum may be used to reinforce the suture line.

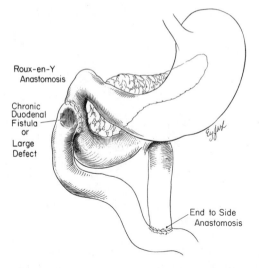

Roux-en-Y
Anastomosis

Chronic
Duodenal
Fistula
or
Large
Defect

End to Side
Anastomosis

Figure 10–3. A Roux-en-Y loop of jejunum may be used primarily where there is substantial loss of duodenal wall or later where a chronic duodenal fistula develops.

circumstances, by a Roux-en-Y loop of jejunum sutured around the defect (Fig. 10–3). This latter maneuver is most often used in the treatment of chronic fistulas. (4) When none of these approaches is feasible, the injured duodenum may be repaired and protected by the performance of a controlled end-duodenostomy followed by antrectomy and gastroenterostomy (so-called "diverticulization of the duodenum") and the insertion of a T-tube in the common bile duct; all of these maneuvers are designed to divert or reduce the flow of bile, pancreatic juice, and chyme from the injured area (Fig. 10–4). (5) If the wound is massive and associated with widespread pancreatic and biliary duct injury, a pancreaticoduodenectomy may be unavoidable.

In all duodenal injuries, the area must be drained adequately and the gastrointestinal tract decompressed by a nasogastric tube or gastrostomy. A

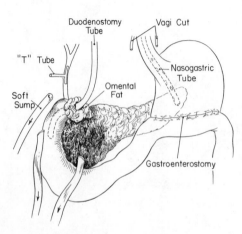

Duodenostomy
Tube

Vagi Cut

"T" Tube

Nasogastric
Tube

Soft
Sump

Omental
Fat

Gastroenterostomy

Figure 10–4. "Diverticulization" of the duodenum in selected severe duodeno-pancreatic injuries.

feeding jejunostomy (catheter or "needle") or the passage of a small polyethylene feeding tube that traverses the stomach into the efferent jejunal loop should be considered at the time of the initial operation if it is believed that the patient is likely to suffer prolonged nutritional depletion.

An intramural hematoma of the duodenum should be suspected in patients who develop high intestinal obstruction after an episode of blunt abdominal trauma. Roentgenograms with radiopaque material may demonstrate a "coiled spring" appearance of the second and third portions of the duodenum. Treatment consists of observation in the first place because most of these hematomas resolve spontaneously within about 10 to 14 days; when symptoms increase, incision of the seromuscular coat, evacuation of the hematoma, and, in a few selected cases, decompression by tube duodenostomy are performed.

SMALL INTESTINE

The small intestine is injured most frequently as a result of penetrating wounds of the abdomen. Surgical treatment involves closure of the holes or resection with anastomosis when the damage is extensive. In the case of all missile wounds, an even number of holes must be counted unless a tangential wound can be demonstrated. A perforation on the mesenteric border of the small intestine may be difficult to visualize. With small bowel injuries, copious peritoneal irrigation and the administration of antibiotics parenterally are adjunctive measures.

In blunt injuries as seen after kicks or seat belt trauma, clinical signs may develop subtly and slowly. Pain may be minimal for a few days, subphrenic gas may not be visible roentgenographically and ileus may only appear very slowly. These signs should be sought in patients who have been wearing seat belts.

LARGE INTESTINE

Wounds of the colon, although less common, are much more serious than wounds of the small intestine. Patients with blunt injuries may develop symptoms over as long as a week, reflecting the gradual ischemia of a colonic wall that leads to ultimate perforation. In suspected penetrating wounds, broad-spectrum systemic antibiotics are administered prophylactically and as soon as possible.

Few situations require as much surgical judgment and experience as do colonic wounds. The final decision in the operating room is influenced by the degree of shock, the number of associated injuries, the age of the patient, the type and extent of the colonic wound, and the degree of fecal spillage.

Simple lacerations and small wounds produced by low-viscosity missiles may frequently be treated by careful debridement and a meticulously performed inverting closure. When none or few of the deleterious factors just listed are present, major damage to the large intestine is best treated by one of the following methods, the choice of which will vary with the experience of the surgeon. (1) Exteriorization of the lesion. Exteriorization is reserved for wounds of the transverse and left colon in which primary repair or resection seems unwise. When the terminal colon is too short to be exteriorized on the abdominal wall following resection of the distal left colon, it may be closed and left in the peritoneal cavity (Hartmann's procedure). The proximal colon is then used as an end-colostomy. When a colostomy is made it should be brought out through a separate incision, never through the site of injury or operative incision. (2) Primary closure or anastomosis followed by the establishment of a proximal colostomy. (3) Primary closure of the colonic wound and exteriorization of the repair with a view to returning this to the abdomen in about seven days if the repair is intact and the patient relatively well. (4) Exteriorization of a defect in the right colon should be avoided; these wounds and extensive injuries of the cecum should be treated by right colectomy and primary ileotransverse colostomy. When there is extensive contamination, prolonged preoperative shock, associated severe retroperitoneal damage, or advanced age, a primary anastomosis should be avoided; resection with a temporary ileostomy and a distal mucous fistula of the transverse colon is far safer.

As in small bowel injuries, extensive irrigation of the peritoneal cavity with saline is indicated. Systemic antibiotics are essential and some surgeons favor peritoneal irrigation with antibiotics. (It should be kept in mind that certain aminoglycosides may cause respiratory difficulties.) In the contaminated abdomen, the surgeon should drain the areas of extensive retroperitoneal damage often seen with injuries to the colon. The skin and subcutaneous tissues are not closed primarily.

RECTUM

Rectal injuries may be deceptively small yet lethal. Blood on the examining glove and air in the pelvic roentgenogram are ominous signs. Wounds of the extraperitoneal rectum should be repaired if possible and a proximal diverting colostomy performed. The rectum is irrigated with saline to reduce its bacterial load. Drainage of the injured area by the presacral route is mandatory. This can be accomplished through an incision anterior to the tip of the coccyx through the fascia propria. In wounds of the anorectum, the sphincter muscles should be repaired and wide drainage established. Perineal injuries in which there is extensive

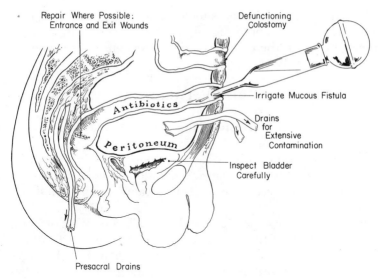

Figure 10-5. Important facets of surgical management in extraperitoneal injuries of the rectum.

crushing of the soft tissues may require a diverting colostomy even though the skin is intact (Fig. 10–5). The presence of associated genitourinary injury should be excluded.

ABDOMINAL INJURY IN PREGNANCY

Occasionally the pregnant woman suffers either blunt or penetrating abdominal injury and decisions have to be made regarding the optimal care of both mother and child. These decisions will depend in part on the stage of the pregnancy and the severity of the injury. In the last trimester of pregnancy, the uterus occupies most of the abdominal cavity and thus fetal injury in penetrating wounds is relatively common. The uterine wall is protective in a sense as evidenced by the fact that concomitant maternal visceral injuries are relatively uncommon. As a generalization, it may be stated that the mother almost always does well if treated vigorously along the usual resuscitative lines but about 50 percent of the infants die and an additional 10 percent sustain injury.

When the period of absence of fetal life is not known, intervention on behalf of the fetus may turn out to be worthwhile. However, the fetus that has not shown any detectable sign of life for more than 20 minutes will abort within a few days. This background has led to some controversy between those who advocate a nonsurgical approach to the injured mother unless her condition shows signs of clinical deterioration and others who think that a penetrating wound should be treated in the same manner as one approaches those in nonpregnant women. Clinical judgment is of vital importance here, but the present tendency remains toward intervention.

CLOSURE OF THE ABDOMEN

Before closure of the incision there should be careful inspection to make sure that no continuing hemorrhage is present. All foreign bodies, tissue fragments, and blood clots should be removed. The abdomen should be irrigated thoroughly with large quantities of saline or an antibiotic solution. In the latter case, care is taken to guard against ventilatory complications.

Laparotomy wounds are usually closed in layers. Wire or nonreactive synthetic sutures placed through all layers may be preferred, because these wounds have a high incidence of dehiscence. When there has been gross contamination, the subcutaneous tissues should be left open initially and closed later by secondary suture or they may be allowed to granulate. In cases of extensive loss of substance from the musculofascial structures of the abdominal wall as occurs with shotgun wounds, closure may be accomplished by mobilization or rotation of flaps of skin and subcutaneous tissue, leaving a potential hernia to be repaired at a later date. If there is appreciable tissue damage around the wounds of entrance and exit, these areas should be thoroughly debrided even though closure is made much more difficult. The penalty for conservatism may be delayed lethal sepsis. Tension must be avoided. When the defect is too large to be covered with autogenous tissue, a synthetic plastic mesh screen may be sewn to surrounding fascia or, when contamination is extensive, coverage with Owen's cloth or similar material and moist occluding dressings may be unavoidable. It is gratifying to see the exposed viscera gradually covered with granulation tissue when meticulous daily dressings are done and the stage developed for later coverage.

Any ileostomy or colostomy that is necessary should be established as far from the main wound as possible.

POSTOPERATIVE CARE

Detailed postoperative care is essential to the successful management of abdominal wounds. The temperature, pulse, respiration, and blood pressure should be checked at regular intervals.

Deep breathing exercises are encouraged to prevent atelectasis. Leg exercises are employed to prevent deep venous thrombosis. The patient is turned frequently from side to side to prevent pulmonary complications. As peristalsis returns, the nasogastric tube should be clamped periodically to determine when nasogastric suction can be discontinued safely. Antacids and perhaps cimetidine are given to produce a pH above 5 in septic and critically ill patients.

Usually, an appreciable loss of fluid occurs into the peritoneal cavity, and the lumen and wall of the bowel. This hidden sequestration of a large volume of fluid requires replacement. Adequate quantities of lactated Ringer's solution should be administered in addition to the other daily fluid requirements. Blood should be given when indicated.

An indwelling urethral catheter serves as an adjunct to accurate measurement of hourly urinary output and helps to provide a guide to the replacement of fluid. In most instances, parenteral antibiotic therapy is continued for up to five days after operation. A combination of antibiotics that is effective against aerobic and anaerobic organisms (such as cephalo-thin, gentamicin, and clindamycin, or selected newer cephalosporins) is widely used until the sensitivity reports from cultures taken at operation are available. Early ambulation is encouraged.

11

Early Management of the Patient with Genitourinary Injury

Early diagnosis is paramount in the patient with genitourinary injury, because a plan of management and successful outcome depends upon it.

DIAGNOSIS

ELEMENTS OF THE HISTORY THAT POINT TO GENITOURINARY INJURY

1. Blunt trauma to the abdomen, lower chest, flank, genitalia, or perineum associated with hematuria, diminished urine output, abdominal or flank mass, or swelling of the genitalia.
2. Penetrating wound of the abdomen, flank, genitalia, or pelvis. Twenty percent of these patients do not have gross hematuria.
3. Deceleration injury. A genitourinary injury should be suspected in any patient who has fallen from a height or who has been in a motor vehicle accident. These individuals are prone to arterial intimal tear and subsequent thrombosis, and, in childhood, avulsion of the ureter at the ureteropelvic junction.
4. Hematuria may be absent. Individuals who have hematuria after slight injury or minor trauma must be suspected of *pre-existing* genitourinary disease.

PHYSICAL FINDINGS THAT SUGGEST GENITOURINARY INJURY

1. Hematoma over fractured 10, 11, 12 ribs.
2. Discoloration, penetrating wound, or mass in the flank.
3. Lower abdominal mass or tenderness.
4. Genital swelling or discoloration.
5. Inability to void urine following trauma.
6. Blood at the urethral meatus.

ROENTGENOGRAPHIC STUDIES

The trauma workup is invaluable as a screening diagnostic procedure. It consists of an excretory urogram and cystogram done at the same sitting, thereby determining the integrity of both the upper and lower urinary tracts (Fig. 11–1). A scout film (KUB) of the abdomen is made. The cystogram is performed first by passing a soft retention catheter of appropriate size (18 F in adults, 12 F in children), and instilling by gravity through an Asepto syringe 250 cc of water-soluble contrast material. A film is taken and while it is being developed an intravenous pyelogram (IVP) is started by injecting the equivalent of 1 cc/lb of 30 percent organic iodine solution in 5 to 10 minutes. A drainage film is made after the static cystogram and then abdominal films are made at 5, 10, and 15 minutes. Delayed films are made as needed, especially if hydronephrosis is present or there is poor visualization of the kidneys.

Urethrography. When there is a history of straddle injury, pelvic girdle disruption, or direct blow to the perineum, urethrography is performed before attempted passage of a urethral catheter. Contrast

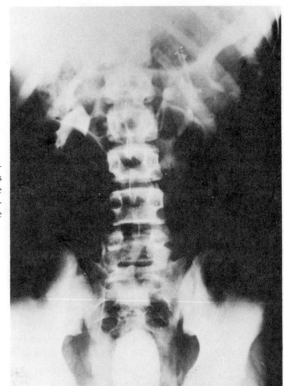

Figure 11–1. The trauma workup. Cystogram and intravenous pyelogram done at same time showing, in this case, an extraperitoneal rupture of the bladder.

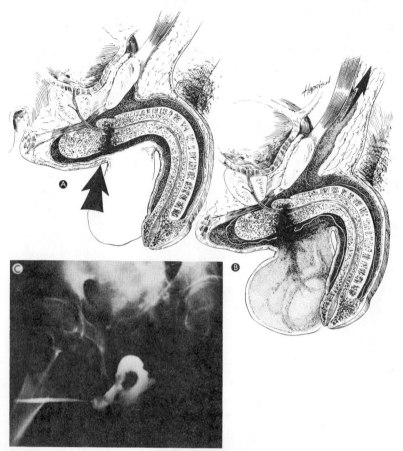

Figure 11–2. Rupture of the urethra inferior to urogenital diaphragm. *A,* confined to Buck's fascia; *B,* confined to Colles' fascia; *C,* roentgenographic appearance. (From Longmire WP: Advances in Surgery, Vol. 10. Year Book Medical Publishers, Inc., 1976.)

material suitable for intravenous use is employed. Injury to the urethra below the urogenital diaphragm must be suspected in patients who have blood at the urethral meatus (Fig. 11–2).

RENAL INJURIES

The kidneys generally tend to be mates in external and internal configuration. Differences in size, position, function, and integrity of the kidneys are sought roentgenographically. Relatively lucent areas in the parenchyma may indicate rupture of parenchyma. Extravasation of contrast material usually indicates adequate function and may delineate important damage to the renal pelvis, ureter, or bladder. Nonvisualization of the kidney by excretory urography is an urgent indication for angiography, because this finding is usually indicative of a major renal artery injury, and prompt surgical attention is necessary if this kidney is to be salvaged (Fig. 11–3). At the time of this writing, renal salvage rate of this injury is very low. Patients whose kidneys show lesser degrees of function may also be subjected to arteriography; these cases will require individual judgment.

When the decision for renal arteriography has been made, the transfemoral route is preferred. A flush aortogram, combined with a celiac artery injection, allows evaluation of possible splenic or hepatic injury as well.

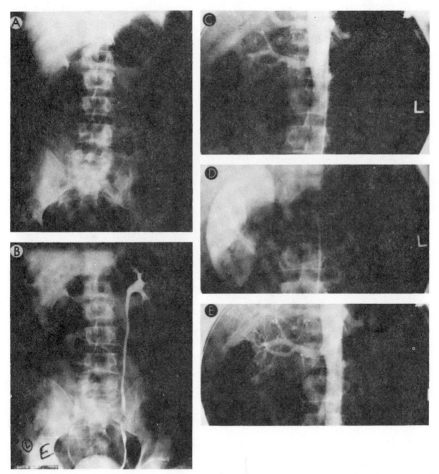

Figure 11–3. *A*, nonvisualizing kidney on the left by excretory urography. *B*, retrograde pyelogram showing normal collecting system; if there is no urine, this is indicative of a vessel injury. *C*, arteriography. *D*, nephrogram phase showing complete block of left renal artery. *E*, postoperative result showing some improvement of vascularization of left kidney. (From Longmire WP: Advances in Surgery, Vol. 10. Year Book Medical Publishers, Inc., 1976.)

Sonography and Computerized Tomography. Gray-scale ultrasonography may be of value in ascertaining the rupture or absence of a kidney or in demonstrating large extravasations of blood or urine. CT is valuable in evaluation of the blunt trauma patient. Its use in the patient with penetrating trauma will increase with shortening of exposure times and with increasing availability.

Retrograde Pyelography. Retrograde pyelography is seldom used in the evaluation of the acute injury, but if facilities for angiography are not available, diagnosis of the likelihood of a vascular lesion in a patient with a grossly abnormal IVP can be made by passing a catheter to the kidney and demonstrating a relatively normal pyelogram and lack of urine output from the affected kidney (Fig. 11–3*B*).

Radionuclide Studies in the Trauma Patient. Although selective angiography best defines the pattern of anatomical injury, renal isotope scanning plays an increasingly important role in the early diagnosis of renal injury in the trauma patient. Integrity of blood flow to the kidneys and extravasation of isotope-laden urine may be detected with minimal risk to the patient. In general, 10 microcuries of technetium 99 DTPA are injected intravenously. Renal presence, assessment of blood flow, and any major renal artery obstruction can be detected within 30 seconds. Although the

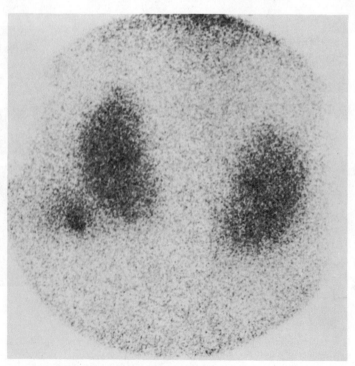

Figure 11–4. Radionuclide (99 technetium DTPA) scan showing bladder flow to both kidneys and extravasation of urine outside the right kidney.

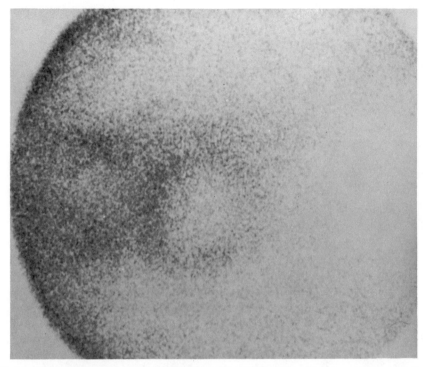

Figure 11–5. Radionuclide scan showing torsion of left testis with clear area representing diminished perfusion.

exact anatomical pattern cannot be defined, major areas of infarction or ischemia can be identified, as well as areas of urinary extravasation. Associated hepatosplenic injury can also be determined, and patients can be selected for angiography on the basis of this abnormal liver and spleen scan. Radionuclide scanning is of particular value in the differential diagnosis of testicular torsion (Figs. 11–4, 11–5).

URETERAL INJURIES

DIAGNOSIS

Isolated ureteral injuries are rare. One should, however, be suspicious of ureteral injury in patients with penetrating wounds of the urinary bladder or wounds near the common iliac artery bifurcation. Renal wounds also are commonly associated with lacerations of the collecting system. The trauma workup with the concomitant cystogram and IVP will usually disclose any extravasation. At exploration, indigo carmine, given intravenously, may show a discoloration of the tissues at the area of injury.

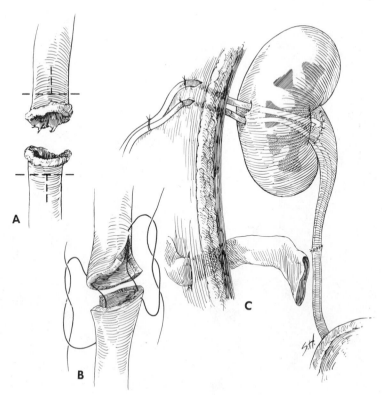

Figure 11–6. *A,* debridement of traumatized ends of severed ureter; *B,* spatulated re-anastomosis, interrupted suture technique; *C,* nephrostomy and stent. (From Urethral injuries due to external violence. J Trauma 17:616–620, 1977.)

TREATMENT

It is important to ascertain in gunshot wounds of the ureter whether the injury was due to a high-velocity or a low-velocity missile. Most civilian weapons, such as 38-caliber and 45-caliber guns, fire low-velocity missiles (less than 2200 ft/sec muzzle velocity). In patients injured by high-velocity missiles, careful debridement is necessary to obtain ureteral healing, because the blast effect and coagulation necrosis make the determination of viability by inspection alone difficult. One must debride back to the bleeding ureter before a spatulated re-anastomosis is done with interrupted 5–0 chromic gut sutures. I would recommend a second reinforcing adventitial-muscular layer of 5–0 silk sutures, placed so as to avoid contact of the suture with urine. A Penrose drain is placed near the anastomosis and a proximal nephrostomy and stent are used for upper and midureteral injuries (Fig. 11–6). Lower ureteral injuries below the pelvic brim are treated by ureteral reimplantation into the bladder, using a tunnel technique and a bladder flap if necessary. In distal and lower ureteral injuries, the stent may be passed up the ureter and brought out through the bladder with a suprapubic tube. Nephrostomy is not necessary in this circumstance.

BLADDER INJURIES

Bladder injuries are usually classified into extraperitoneal and intraperitoneal ruptures (Figs. 11–7, 11–8). Intraperitoneal ruptures usually occur when a patient with a full bladder sustains a violent external blow to the abdominal wall. This occurs in sudden deceleration injuries, such as falls and motor vehicle accidents. The fluid-filled container (bladder) transmits the sustained force equally in all directions and the bladder usually ruptures at its weakest point, the dome. The diagnosis is usually made by passing a small 18 F retention catheter and performing cystography and postevacuation films. One must be certain to instill at least 250 cc of contrast material into the bladder in order not to miss a rupture that has been sealed off following evacuation of the bladder contents into the peritoneal cavity. Loops of bowel outlined by the peritoneal contrast material are frequently seen (Fig. 11–8). The patient may complain of severe lower abdominal pain and may have signs of peritoneal irritation, such as rebound tenderness or lower abdominal muscular rigidity. An inability to void more than a few ccs of urine is seen on occasion.

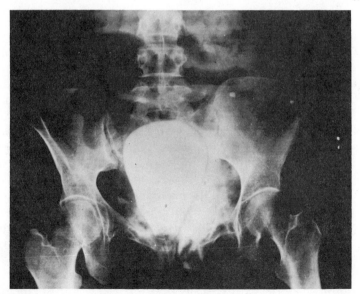

Figure 11–7. Extraperitoneal rupture of the bladder. Note that the bladder shadow is on the symphysis; note the teardrop configuration of bladder. Note also the flame-shaped extravasation of contrast material alongside the bladder.

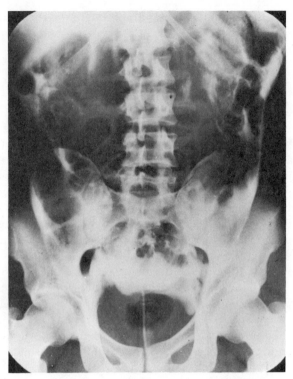

Figure 11–8. Intraperitoneal rupture of the bladder showing loops of bowel outlined by contrast material.

The inability to void, however, is particularly marked in rupture of the urethra whether superior or inferior to the urogenital diaphragm. The treatment of the bladder injury is closure of the rupture, cystostomy through an uninjured area of the bladder, and extraperitoneal drainage for seven to ten days until satisfactory voiding from below is demonstrated by cystography. The suprapubic tube and drain are then removed. Alternatively, if the bladder wound is not contaminated with foreign material, the surgeon may prefer to perform a layered closure of the bladder (three layers) with absorbable suture and to provide for drainage simply with an indwelling urethral catheter.

Extraperitoneal ruptures of the bladder occur often in association with pelvic fracture. Conversely, only about 5 percent of pelvic fractures result in extraperitoneal bladder rupture from a pelvic bone fragment. The patient often complains of severe lower abdominal pain and may have discoloration in the area of the pelvic fracture. The diagnosis is accomplished by cystography. A typical sunburst pattern and extravasation of the contrast material extravesically is seen (Fig. 11–7). Also, the bladder shadow on the cystogram is seen to descend to the level of the symphysis. This helps to differentiate extraperitoneal rupture of the bladder from rupture of the urethra superior to the urogenital diaphragm (Fig. 11–9). The patient with a ruptured urethra usually cannot void, unlike the patient with extraperitoneal rupture of the bladder.

INJURY TO THE URETHRA SUPERIOR TO THE UROGENITAL DIAPHRAGM

This is an injury that is associated with severe external violence. The patient usually complains of lower abdominal discomfort and severe pelvic pain if he is conscious, as there has often been a pelvic fracture associated with the lesion. In rectal examination of the male the prostate is difficult to palpate; this was originally described by Vermooten in 1938 as the "floating prostate." Urethrogram shows extravasation, and the trauma series will often reveal a bladder full of contrast material floating high in the pelvis (Fig. 11–9). The bladder silhouette is often two to three inches above the pubis. This varies greatly, depending on the magnitude of the injury, and helps differentiate this lesion from extraperitoneal rupture of the bladder. The patient is unable to void as a rule, or voids only a drop or two at most, if there is a large pelvic collection of urine. Immediate management consists of the placement of suprapubic cystostomy (Fig. 11–10). A few patients need intermediate treatment after a few days, but most such lesions are complete ruptures. The patients should have initial cystostomy

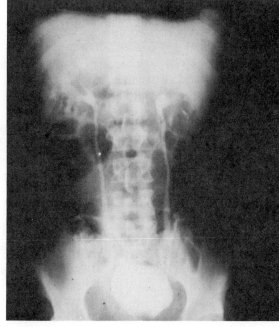

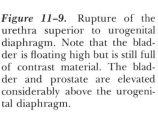

Figure 11–9. Rupture of the urethra superior to urogenital diaphragm. Note that the bladder is floating high but is still full of contrast material. The bladder and prostate are elevated considerably above the urogenital diaphragm.

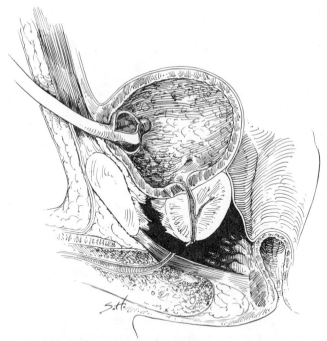

Figure 11–10. Proper placement of a cystostomy tube high in the bladder away from the trigone, creating an oblique tract through the abdominal wall.

and definitive reconstruction of the urethra after the prostate has descended to the urogenital diaphragm three to four months after the injury.

Considerable controversy has existed over the years regarding immediate reconstruction over interlocking sounds as opposed to cystostomy and delayed reconstruction. I definitely favor initial cystostomy the night of the injury and delayed reconstruction. Attempts to manipulate the urethra and restore continuity in the absence of expertise and in the absence of supporting blood bank facilities are fraught with danger. Complications that follow, such as impotence, incontinence, and urethral stricture, are minimized by initial cystostomy and delayed reconstruction. A few patients in whom bony fragments impede physically the descent of the prostate may require exploration and attempted restoration of continuity within a week of the injury, but this need not be done at the time of the injury when the patient's condition is unstable or critical. Initial cystostomy will suffice. Later reconstruction will be done by a transpubic or perineal route.

INJURY OF THE URETHRA INFERIOR TO THE UROGENITAL DIAPHRAGM

Rupture of the urethra inferior to the urogenital diaphragm usually results from straddle injury. Occasionally it may be from a blow or a kick to the perineum. There is usually a history of extreme pain on voiding or complete inability to void in those cases in which there is complete transection. At times there will be a drop of blood at the meatus secondary to spasm of the bulbocavernosus muscle at the time of injury. When there is a history of a straddle or similar injury, urethrography should be performed first. Immediate repair with an oblique spatulated interrupted suture anastomosis has been advocated by Zinman et al. Very satisfactory results can be obtained in these cases (Fig. 11–11). In other instances, when the lesion is seen to be minimal following urethrography, simple passage of

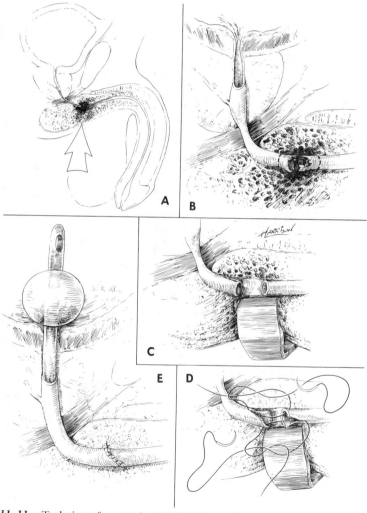

Figure 11–11. Technique for spatulated oblique immediate reanastomosis of the urethra in injuries below the urogenital diaphragm. *A*, rupture of urethra below urogenital diaphragm; *B*, debridement back to freshly bleeding tissue; *C*, spatulation to increase caliber of reanastomosis; *D*, dexon or chromic gut (4 zero) closure; *E*, stenting catheter through oblique anastomosis silastic catheter of appropriate size (18 F suggested). (From Harrison JH et al.: Campbell's Urology, 4th ed., W. B. Saunders, 1976.)

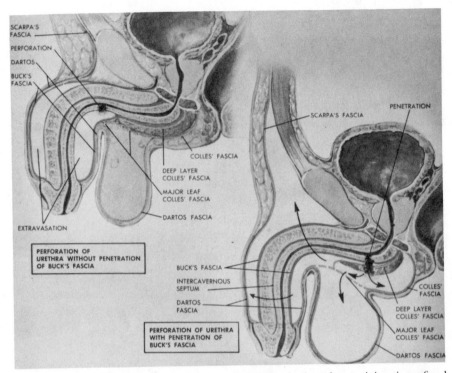

Figure 11–12. The extent of extravasation of bladder of urine when an injury is confined by Buck's fascia (*left*), and when the injury has ruptured through Buck's fascia and is confined by Colles' fascia (*right*). (From Netter FH: The CIBA Collection of Medical Illustrations, Vol. 2, Reproductive System. CIBA Pharmaceutical Co., 1970.)

a retention urethral catheter to the bladder will suffice. The catheter is usually left in for ten days and a voiding cystourethrogram performed at the time of its removal. If no extravasation results, the catheter is left out. If minimal extravasation is still present, the catheter is replaced for an additional four to five days and the procedure repeated. Rupture of the urethra inferior to the urogenital diaphragm results in a lesion confined either by Buck's fascia or Colles' fascia. If the lesion is confined by Buck's fascia, the distribution of extravasated blood or urine or both is essentially that of a sleeve of the penis (Fig. 11–12). If the lesion has ruptured through Buck's fascia and is confined by Colles' fascia, there may be a typical butterfly extravasation of urine seen in the scrotum and perineum, limited by the fusion of Colles' fascia with the inferior layer of the urogenital diaphragm, thus confining the extravasation to the anterior half of the perineum (Fig. 11–13). Occasionally in these patients extravasation of blood or urine may be limited in its spread into the thigh by the fusion of Scarpa's fascia with the fascia lata, but it will proceed in the abdominal wall superiorly to the axillae, where its spread is again limited by the fusion of Scarpa's fascia with the coracoclavicular fascia (Fig. 11–14). Immediate management has result-

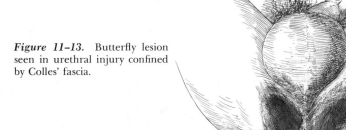

Figure 11–13. Butterfly lesion seen in urethral injury confined by Colles' fascia.

ed in fewer cases of the extensive dissection of blood and urine just described. Emergency surgical management consists of appropriate urinary diversion, usually by suprapubic cystostomy, but reconstruction is delayed in cases recognized after 48 hours. In cases recognized within 24 hours, the author prefers exposure of the injured urethra through the perineum and immediate reconstruction by elliptical anastomosis over an indwelling catheter, which is left in place seven to ten days as a stent as described above.

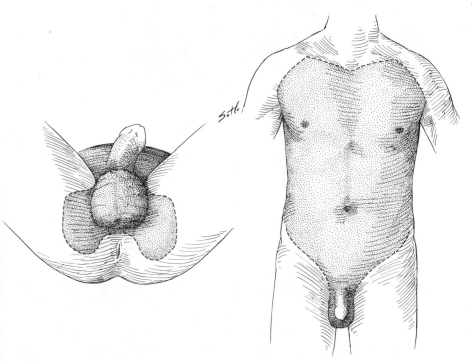

Figure 11–14. Attachments of Colles' and Scarpa's fascia that limit the extent of extravasation of the bladder and urine in a rupture of the urethra inferior to the urogenital diaphragm.

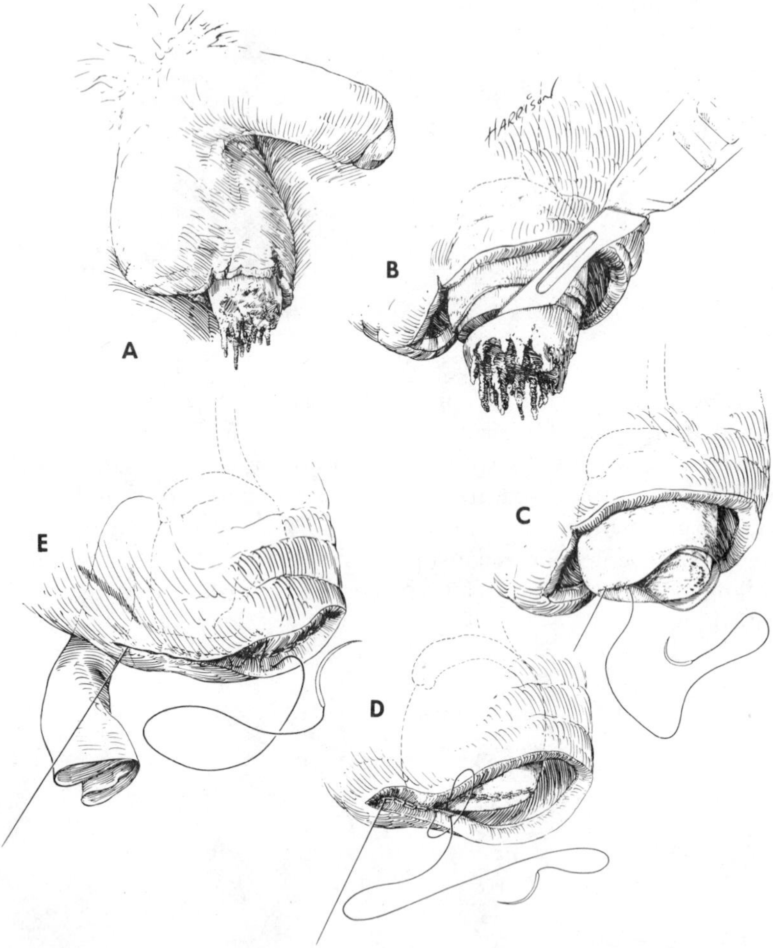

Figure 11–15. Debridement and tight closure of the tunica albuginea of the testis to preserve testis tubules. *A,* Contaminated testicular wound; *B,* Sharp debridement to healthy testis; *C,* Complete closure of tunica albuginea of testis; *D,* Drain in scrotum only; tunica albuginea of testis tightly closed.

INJURIES TO THE GENITALIA

Penetrating wounds should be explored. With injury to the testis, careful debridement of all necrotic and foreign material is necessary followed by thorough cleansing and closure of the tunica albuginea of the testis. A drain should not be placed inside the tunica albuginea of the testis, as subsequent sloughing and extravasation of the tubules will result (Fig. 11–15). Fractures or ruptures of the corpus cavernosum should be treated by debridement and closure with interrupted absorbable sutures, such as chromic gut. The use of nonabsorbable sutures may result in the formation of tender nodules beneath the penile skin that may be disturbing to the patient. Immediate repair is indicated to diminish further extravasation. Late cases, when the hematoma appears to be confined and no longer expanding, require surgical judgment. Many patients' injuries do not require exploration and closure; others require drainage of a pendulous hematoma and closure of the rupture of the corpus cavernosum.

Materials such as rings and tools, which have been used for masturbation and which remain on the penis because the patient is unable to remove them, are best removed under general anesthesia. If it is not possible to remove them by simple cleansing with soap and water with the patient anesthetized, metal-cutting tools (usually found within the engineering department of any major hospital) can be used. Psychiatric consultation is recommended but is frequently refused by the patient.

MANAGEMENT OF THE SEXUALLY ASSAULTED PATIENT (MALE)

The patient alleging sexual assault presents a medicolegal challenge that demands astute examination and treatment with special emphasis on proper collection of evidence. (See the form on pp. 180–181.)

INSTRUCTIONS

1. Moisten a cotton gauze pad with a portion of the sterile saline in a culture tube labeled "acid phosphatase." Wipe the perianal area and place the gauze pad in the envelope provided.

2. Carefully insert a cotton swab into the anal canal without touching the perianal area. Prepare two slides with the anal swab and spray immediately with fixative. Allow to dry about two to three minutes and place the slides in a slide tray (for spermatozoa search).

3. Place this same swab in a culture tube containing normal saline (for acid phosphatase).

4. Obtain a blood sample from the patient (for comparison with semen type and for VDRL).

5. Oral-genital: In these cases, carefully swab the mouth of the patient, especially the gums and pharynx, with a cotton swab and smear on a microscope slide. Spray with fixative.

6. Place this same swab in a separate culture tube containing normal saline (for acid phosphatase).

7. Label all containers, especially when additional samples such as fingernail scrapings are obtained. Labels should have patient's name, age, race, sex, hospital identification number, date and time of collection, collector's name, anatomical source of specimen.

8. Place all specimens in locked drop box marked for pickup by a criminal investigation laboratory.

9. Rape is *not* a diagnosis; it is a matter of jurisprudence. If the word "rape" is recorded, use the preface "alleged" or "suspected."

AUTHORIZATION BY PATIENT FOR EXAMINATION, COLLECTION OF EVIDENCE AND RELEASE OF INFORMATION

I hereby authorize __(hospital)__ to collect specimens including blood, urine, tissue, and clothing as needed. I understand that copies of all medical reports will be supplied to the police agency and the Office of the District Attorney. I authorize the police agency to obtain photographs for documentation of injuries.

Witness: _____ Patient: _____

Date: _____ Address: _____

Parent/Guardian: _____

Address: _____

(Above information is to be obtained by admitting nurse)

Brief Description of Assault:

Date: Time:

Form for authorization by patient for examination, collection of evidence and release of information, whether male or female.

MANAGEMENT OF THE SEXUALLY ASSAULTED PATIENT (FEMALE)

The patient alleging sexual assault presents a medicolegal challenge that demands astute examination and treatment with special emphasis on proper collection of evidence. (See the form on pp. 180–181.)

INSTRUCTIONS

1. Immediately inform the appropriate law enforcement agency if a representative is not in attendance.
2. Triage the alleged victim ahead of nonemergency patients.
3. Obtain written and witnessed consent for:
   a. Examination

    b. Collection of specimens and release of information to authorities

    c. Photographs (be sure to check with police to see if they wish to make official photographs)

4. A female nurse should be present during history taking, examination, and treatment. A female chaperone, counselor, etc., can be present for emotional support.

5. Record:

    a. Date and time of alleged assault

    b. Date and time of examination

    c. Name of policeman, badge number, name of chaperone

6. Collect evidence. All labels should have patient's name, age, race, sex, hospital identification number, date and time of collection, collector's name, anatomical source of specimen.

    a. Obtain and label two tubes of clotted blood (one for VDRL, one to hold for forensic pathology laboratory).

    b. Scrape and trim fingernails into envelope and label it.

    c. Comb and collect free pubic hair into envelope and label it.

    d. Cut off a few pubic hairs into envelope and label it.

    e. Collect any loose hair or dried blood and label it.

    f. Examine a saline wet mount of vaginal contents and cervical mucus for sperm. Present? Motile?

    g. Prepare four dry slides of vaginal contents and place in ether-alcohol fixative. If the vagina is dry, wash with 3.0 cc of normal saline and prepare slides from the washing.

    h. Collect vaginal aspirate or washings into test tube (for acid phosphatase determination).

    i. Do cervical culture for *N. gonorrhoeae.*

    j. Place cotton swab wet with vaginal secretions into dry test tube (for semen typing).

    k. If indicated:

        1. Urine for Pregnosticon

        2. Wet prep, dry preps, culture from mouth or rectum

        3. Urine for urinalysis if bladder trauma is suspected.

        4. X-ray (if fracture, dislocation, etc., are suspected)

        5. Photographs

7. Rape is *not* a diagnosis; it is a matter of jurisprudence. If the word "rape" is recorded, use the preface "alleged" or "suspected."

8. Three elements define rape:

    a. Carnal knowledge — slightest penile penetration of the labia minora (Hymenal penetration or ejaculation are not requirements.) Oral or anal intercourse without consent is also considered rape.

   b. Force — strength, threat, coercion

   c. Commission without consent — a woman with mental deficiency or a woman under the influence of drugs or alcohol may be incapable of giving consent.

9. Each state designates a minimal age at which a woman may consent to coitus. Statutory rape is sexual contact with a woman before the age of consent.

10. Sodomy is a common law crime encompassing many so-called "unnatural" sexual acts. Sexual molestation is often used to designate forced sexual acts other than coitus.

SUBJECTIVE

During the investigation, previously "insignificant" data may acquire importance. Documentation of the following facts, affirmative or negative, is recommended at the initial examination.

1. Patient's complaint — direct quote
2. Age
3. Gravidity, parity, date of termination of last pregnancy
4. Age of onset of menses (menarche)
5. Date of last menses
6. Last menses normal? If not, describe
7. Symptoms of pregnancy? If yes, describe
8. Most recent coitus prior to alleged assault: (date, time, whether a condom was used)
9. Current method of contraception, if any
10. Does patient state she is (was) virgin prior to alleged assault?
11. Vaginal tampons used? Age begun?
12. Douching practiced? Most recent?
13. During alleged assault:
   a. Did penis penetrate vulva?
   b. Did assailant experience orgasm?
   c. Did assailant wear condom?

14. Since alleged assault has patient:
   a. Douched?
   b. Bathed or showered?
   c. Defecated?
   d. Urinated?

15. Has patient knowledge of:
   a. Any present illness?
   b. Any drug allergy or other allergy? Describe
   c. Any medication being taken continually?

16. Has patient had a venereal disease past or present? Describe therapy

17. History of emotional illness? Describe

18. Previous vaginal surgical procedures? Describe

19. In 24 hours before alleged assault, did patient use alcohol or illegal drugs? Describe date, time, amount. If patient is a known habitual abuser, record frequency of use, duration of use, and usual amount of intake.

OBJECTIVE

Physical examination should include these recorded observations:

1. General appearance
2. Emotional status
3. Apparent influence of alcohol or drugs
4. Clothing (stain, tears, missing buttons, dirt, gravel, grass, leaves, etc.)
5. Body surface (bruises, scratches, lacerations, rope imprint, teeth imprints, pressure imprint, point tenderness)
6. Mouth (bruises, bites, lacerations)
7. Fingernails (length, broken, material beneath nails)
8. Pubic hair (matted, foreign hair)
9. Vulvar (bruise, laceration, hematoma, tender)
10. Speculum examination and bimanual examination. *Do not use lubricant.* Describe vaginal mucosa and vaginal secretions. Examine and describe cervix, uterus, adnexa, and rectovaginal region and any evidence of trauma or other abnormalities. Pediatric patients may require general anesthesia.

TREATMENT

1. Serious hemorrhage necessitates control and resuscitation with replacement of any deficit of fluid or blood volume. An experienced gynecological surgeon should be summoned if extensive laceration is suspected.

2. If skin is broken, ensure tetanus immunization and provide prophylaxis in accord with immunization status (see Chapter 5).

3. The symptoms associated with most minor trauma are relieved by cold compresses, elevation of hips, and mild analgesia.

4. Postcoital prevention of pregnancy should be attempted in unprotected victims in the ovulatory stage of the menstrual cycle. Immediately begin diethylstilbestrol, 25 mg orally b.i.d. and continue for 5 days. An antiemetic of choice is of benefit prophylactically. 1.5 mg Estinyl t.i.d. for 5

(Text continued on page 182)

Medicolegal Information to Obtain

 Police Case No.:

 Police Jurisdiction:

 Police Officer with Patient:

 Badge No. of Police Officer:

 Patient's Name:

 Emergency Case No.:

 Admitted to Hospital/Emergency Department (date):

                (time):

Examination

 Name of Patient: Age:

 BP: Pulse: T°: Wt.: Ht.:

Demeanor or emotional status of patient:

Describe any clothing stains or foreign matter:

Body bruises: (Yes)   (No)

Scratches/lacerations: (Yes)   (No)

 Describe:

Mouth:

Genital area:

Anal examination:

During alleged assault:

 Did penis penetrate rectum?

 Assailant have orgasm?

 Assailant wear condom?

Since alleged assault, has patient:

180

Showered or bathed?

Urinated?

Defecated?

Is patient taking any medication?

Any pre-existing illness or drug allergy?

Physician's Signature:

Evidence Collection

Name of Patient:

Blood specimens obtained: (Yes)   (No)

    Forensic pathology laboratory

    Serology

Rectal swabs obtained: (Yes)   (No)

Oral swabs obtained: (Yes)   (No)

Items of clothing taken: (Yes)   (No)

    Describe:

X-rays taken: (Yes)   (No)

    Describe:

Physician's impression:

Recommendations:

I hereby certify that this is a true and correct copy of the official examination of this patient.

Physician's Signature:

Date:

Time:

An example of a useful form in cases of alleged rape.

days is effective with few side effects. (Estinyl is available in the form of a 0.5 mg tablet.)

    5. Prevention of venereal disease (Applicable to males, also.)

        a. If patient is *not* allergic to penicillin: Adult — 1 gm of Benemid orally followed in 30 minutes by 4.8 million units of procaine penicillin intramuscularly. Observe patient additional 30 minutes for possible hypersensitivity reaction.

        b. If patient is allergic to penicillin: Adult — Erythromycin or tetracycline 500 mg orally q.i.d. for 15 days.

6. Any emotional disturbance sufficient to require consideration of sedative medication warrants the offer of psychiatric help at time of initial examination.

FOLLOW-UP PROGRAM

Strong recommendation must be given for psychological counseling. Follow-up must also be given for possible pregnancy and venereal disease. Counseling is especially important for rape victims who are children. In some areas hospitals are responsible for reporting all types of child abuse, including sexual abuse, to child protective agencies.

Chapter

12

Head

An injury to the head may involve either the scalp, skull, or brain alone. Injuries in which the brain is involved are an immense problem. Severe head trauma ranks behind only heart disease, neoplasm, and stroke as the leading cause of death. Seventy percent of individuals with injuries as a result of vehicular accidents will have a head injury alone or as a part of multiple trauma. It is evident from the figures indicating the magnitude of the problem that the initial care of the patient with a head injury often is not the responsibility of a person specifically trained in the management of neurosurgical problems. The fact that the functional outcome after a severe head injury is strongly influenced by the quality of care initially received emphasizes that the individuals who are likely to be entrusted with the care of such patients should be aware of proper techniques.

PRIMARY CONSIDERATIONS

RESPIRATORY EXCHANGE AND SHOCK

Hypoxia from respiratory obstruction or ischemia from a decrease in cerebral perfusion pressure due to peripheral vascular collapse can increase neuronal damage and can aggravate the brain's reaction to a primary injury. Although respiratory difficulty and systemic hypotension can occur terminally in the patient with a severe head injury, it is hazardous to attribute these to the effects of a head injury at the outset. The upper airway should be cleared of blood and mucus. If no other injuries are suspected, the unconscious patient may be transported in the semiprone position so that secretions tend to flow from the mouth and the tongue falls forward rather than back, where it could obstruct the posterior oropharynx. If other injuries are likely to be present, the patient is best transported supine on a backboard with the neck supported and an adequate airway in place. In both instances, 100 percent oxygen should be administered en route to the hospital. When the patient arrives at the hospital, if signs of airway obstruction persist or if arterial blood gases are abnormal, immediate endotracheal intubation should be performed, and mechanical ventilation utilized if required.

As a rule, head injuries do not result in hypotension. The exceptions are: (1) terminally in the patient with irreversible increased intracranial pressure, (2) in the infant or child with a large scalp laceration, (3) in the infant with a large subdural hematoma, (4) in the patient who is deeply intoxicated, and (5) in the patient with a spinal cord injury in whom hypotension is likely to be accompanied by bradycardia. When these exceptions are not present, shock should be the signal for an immediate search for concomitant thoracic or intra-abdominal injuries or fractures of long bones.

Blood pressure, pulse, and respirations should be recorded immediately and frequently. Any change in the vital signs may indicate a rise in intracranial pressure; the cause for this should be sought promptly. A rapid rise in intracranial pressure is likely to result in an elevation of the blood pressure with a slowing of the pulse and of the respiratory rate, the classic triad of intracranial hypertension. If a further elevation in intracranial pressure occurs with additional compression of the cerebral circulation, decompensation will take place. This deterioration will be reflected by a fall in the blood pressure accompanied by a rapid pulse and respiratory rate. If events have progressed to this point, the patient's death will ensue shortly.

ASSESSMENT OF NEUROLOGICAL STATUS

Once it has been determined that there is no respiratory or cardiovascular embarrassment, a neurological evaluation should be carried out. The most common neurological deficit that occurs with a head injury is an altered state of consciousness. An accurate assessment of the state of consciousness and a comparison of the initial examination with subsequent examinations are the most reliable means for evaluating the progress of the patient with a head injury.

The state of consciousness is evaluated by utilizing the response of the patient to various stimuli. If the stimulus and the response are meticulously recorded, the evaluation can be repeated and compared later by the same examiner or others. The most commonly used stimuli are vocal and noxious. The response to each provides a reliable and reproducible estimate of the level of consciousness and how it may be changing. The level of consciousness is obviously higher initially in the patient who follows commands but who later responds only to a painful stimulus with nonpurposeful movements. The rapidity with which this change has occurred also indicates how quickly definitive treatment must be started.

In assessing the level of consciousness, the use of terms such as comatose, semicomatose, and stuporous is imprecise. To be more objective, the use of the Glasgow Coma Scale, a tool originally designed to compare various forms of treatment, has been helpful. This scale requires only a recording of the best possible responses to vocal or noxious stimuli as characterized by eye opening, verbalization, and motor activity (Fig. 12–1). As an example, the patient in coma, according to this scale, does not open his eyes spontaneously to sound or to pain, does not give any comprehensible verbal response when asked simple questions, and does not obey the command to grasp a hand.

Following an assessment of the level of consciousness, any sign of focal central nervous system damage should be sought. The response of the pupils to light is especially important, because an abnormality may signal a dangerous shift in the brain. A dilated pupil on one side that is poorly responsive to light generally indicates compression of the oculomotor nerve by the medial portion of the ipsilateral temporal lobe, which is being displaced over the edge of the tentorium by an expanding intracranial mass. Tentorial herniation of the temporal lobe may also result in a hemiparesis on the opposite side caused by compression of the corticopyramidal tract within the brain stem. Infrequently, an ipsilateral hemiplegia may occur with compression of the contralateral cerebral peduncle against the tentorial edge.

The position of the eyes should be observed. Any abnormalities such as a forced gaze or disconjugate movements should be noted. The integrity of the brain stem should be evaluated in the patient who is in coma. Closure of the eyelids when the corneas are touched with a wisp of cotton indicates an intact corneal reflex. Conjugate deviation of eyes in a direction opposite to that in which the head is being sharply rotated indicates the presence of the oculocephalic reflex (doll's eye movement). The latter test should not

Eye opening	Spontaneous	4
	To speech	3
	To pain	2
	None	1
Verbal response	Oriented	5
	Confused conversation	4
	Inappropriate words	3
	Incomprehensible sounds	2
	None	1
Best motor response	Obeys commands	6
	Localizes pain	5
	Flexion withdrawal	4
	Flexion abnormal	3
	Extends	2
	None	1
Score or responsiveness sum	3–15	

Figure 12–1. Glasgow Coma or Responsiveness Scale.

be performed before cervical spine x-rays have demonstrated the absence of an accompanying spinal fracture.

An attempt to examine the optic fundi should be made. This should not be pursued, however, to the point of using mydriatic drugs that affect the more important pupillary response. Even though the intracranial pressure may be elevated, insufficient time will have elapsed for papilledema to develop in most cases.

Muscular tone and strength in the extremities should be evaluated. Reflexes should be compared bilaterally and plantar responses tested. The sensory examination may be of little value, but in the patient who is moving spontaneously, the absence of a response to pinprick may indicate an accompanying spinal cord injury.

The head should be inspected for evidence of a compound fracture or a depressed fracture. A basal skull fracture may be presumed when nonclotting blood is found in nares or in the external auditory canals, indicating rhinorrhea or otorrhea, or when mastoid or upper eyelid ecchymosis develops.

Many hospitals that treat large numbers of patients with head injuries employ a flow sheet for each patient. Especially in the unconscious patient, a graphic record of parameters, such as vital signs, Glasgow Coma Scale score, and brain stem reflexes, and of drugs and fluids and their amounts will enable a change in the patient's neurological status to be more readily appreciated. When a flow sheet is not available it remains important to record as carefully as events permit the results of frequent neurological examinations.

Not all patients with head injuries need to be admitted to the hospital for observation. If the patient is able to recall the events immediately preceding and following the injury, if the level of consciousness and the neurological evaluation are normal, and if the patient is accompanied by a responsible adult, he may be discharged. Before the patient leaves, the person accompanying the patient should be informed in writing of warning symptoms that suggest an impending complication of the head injury. These include:

1. Unusual behavior, sleepiness, stupor, difficulty in arousing the patient after sleep.
2. Walking off balance or constant falling to one side or the other. Paralysis of an arm or leg.
3. Unusual movements of the eyes.
4. Vomiting with or without nausea.
5. Severe headache, not relieved by aspirin.
6. Fevers, shaking chills.
7. Bleeding from nose or ears.

If any of these symptoms are noted, the responsible individual should be instructed to call the patient's family physician or bring the patient back to the emergency department immediately.

MANAGEMENT OF INITIAL TREATMENT AFTER AIRWAY AND SHOCK

1. Protect wounds with generous sterile dressings.
2. Do not manipulate or disturb foreign bodies.
3. Apply adequate compression with gauze or elastic bandage.
4. Patients with multiple injuries and cranial trauma should not be rushed to the x-ray department. If a depressed fracture or a penetrating wound is suspected, x-rays should be obtained in the emergency department before the wound is closed. Careful observation of vital signs and level of consciousness is more important in the seriously ill patient than an exact roentgenographic diagnosis.
5. Consider the possibility of cervical spine injury.

SIMPLE WOUNDS

In general, the management of simple wounds involving only the tissue of the scalp consists of (1) protecting the patient from further soft tissue injury, hemorrhage, and infection; (2) establishing an accurate diagnosis; (3) performing thorough cleansing and debridement; and (4) making a snug closure.

Control of Bleeding. After the scalp area has been shaved, cleansed, and surgically prepared and draped, the wound may be examined with a sterile gloved finger. Bleeding from the margin is controlled by grasping the galea with hemostats and reflecting it over the scalp, or by compressing the scalp against the intact skull with the fingertips. Self-retaining retractors, spread taut, also reduce scalp bleeding and aid in inspection and debridement. Attempting to clamp and ligate individual scalp bleeders as may be done elsewhere will result in undue blood loss because of the vascularity of the scalp.

CLOSURE OF SCALP LACERATIONS

For closure of lacerations in the emergency department or operating room, the essentials are adequate lighting and instruments, local anesthesia (1 percent procaine or Xylocaine) and, frequently, an assistant to help control bleeding. All open fractures require the facilities and assistance available in a major operating room, for it may be necessary to remove debris or bone and to control hemorrhage from the dura mater and brain.

1. Be sure the patient's general condition warrants closure of the wound.
2. Shave scalp widely around the wound.

3. Cleanse the skin around the wound with soap and water, and irrigate the wound with sterile salt solution.

4. Infiltrate the margins of the skin around the wound with 1 percent procaine or Xylocaine.

5. Debride obviously devitalized tissue at the margins of the laceration.

6. Gently explore the exposed surface of the skull for fractures with a gloved finger or hemostat.

7. Close small wounds snugly with one layer of interrupted sutures. When the galea is lacerated (the wound will gape), it should be closed first with interrupted sutures. The scalp laceration can then be closed with through-and-through sutures 1 centimeter apart. These are tied tightly, which usually controls bleeding.

8. Tetanus prophylaxis is indicated.

9. Antibiotic therapy in the emergency department is indicated for all open fractures, fractures involving the paranasal sinuses, and cerebrospinal fluid leaks.

CONVULSIONS

Convulsions following head injury may be associated with intracranial hemorrhage, cortical contusions, and anoxia. Focal Jacksonian seizures and generalized seizures require special studies to prove or disprove the presence of an expanding lesion or mass lesion. The convulsing patient is subjected to systemic hypoxia because secretions collect in the respiratory tree as the result of an impaired cough reflex and because the spasmodic contractions interfere with respiration. Moreover, at such times the brain requires larger amounts of oxygen than during normal activity.

Prophylactic anticonvulsants should be administered initially to all patients who have experienced severe head trauma. Phenytoin (Dilantin), 200 mg twice daily, or phenobarbital, 30 to 45 mg three to four times daily, or both, may be given. Rapidly repeated seizures may be brought under control with phenytoin (Dilantin) given intravenously in doses of 250 mg every 30 minutes until 2½ times the daily maintenance dose (1000 mg) is reached, with the full dose not to be given in less than 90 minutes. The injection should be at the rate of 50 mg/minute while vital signs are monitored. Dilantin should not be given by the intramuscular route or through a central venous catheter. If seizures continue, sodium amobarbital (Amytal) may be used in conjunction with Dilantin or started before the full dose of Dilantin has been given. A 10 percent aqueous solution is injected at the rate of 1 ml/minute until the seizures stop or until 500 mg have been given. This can be repeated in 30 minutes if the dosage of the first 500 mg fails.

RESTLESSNESS AND PAIN

Restlessness or thrashing about in bed is a fairly common symptom of brain injury and cerebral hypoxia. Its development in a previously quiet patient may be the first indication of increasing intracranial pressure and should not be confused with an improvement in the level of consciousness. Restlessness can often be controlled by correction of the cause. Cerebral anoxia is a frequent cause, and primary attention should be given to this. On the other hand, a distended urinary bladder or painful bandages or casts may induce restlessness. A considerate nurse can often eliminate the necessity of mechanical restraints. A chest restraint, permitting free movement of the arms and legs, will usually prevent the restless patient from falling out of bed. Encasing the hands in padded dressings will protect catheters and dressings and encourage rest.

Headache is rarely complained of early after a head injury. When severe and accompanied by agitation, headache may be a sign of an epidural hematoma that has stripped the dura mater from the inner table of the skull.

Pain from associated injuries can usually be controlled with aspirin 600 mg or codeine 15 or 30 mg. More potent narcotic analgesics are likely to depress the level of consciousness and therefore should not be used.

HYPERTHERMIA AND HYPOTHERMIA

Temperature regulation may be deficient with head trauma. Most commonly the deficiency is related to the loss of superficial vasodilation and sweating resulting in hyperthermia. This increases the metabolic demands of a brain that already may be suffering from an inadequate flow of blood. If the temperature of the body is lowered to normal or subnormal levels, the needs of the brain can be met even if the cerebral circulation is reduced by the injury. Should the rectal temperature be elevated above 101° F, aspirin suppositories may be used. For temperature above 103° F, major portions of the body may be exposed, tepid water sponging carried out, and the cooling blanket used to control the fever.

FLUID BALANCE

Nervous system tissue, like other tissue, responds to injury by swelling. Since the brain is encased within the skull and dura, swelling causes an elevation in intracranial pressure that may increase to the point at which it equals the systemic arterial pressure. At that point, circulation through the brain ceases, and tissue death ensues. Swelling to this degree is not inevitable in all head injuries. Protective measures, nonetheless, should be taken in all patients to limit its occurrence and thereby lessen morbidity. Since swelling is gradual, starting a few hours after injury and reaching a maximum in 36 to 48 hours, these measures can have considerable value.

Fluid intake should be limited to replacing insensible water loss and urinary output. This usually requires between 1800 to 2000 ml/24 hrs of which at least 150 mEq of sodium chloride should be included. For intravenous administration the isotonic solution that has the least effect on intracranial pressure is 2½ percent glucose in ½ normal saline. Normal electrolyte concentrations and osmolality must be maintained. In order to prevent dehydration, the fluid volume should be increased if the serum sodium or osmolality increase above the normal range. Further, a urine output that falls below 500 ml/24 hrs or a blood urea nitrogen level that rises above 30 mg percent are indications that more fluid is required.

STEROIDS AND DIURETICS

Adrenal corticosteroids currently are widely used in patients with head injuries. Their effectiveness may be related to stabilization of the blood-brain barrier, thereby reducing cerebral edema. Dexamethasone (Deca-dron), or the equivalent of methylprednisolone sodium succinate (Solu-Medrol), can be started in the emergency department with a minimum loading dose of 10 mg given intravenously, followed thereafter by 4 mg every 6 hours for 36 to 72 hours. The steroid may then be tapered as the patient's condition warrants. In conjunction with the steroid, antacids should be administered. If a history of peptic ulcer disease or tuberculosis is obtained, the steroid should be discontinued. It need not be tapered under these circumstances.

Hyperosmolar diuretics, with mannitol being the first choice, increase serum osmolality by containing molecules that do not readily cross the blood-brain barrier, thereby creating a gradient along which water moves from the brain to the blood. The administration of 500 ml of 20 percent mannitol over 15 minutes will produce a rapid decrease in intracranial pressure. It is particularly effective when a mass lesion threatening tentorial herniation is present and additional time is required to remove the lesion. When mannitol is used on a more long-term basis, the degree and duration of response can be variable and serious electrolyte disturbances and dangerous increases in serum osmolality can result. It is appropriate that the use of mannitol under these circumstances be restricted to head injury centers that have equipment and trained personnel for monitoring intracranial pressure. Because of the brisk diuresis produced by mannitol, a urinary catheter is essential.

MONITORING OF INTRACRANIAL PRESSURE

Establishing that further neurological deterioration has occurred in the patient who is unconscious with brain stem reflexes but responding to painful stimuli with only reflex movements is difficult. Often such patients will have an elevated intracranial pressure caused by cerebral swelling. In an effort to avoid the deleterious effects of further increases in the intracranial pressure in such situations, in many neurological centers the intracranial pressure is monitored. This is most commonly done by means of an intraventricular catheter connected to an extracranial pressure transducer and polygraph. Before the procedure is undertaken, the absence of a localized mass lesion must be demonstrated. This is most expeditiously done with a CT scan. The procedure is not without risk. The introduction of the catheter may produce an intracerebral hemorrhage, and the presence of a foreign body in the ventricle may result in an infection. Furthermore, a specialized knowledge is required to interpret the variations that may occur in the waveforms of the intracranial pressure. For these reasons the monitoring of intracranial pressure should be done only by a neurosurgeon.

SPECIAL STUDIES

ROENTGENOGRAMS

Skull x-rays can be helpful. They should be obtained *after* the patient's general condition has been stabilized. If the midline pineal gland is calcified, a shift on the anteroposterior view signifies a mass lesion. A fracture crossing a vascular groove, such as that for the middle meningeal artery, will indicate a potential source for an epidural hematoma. A single linear fracture depression usually does not exceed 1 to 3 mm and requires no surgical intervention. Closed comminuted fractures with fragments of bone depressed more than 3 mm should be elevated so as to lessen the likelihood of epilepsy developing. Most depressed fractures of the skull are associated with open wounds. Fractures of the base of the skull are the most common type of skull fracture but are the most difficult to visualize on plain x-rays. Their presence, however, can be presumed when other signs are detected. Air within the skull, indicating a tear in the coverings of the brain, and the presence of a foreign body such as a missile fragment may be demonstrated by plain skull x-rays.

COMPUTERIZED AXIAL TOMOGRAPHY (CT)

The CT scanner has altered the evaluation of the patient with an acute head injury because it can demonstrate the size and location of recent intracranial hemorrhage. Localized cerebral swelling will produce a shift in the ventricles, and generalized swelling is likely to reduce the size of the ventricles. While no diagnostic procedure should displace clinical observation, information acquired noninvasively may provide a rapid determination of the need for surgical intervention.

CEREBRAL ARTERIOGRAPHY

If a CT scanner is not available, cerebral arteriography is indicated to exclude an expanding intracranial lesion only when the patient's condition precludes serial clinical evaluation or when a course of progressive neurological deficit has been established. Arteriography should be undertaken only by trained individuals.

LUMBAR PUNCTURE

This test is contraindicated in obvious head injuries, especially in the acute state. The removal of cerebrospinal fluid at the time of the test and its continued drainage through the dural fistula into the extradural space at the site of puncture may alter cerebrospinal fluid dynamics and may thereby promote dangerous brain shifts. This risk outweighs the potential benefit of any information that may be gained.

DEFINITIVE TREATMENT

Before any medical or surgical therapy is undertaken that may potentially further complicate the patient's neurological status, it is imperative that a neurosurgeon be contacted at least for discussion. Only under the most dire of circumstances should operative intervention be undertaken — except, of course, by a neurosurgeon.

ANESTHESIA AND HEAD INJURIES

Indications for anesthesia are the same, whether the lesion is open or closed. Local anesthesia is preferable except in the restless patient. Volatile anesthetics such as halothane should not be used because of their cerebral vasodilating effect, which will increase the cerebral blood volume, and in the patient with a mass lesion may result in a dangerous elevation of the intracranial pressure. Various combinations of nitrous oxide, barbiturates, narcotics, and tranquilizers are preferable because of their minimal effect on intracranial pressure.

OPEN FRACTURES OF THE SKULL

In the operating room and after cleansing and draping of the scalp, the following procedures should be carried out in addition to the therapy outlined for simple lacerations:

1. Remove foreign bodies (distant metallic foreign bodies are occasionally not removed).
2. Remove all macerated brain tissue with a suction tip.
3. Elevate depressed fragments of the cranium.
4. Remove loose fragments of bone.
5. Make hemostasis complete to prevent hematoma formation.
6. Close the wound in layers. It is especially important to close the dura mater.
7. Culture the wound and continue antibiotics started in the emergency department.
8. Obtain postoperative skull x-ray (before the wound is closed if possible) to make sure debridement was adequate.

EPIDURAL HEMATOMA

The patient with a head injury in whom an epidural hematoma is evolving will frequently have a history of having lost consciousness transiently after striking the head. This will then be followed by a period of intact consciousness, referred to as the lucid interval, which may last from a few minutes to a few hours. This interval will then be superseded by a progressive deepening level of consciousness, dilation of the pupil on the same side as the hematoma, compression of the upper midbrain with a contralateral hemiparesis or decerebrate posturing, and ultimately death with further brain stem compression.

Surgical treatment of extradural hemorrhage prior to loss of consciousness will permit complete cure; thereafter, the mortality is directly related to the severity of neurological damage.

The following dicta may be useful:

1. The temporal area, which is the region of the middle meningeal artery, is most frequently involved; the areas of the transverse and sagittal dural sinuses are less frequently involved.
2. Fracture lines seen in roentgenograms and in the area of scalp contusion help in localization (contrecoup fractures or middle meningeal artery tears to occur).
3. Drill in the temporal region 3 cm anterior to the external auditory meatus.
4. Nick the dura to look for subdural hematoma.
5. When clot is located, enlarge the bone opening and evacuate the clot by suction, scoops, and irrigation.

6. Control bleeding:
   a. Control bleeding from middle meningeal artery by electrosurgical coagulation or by plugging the foramen spinosum with cotton alone or impregnated with bone wax. Use of a toothpick to plug the foramen also has been described.
   b. Speed is not important, but transfusions may be required.
7. Suture dura mater to the pericranium.
8. If signs of brain stem compression persist, explore to determine whether the temporal lobe is herniated through the incisura. If herniated, the prolapsed structures should be elevated: rarely does the tentorium need to be sectioned.
9. If no hematoma is found, drill the opposite side.

Craniotomy for extradural hematoma performed in the emergency department may occasionally be justified in a patient admitted in extremis with a history and findings indicative of an extradural clot. A drill hole is placed without the scalp having been shaved and without sterile technique, if necessary. The establishment of an adequate airway is the only step that takes precedence over evacuation of the clot.

After the clot has been evacuated, the patient is transferred to the operating room, where hemostasis and closure are performed. Even a patient in extremis can usually be temporarily resuscitated by the intravenous administration of mannitol. The resultant brain shrinkage provides about a 30-minute period of grace in which to prepare the operative site, put in a burr hole, and evacuate the clot.

SUBDURAL HEMATOMA

One of the most common types of post-traumatic intracranial hemorrhage is the subdural hematoma. Symptoms may appear as early as within the first minutes or as late as six to eight weeks after injury. Acute subdural hematomas are defined as hematomas that cause significant progressive neurological deficit within 48 hours of injury. When first seen, the patient with an acute subdural hematoma is usually unresponsive with a focal neurological deficit. The diagnosis is made when an acute subdural is suspected in the severely head-injured patient who shows any deterioration in neurological status. Evidence for the diagnosis is strengthened by the presence of a shift of a calcified pineal gland on plain skull x-rays, an area of high attenuation over the surface of the brain and a shift of the ventricles on the CT scan, and a clear space between the brain and the inner table of the skull on cerebral arteriography.

Treatment consists of removal of the hematoma through a large craniotomy with control of bleeding points, decompression by removal of large areas of the skull and relaxation of the compressing dura mater, and, when necessary, internal decompression by excision of portions of the frontal or temporal lobes. Drainage of the hematoma through perforator openings is never satisfactory, since the major portion of the hematoma is solid clot and the problem is a combination of mass from clot and from the reaction of the brain to a severe injury.

INTRACEREBRAL HEMATOMA

Post-traumatic intracerebral hematomas are most often seen in patients with severe head injuries. The symptoms of an intracerebral hematoma are similar to those of an acute subdural hematoma; and frequently the two will occur in conjunction. As with acute subdural hematomas, a CT scan or cerebral arteriography will localize the intracerebral hematoma.

Effective treatment for an intracerebral hematoma in a head-injured patient whose condition is deteriorating neurologically is a craniotomy or craniectomy with incision of the hemisphere over the most superficial area of the hematoma and evacuation of the clot. Simple aspiration of the lesion is not adequate, because most of the hematoma is usually solid. Often the evacuation must be accompanied by an excision of part of the involved brain in order to remove devitalized tissue and to obtain an effective decompression.

SUBARACHNOID HEMORRHAGE

The most common type of intracranial hemorrhage following a head injury is a subarachnoid hemorrhage. It usually causes symptoms and signs of meningeal irritation such as headache and a stiff neck. Occasionally, it will result in markedly agitated behavior in the young patient. It has little surgical significance because the blood is rapidly diluted by the circulating cerebrospinal fluid, usually within three to five days. Infrequently, the subarachnoid blood may obstruct the circulation or the absorption of the cerebrospinal fluid, resulting in a communicating hydrocephalus. If this occurs, it may manifest itself as a progressive dementia and a gait disturbance in a patient who has had a head injury weeks before.

LEAKAGE OF CEREBROSPINAL FLUID

Fortunately, most cranial cerebrospinal fluid fistulas close spontaneously. Unless roentgenograms reveal a definite protrusion of bone into the subdural space or a marked depression in the frontal sinus area, one is justified waiting with the anticipation that within 10 to 12 days the fistula will close. During this time the patient should be under observation and should be given prophylactic antibiotics. If the rhinorrhea or otorrhea persists for more than 14 days, surgical repair of the dural tear is necessary.

13

Spine and Spinal Cord

From 10,000 to 20,000 new spinal cord injuries occur each year. Forty percent of the spinal injuries are caused by vehicular accidents, 20 percent are due to falls, and 40 percent are due to recreational, industrial, agricultural, or gunshot accidents. According to the National Spinal Cord Registry, in 1975 there were approximately 200,000 patients with spinal cord injuries living in the United States. The cost of supporting such a patient during his lifetime who is injured in early adulthood may be greater than one million dollars. Therefore, the loss and hardships from this type of injury placed upon the patient, his family, and society cannot be overemphasized.

Unfortunately, nothing at the present can be done to reverse the disruption of central nervous system tissue that occurs at the time of injury. Consequently, the management of these patients is aimed at preventing the progression of the cord injury, either by relieving compression or by stabilizing the patient's condition in order to facilitate the cord's own healing process. A discussion of this management can be divided into stabilization, evaluation, treatment, and ancillary problems.

STABILIZATION OF THE SPINE

IMMOBILIZATION OF THE SPINE

The management of spinal cord injuries begins at the scene of the accident. Any trauma patient who is unconscious could be harboring a spinal injury and should be treated accordingly. When a spinal injury is suspected, immediate immobilization of the spine is mandatory. It has been well documented that motion of the spine in a patient with an injured cord accentuates the pathology. In the early phase of the management, immobilization can be accomplished with sandbags, cervical collar, or skeletal tongs and traction for a cervical injury. A thoracolumbar injury can be immobilized by keeping the patient supine on a firm backboard.

Providing Optimal Oxygenation and Perfusion

During the initial management, one should provide optimal oxygenation and blood flow to the injured spinal cord. A neurological deficit can be created or made worse by tissue hypoxia caused by either ventilatory or circulatory problems. Strict attention should be paid to maintaining a good airway and oxygenation and to providing the support necessary to maintain the blood pressure within normal limits. During the patient's initial treatment, intravenous lines should be inserted for fluid administration in the event of hypotension. This may be necessary because of actual blood loss from associated injuries or because of vasomotor paralysis from the cord injury itself. Disruption of descending sympathetic pathways results in loss of vasomotor tone and subsequent hypotension (Table 13–1).

Cervical cord injuries also cause paralysis of intercostal respirations. Under these circumstances, respiratory distress can develop rapidly and sometimes lead to apnea. *Careful* nasotracheal intubation should be performed and ventilatory support provided if oxygen administration alone does not adequately oxygenate the patient.

Gastrointestinal Decompression

A nasogastric tube should be inserted in order to prevent abdominal distention secondary to a paralytic ileus. If untreated, this can result in unwanted vomiting with aspiration and respiratory embarrassment. If ileus develops, the nasogastric tube should be placed on continuous suction or gravity drainage for one to two days and intravenous fluids provided.

Bladder Catheterization

A Foley catheter should be inserted as soon as possible after the diagnosis of a cord injury is made. Retention of urine can develop within hours; this can lead to bladder overdistention and subsequent hypotonia. Because of sensory paralysis, this may cause no discomfort. Shortly after the catheter is inserted, a program of intermittent catheterization should be started to maintain a sterile urine, a toned bladder, and a normal upper urinary tract.

TABLE 13–1. VITAL SIGNS IN CNS TRAUMA

Head injury	BP ↑	P ↑
Increased intracranial pressure	BP ↑	P ↓
Hypovolemic shock	BP ↓	P ↑
Spinal cord injury	BP ↓	P ↓

EVALUATION

The evaluation of a cord-injured patient includes the clinical examination and the diagnostic roentgenographic study of the spine.

CLINICAL EXAMINATION

As with any medical or surgical emergency, a good history from the patient may provide information that is invaluable in arriving at a diagnosis and plan of treatment. One should therefore closely question the patient about his own feelings of pain and his ability to move at the scene of the accident and during transport. A past medical history should be obtained with emphasis on the presence of cardiac and pulmonary disease. These may well affect the patient's response to the immediate therapeutic interventions.

The principal symptom of fracture of the spine is acute local pain that may remain localized or radiate into the arms, torso, or legs. If pain is present, a detailed examination should be performed without moving the patient's spine. Inspection of the patient for external signs of trauma may help in localizing the spinal injury. For example, injuries to the forehead and chin may cause hyperextension of the cervical spine. A blow to the vertex of the head may cause compression-fracture of the cervical spine. Abrasion or lacerations over the posterior trunk can be a sign of thoracic and lumbar injuries. Palpation of the spine — without moving the patient — may reveal deformities of spinous processes, local tenderness and pain, edema, and muscle spasm. All of these may be of localizing value.

In the neurological examination the motor and sensory function of the cord must be assessed, as well as reflex changes and autonomic function. The motor examination is done by testing each major muscle group in each extremity individually. The function of the muscle should be recorded according to one of the various grading systems. Such grading is usually based on whether the muscles function normally, are weak but function against resistance, function against gravity but not resistance, do not function against gravity, show a trace of movement, or are paralyzed (Table 13–2). It is only through accurate initial recording of this information that one can determine whether the patient's condition is improving or deteriorating.

The sensory examination must determine any deficit of pain, temperature, and fine touch (spinothalamic function) as well as proprioception, deep sensibility, and vibration (posterior column function). A level of sensory deficit should be determined and correlated with the motor level of deficit. Reflex changes should be ascertained carefully. This may provide information on whether certain spinal roots are spared from injury. In evaluation of lumbar and sacral injuries, the reflex examination is of utmost importance because the surgeon is dealing with nerve root injury of

TABLE 13–2. SPINAL MOTOR INDEX–UNIVERSITY OF MARYLAND*

			Possible Total
Date			
Time			
Diaphragm		S	2
Deltoids	(R/L)	5	10
Biceps	(R/L)	5	10
Triceps	(R/L)	5	10
Flex, dig. prof.	(R/L)	5	10
Abd. dig. minimi	(R/L)	5	10
Intercostals		S	2
Upper abdominal		S	2
Lower abdominal		S	2
Iliopsoas	(R/L)	5	10
Quad. femoris	(R/L)	5	10
Ext. dig. (Toes)	(R/L)	5	10
Gastrocnemius	(R/L)	5	10
Anal		S	2
			100
Sensory Level	(R/L)		

*Diaphragm, intercostals, upper and lower abdominals, and anal tone are graded S (for Strong, = 2), W (for Weak, = 1) or 0 (for absent, = 0). Extremity muscles are graded 5 through 0.

the cauda equina rather than the cord itself. Autonomic dysfunction may be assessed by checking for diminished sweating, vasomotor instability, loss of bladder and rectal control, and priapism.

The initial clinical examination should determine whether the injury has resulted in an apparently complete lesion of the spinal cord or an incomplete lesion. A complete lesion is one in which there are no clinical signs of any cord function below the level of the injury. Incomplete lesions have some preservation of cord function, such as sacral sensory sparing, minimal motor function in the legs, and preservation of a sense of position. The importance of this differentiation lies in its prognostic value. A lesion that is complete on admission and remains complete over the next 24 hours involves an extremely poor prognosis with regard to return of function. An incomplete lesion at least indicates the possibility of some return of function.

ROENTGENOGRAPHIC EXAMINATION

Techniques. After the patient's condition has been stabilized and a clinical motor and sensory level of injury has been determined, roentgenographic examination must be done to delineate the exact site and nature of bony injuries. This is usually done in the emergency department with the patient lying supine on the stretcher. Portable lateral and anteroposterior

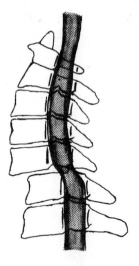

Figure 13-1. Flexion injury resulting in bilateral dislocated (locked) facet joints.

views of the suspected area of injury are generally easily obtained and demonstrate the injury. In the cervical region, an open-mouth view of the odontoid may be of considerable help in assessing for fractures of C1 to C2. Occasionally, polytomography of the injured area is necessary to identify properly the type and extent of bony damage. The roentgenograms should be examined closely for contour and alignment of the vertebral bodies, displacement of bone fragments into the spinal canal, and linear or comminuted fractures of the laminae, pedicles, or neural arches.

Types of Fractures. The roentgenographic appearance of a spine injury depends on the mechanism of injury and the force with which it occurs. In the cervical spine, flexion injuries can result in bilateral dislocation of the facet joints (Fig. 13–1), simple anterior wedge compression of

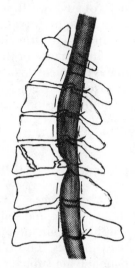

Figure 13-2. Flexion injury resulting in a comminuted wedge fracture and dislocation.

the vertebral body, or teardrop wedge fractures (comminuted) of the vertebral body (Fig. 13–2). Flexion-rotation injuries often lead to a unilateral facet dislocation. Vertical compression injuries to the cervical spine can cause bursting fractures of the vertebral bodies. These may also occur in the thoracolumbar region (Fig. 13–3). Finally, it should be noted that a patient may have a significant neurological deficit with a normal-appearing cervical spine x-ray. If this occurs, tomography and flexion and extension views should be obtained with a physician covering the procedure. These views may demonstrate instability caused by soft tissue injury. Thoracic and lumbar fractures may occur by the same mechanisms as those in the cervical area. The most frequently injured vertebrae in this area are the thoracolumbar junction at T11 to L2.

Myelography.   The use of myelography in the immediate diagnostic work-up of a spinal cord injury is controversial. The purpose of the myelogram is to identify any surgically correctable compression of the cord that, if treated, may result in a better recovery for the patient. Compression may be demonstrated by either a total block of flow of the contrast material or by a specific filling defect in the dye column. The type of optical myelographic material to use is also debated. We prefer Pantopaque via a C1 to C2 puncture in the prone position. Others prefer gas myelography via the traditional lumbar route. Whichever method and technique is employed, myelography is generally performed after the spine has been realigned by means of skeletal tongs and traction.

TREATMENT

The initial aim of treatment of spinal injuries is realignment of the spine and subsequent immobilization of the spine in its normal anatomical position.

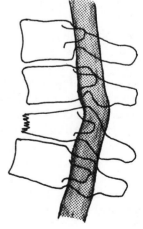

Figure 13–3. Thoracolumbar compression fracture and dislocation.

CERVICAL INJURIES

In fractures of the cervical spine, realignment of the spine is best accomplished by skeletal tongs and traction. There are numerous types of skeletal tongs (Crutchfield, Gardner-Wells, Halo), all of which are effective. After the tongs are inserted, weights are applied for traction in 10- to 20-pound increments, depending on the age and weight of the patient. As the traction is increased, the head and neck can be appropriately and gently positioned — with mild hyperextension or flexion — in order to adequately align the spine. Frequent x-rays should be obtained during this time in order to assess the result of each maneuver. If adequate realignment cannot be achieved by this method, open surgical reduction should be performed. This is particularly true with locked, dislocated facet joints.

After the spine is realigned by this closed technique, a myelogram (as described) may be performed. The percentage of cervical spine injuries that warrant an emergency decompression operation is probably less than 10 percent. It should also be noted that the majority of those patients who undergo emergency operation will *not* improve neurologically, especially if the cord lesion is complete. Nevertheless, since some patients may have significant improvement, any patient with demonstrable cord compression should be considered for emergency operation. Decompression does *not* necessarily mean laminectomy. If myelography reveals anterior cord compression from *extruded* intervertebral disc material or posteriorly displaced bone fragments, an anterior discectomy or corpectomy with fusion may be required. If spinal block or compression is due to fractured lamina arches or disrupted ligamentatum flavum, then a laminectomy is in order. Thus the procedure chosen is designed to relieve the specific compression, not just to unroof the spine.

Once the spine is aligned and no compression is demonstrated, attention must be turned toward achieving permanent stabilization of the spine. This can be accomplished either by elective surgical stabilization or by prolonged skeletal traction. The advantages of an early surgical procedure are early mobilization and rehabilitation. This helps prevent the complications associated with prolonged bed rest (especially when the patient is kept prone or supine) and also allows an early retraining program to be started if the patient can be gotten out of bed. However, nonsurgical stabilization can be just as effective. The patient who is quadriplegic or has marked neurological deficit may be maintained in skeletal traction on a frame or regular bed for approximately six weeks. After that time, he may be placed in a cervical brace and the process of mobilization is begun. If a neurological deficit is absent or minor, the patient may be put into traction with a Halo vest apparatus that will give immobilization and allow the patient to be ambulatory. Effective stabilization requires that the patient remain in this device for three to six months.

THORACOLUMBAR INJURIES

The treatment of fracture of the thoracic or lumbar spines is based upon the same principles as that of the cervical injuries. If a myelographic block is present or if bone fragments are compromising the canal, a decompressive-stabilization procedure should be performed with some urgency. The realignment of the spine using surgically inserted Harrington rods may by itself restore the canal to its normal dimensions and thus decompress the cord or nerve roots. However, a direct decompressive procedure such as laminectomy, hemilaminectomy, or posterolateral decompression is often required to remove bone fragments or disc material from the canal. These procedures should be performed in conjunction with a rodding procedure.

If no myelographic block or compression is present with the thoracolumbar fracture, an elective stabilization procedure should be done to allow early mobilization and rehabilitation and to prevent chronic spinal deformity and pain that is often associated with these types of fractures.

OPEN INJURIES TO THE SPINE

Open injuries to the spine and spinal cord are not common in the civilian experience. In addition to the risk of neurological damage, the patient is also threatened with hemorrhage, infection of the wound, and meningitis. The soft tissue injury should be explored and debrided carefully.

An operation on the spine itself is indicated if there is a cerebrospinal fluid leak or evidence of bone or foreign bodies in the spinal cord causing cord compression in a patient who has a possibility of neurological recovery. The laminectomy done for this reason should provide adequate exposure to allow a thorough exploration of the canal for fragments and room to effect a watertight dural closure to stop the spinal fluid leak.

NONSURGICAL THERAPY

The nonsurgical treatment of spinal injuries is primarily supportive and preventive. Several such modes of therapy are available but are of debated efficacy.

Steroids. Acutely, steroids are thought to minimize the amount of cord edema and the deleterious consequences of edema. Dexamethasone (1 mg/kg/day) or methylprednisolone (5 mg/kg/day) should be given for approximately five to seven days. An antacid or cimetidine should be given concomitantly to reduce the possibility of gastrointestinal hemorrhage.

Hyperbaric Oxygen. The use of hyperbaric oxygen therapy for cord injuries has been reported to have some beneficial effects. This remains controversial and is experimental at this point. The thrust of medical treatment of cord injuries is to optimize the conditions in which the cord may recover. Good oxygenation should be provided through active pulmonary therapy, oxygen administration, and assisted ventilation if necessary.

Supportive Therapy. Physical therapy beginning on admission should consist of frequent movement of all extremities through a wide range and regular turning and repositioning of the patient to prevent pulmonary emboli, pneumonia, or bedsores. Maintaining adequate systemic blood pressure is also important in order to optimize spinal cord blood flow.

Prevention of Complications

Preventive medical treatment consists mainly of good nursing care to ward off the threat of infection, which in itself can prevent cord recovery and threaten the life of the patient.

Skin Care. Special measures for skin care should be initiated as soon as the patient arrives in the emergency department. It is imperative to change the position of paralyzed, anesthetic body areas at least every two hours. Specialized foam or rubber mattresses or rotating frames should be employed. Anesthetic skin should be washed, massaged with alcohol, and powdered at least once a day. Bed coverings should always be dry. Meticulous perineal and sacral skin care is obligatory.

Bladder Care. After the acute phase of injury, the patient should be started on a program of intermittent sterile catheterization to prevent bladder dysfunction secondary to overdistention and to prevent infection. Early urological consultation should ensure a proper regimen with continuity of bladder care and administration of appropriate antimicrobial agents.

Gastrointestinal Care. The patient should be started on a reasonable regimen of stool softeners and laxatives to maintain good gastrointestinal function. Gastrointestinal hemorrhage or perforation can be a fatal complication of the cord-injured patient. Consequently, antacids should be continued whether the patient is receiving steroids or not.

Abdominal disease accounts for 10 percent of all fatalities in the cord-injured population. A perforated viscus with peritonitis is the most common. Although the sensory deficit makes the routine abdominal examination virtually useless, certain clinical signs should raise the index of suspicion; by heeding these signs, the surgeon possibly can prevent a catastrophic complication. Persistent nausea and vomiting or tachycardia or bradycardia when the pulse has been normal may be a sign of intra-abdominal problems. Pain in the shoulders and clavicular regions may be referred pain from diaphragmatic irritation from free air or inflammation. If any of these signs appear, one should begin a diagnostic work-up to rule out an intra-abdominal lesion.

REHABILITATION

The most important goal in the management of a patient with a spinal cord injury is to make the patient as functional and independent as his neurological deficit allows. A physical and psychological rehabilitation program should be started as early as possible. Even in the acute phase, the physical therapist should begin exercise programs and instruct the patient and family in detail. Psychologists and social workers should begin working with the patient and his family in regard to social, sexual, occupational, and financial adjustments. The physicians who are caring for the patient should keep the patient's rehabilitation potential in mind when deciding on the type of operation or external braces. Anything that might impede the patient's rehabilitation program should be avoided *if possible.* After the acute phase, the patient should be transferred to a rehabilitation center without delay.

CONCLUSION

The majority of spinal cord injuries are accidental and preventable. Nothing can be done directly to correct CNS tissue disruption that occurs at the time of injury. Furthermore, the cord does not regenerate itself. Consequently, the best treatment of spinal cord injury is its prevention. Physicians in all medical disciplines and other medical personnel need to encourage and promote public and personal safety standards whenever possible. Otherwise, we will continue to experience the high incidence of needless death and disability secondary to spinal injuries.

14

Face

With the exception of a compromised upper airway, hemorrhage, or intracranial injury, facial injuries are located far down the list of therapeutic priorities in patients with multiple system injuries. In the patient with suspected multiple system injury, the early administration of a general anesthetic agent for repair of the facial injury interposes time and prolonged sedation between the examiner and a possible life-threatening injury. That time is frequently needed to complete diagnostic measures and to perform repeated examinations to define a subtle or evolving injury in the central nervous system, thorax, or abdomen. Therefore, too early detailed involvement in definitive repair of the facial injury before more serious injuries have been ruled out is contraindicated. Fortunately, deformities caused by facial injuries can often be prevented by simple, early manipulations performed under local anesthesia, or they can await repair under general anesthesia some days after their occurrence.

INITIAL TREATMENT

AIRWAY

Severe injuries of the face require immediate investigation of the upper airway. Foreign material in the oropharynx such as blood, vomitus, teeth, and broken dentures is relatively common in the posterior pharynx and must be removed promptly. Retrodisplacement of the tongue as a result of injury to the central nervous system or collapse of the mandibular arch as a result of fractures must be relieved. Laryngeal edema, either not present or asymptomatic at the initial examination, may evolve within hours after blunt or sharp trauma to the tongue, pharynx, and larynx. Respiratory support is necessary in the case of brain stem injury or severe cerebral injuries.

Supportive emergency measures include (1) anterior traction on the fractured mandible and tongue; (2) frequent pharyngeal suction; (3) endotracheal intubation (cricothyroid laryngotomy may be indicated if the treating physician is unable to intubate the patient; see Chapter 15); (4)

emergency tracheostomy (rarely required for facial injuries alone); and (5) mechanical ventilatory support (Ambu bag, respiratory). Emergency tracheostomy requires good lighting, proper instruments, and at least one assistant.

HEMORRHAGE

Hemorrhage in the facial areas should be treated with direct pressure, because clamping of the larger vessels under ordinary emergency department conditions involves the risk of clamping one of the facial nerves or their branches, resulting in paralysis. Since shock is rare in patients with facial injuries only, its presence should prompt a thorough search of other body areas for injuries that are more commonly related to shock.

INTRACRANIAL INJURY

Intracranial injuries should always be suspected in patients with facial injuries. Therefore, all patients must have baseline and serial neurological examinations recorded as recommended in Chapter 12. Pain associated with facial injuries is often mild, even when the injury is extensive, so it is rarely necessary to use narcotics. In fact, administration of narcotics is often contraindicated because they interfere with monitoring of the status of the central nervous system and abdomen.

EXAMINATION AND DIAGNOSIS OF SOFT TISSUE INJURIES

Lacerations, avulsions, and abrasions about the head and neck are usually evident. However, what is thought to be an avulsion with skin loss may not always be so in reality. This is especially true in the face and scalp, where skin edges retract due to elasticity and the thin skin tends to roll up into small amounts of tissue. Intraoral lacerations (produced by broken dentures or pipe stems or tongue bites) must be looked for immediately. Bleeding from these injuries is often brisk and, if the patient's mental status is depressed, they may be the cause of blood in the trachea. Bleeding about the head and neck can be controlled with pressure. Devitalized tissue should be removed, since this is the most common source of facial wound infection. As much viable tissue as possible should be saved.

The following soft tissue injuries will likely require operating room repair under optimal conditions: (1) ocular or severe eyelid injury, (2) parotid gland or duct injury, (3) facial nerve injury, (4) nasolacrimal injury with interruption of the canaliculus, sacculus, or nasolacrimal duct,

(5) alveolar process and severe tooth injuries, (6) moderate soft tissue loss, and (7) extensive lacerations requiring debridement and accurate closure.

Both vertical and horizontal lacerations of the eyelids can produce serious sequelae. Laceration of the globe can occur through a lid laceration with the conjunctiva intact. In vertical lacerations, notching and contracture can cause severe deformity if the repair is not performed with care. Horizontal lacerations in the upper lid may result in division of the levator muscle or its tendinous insertion, or in lacerations of the globe at or above the conjunctival fornix. When ptosis is not caused by laceration of the levator muscle, intraorbital nerve damage, frequently at the level of the superior orbital fissure (superior orbital fissure syndrome), should be suspected.

Even if the eyelid is uninjured, it must be opened and the globe examined before the possible development of hematoma or edema makes the examination difficult. Vision should always be recorded when the patient is first examined. If vision-testing charts are not available the examiner can compare vision by holding up a hand or fingers, alternately covering one eye and then the other. Once involvement is ascertained, further manipulation of the eye or eyelids is contraindicated. Improper handling of the injured eye may convert a relatively trivial injury into an extremely serious one that may result in blindness. In addition, the physician should be aware of the possibility of associated intracranial injury. A penetrating wound in the region of the eye not infrequently involves the cranial cavity because the roof of the orbit is fragile.

Except to determine the presence of ocular injury, examination of the eye should be deferred until adequate anesthesia, good lighting, and satisfactory facilities are available, ideally by an ophthalmological consultant. A facial nerve block with local anesthesia should be employed so that the patient cannot squeeze his eyelids together, thus causing herniation of ocular contents. The orbital rim should be palpated. Extraocular movements should be tested and recorded. Diplopia suggests injury to cranial nerves or the orbit.

Deep lacerations from the midportion of the cheek back to the ear should arouse strong suspicion that injury has occurred to the facial nerve, parotid gland, or parotid duct. Careful examination for injuries to these areas is indicated. It is mandatory to test the major branches of the facial nerve prior to injections of local anesthesia. Transoral probing of the parotid duct will facilitate diagnosis of a parotid duct injury. Nasolacrimal injury should be suspected when blunt or sharp trauma has occurred near the medial canthus. Fluorescein may be used to evaluate the integrity of the ducts by placement of the dye in the conjunctival sac and observation of its appearance in the nostril. In case of doubt, such injury should be assumed to exist and repair planned accordingly.

The alveolar process may be fractured or displaced without fractures to the facial skeleton, causing severe injuries to the teeth. Alveolar injuries can be diagnosed both by observation and palpation. Their importance lies in the embarrassed vascularity in the displaced position of the alveolar process. Teeth may be displaced or fractured by the injury. Management of dental injuries is based on the blood supply to the dental pulp, which enters a tooth by small vessels through a constricted opening in the apex of the root. Vitality (intact blood supply) is readily disrupted by displacement of a tooth or exposure of the dental pulp through a fracture in the crown or root. Loss of vitality, however, can occur without physical displacement. Diagnosis of the presence or absence of dental vitality is frequently impossible immediately after an injury. Periapical and dental occlusal x-rays of the teeth are necessary for evaluation. Routine facial bone x-rays are not sufficient.

FRACTURES

The facial skeleton is constructed so that, through sequential small bone failures, it can absorb a tremendous amount of impact energy while affording maximal protection against concussion of the cranial vault. Recognition of these small bone fractures is essential if healing is to occur with maintenance of proper contours of the face and its associated structures. Diagnosis of these fractures involves a combination of clinical inspection, palpation, and roentgenographic examination. Careful clinical examination of the face will detect fractures with significant displacement of fragments.

The essential signs in the clinical evaluation of fractures are (1) presence of dental malocclusions; (2) limitation of mandibular excursion; (3) sensory loss in the distribution of the mental, infraorbital, and supraorbital nerves; (4) presence of diplopia; (5) limitation or lag in ocular movements; (6) asymmetry of the cheek prominences; (7) discontinuity of the orbital rim; (8) ocular proptosis or enophthalmos; (9) asymmetry, hypermobility, and crepitus at the nasal bridge; and (10) displacement of the nasal septum.

FRACTURES OF THE MANDIBLE

Malocclusion, particularly an opening between the biting surfaces of the teeth when the patient closes the jaws, is present in the great majority of fractures of either the mandible or maxilla (Fig. 14–1). With minor displacement of the fracture fragments, the malocclusion may be subtle and the patient may volunteer that the teeth do not feel right when closing the jaws. Hypesthesia or anesthesia in the distribution of the mental nerve indicates an injury to the inferior alveolar nerve from a fracture of the body of the mandible. Bleeding from a laceration along a tooth socket

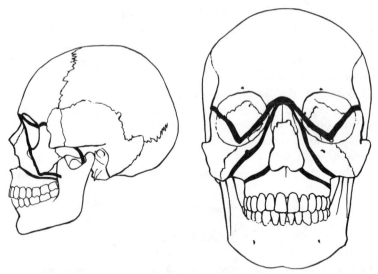

Figure 14–1. Schematic representation of fracture lines in maxillary fractures that defines the LeFort I, II, and III classifications.

involved in a fracture, or tenderness and swelling, may further localize the site of fracture. The mandible is like a hoop or a teacup and seldom fractures in only one location. Therefore, one should look for signs of more than one fracture such as a body fracture on one side of the mandible with fracture of the subcondylar area on the other side.

FRACTURES OF THE MAXILLA

The usual malocclusion of a displaced maxillary fracture is an open anterior bite. Hypermobility in maxillary fractures can be demonstrated by grasping the anterior maxilla with the thumb and index finger of one hand while stabilizing the forehead with the other hand. The degree of maxillary fracture can be defined clinically by noting the concomitant mobility or lack of mobility at the nasal bridge and zygomas. An open anterior bite deformity in which the maxilla is immobile implies that the maxilla is impacted or that a fracture of the mandible exists, frequently in the mandibular neck region. Fractures of the mandible and maxilla may coexist. Roentgenographic examination will help answer these questions.

FRACTURES OF THE ORBIT AND ZYGOMATIC ARCH

With the exception of the uncommon massive disruption of the bony orbit and fractures of the superior orbital rim, fractures in and around the orbit occur: at or near the suture lines of the zygomatic bone along the orbital rim, as an inward fracture of the zygomatic arch alone, or as an isolated fracture of the orbital floor (blowout fracture). Along with asymmetry of the cheek prominences, palpation of the orbital rim will detect discontinuity in the displaced zygomatic or malar fracture. Depression of the zygomatic arch is readily detected in significant displacements of this isolated fracture. If the examination is not performed early, soft tissue swelling may hinder the detection of these fractures by clinical examination. If the zygomatic arch is sufficiently depressed, jaw opening may be limited because of the mechanical stop placed in front of the coronoid process of the mandible.

Hypesthesia or anesthesia in the distribution of the infraorbital nerve indicates injury to that nerve in the floor of the orbit. When this occurs without evidence of direct trauma to the nerve, without zygoma asymmetry, or without discontinuity of the orbital rim, a blowout fracture should be suspected. Enophthalmos detected before lid swelling occurs is further evidence of a blowout fracture.

Double vision must be specifically tested for and quantitated. Lid swelling makes this difficult and therefore diplopia should be evaluated as soon as possible. Double vision can occur as a result of dropping or displacement of the orbital contents in fractures occurring high along the lateral orbital rim, entrapment of periorbital fat around the inferior rectus muscle in fractures of the orbital floor, or as a result of nerve paralysis or muscle contusion with or without a fracture of the orbit. Diplopia, therefore, can occur in zygomatic, blowout, and LeFort III fractures, but may not necessarily be causally related to the fracture.

FRACTURE OF THE NOSE

Nasal fractures are usually more evident clinically than roentgenographically. Nevertheless, x-rays should be taken if such injury is suspected. The injury may depress the dorsum of the nose, displace it to one side, or may simply result in epistaxis and marked swelling over the nose without apparent skeletal deformity. Crepitus and hypermobility of the nasal pyramid are usually evident in these fractures. Inspection for hematoma or dislocation of the septum should be done. In any injury of the naso-orbital complex, inspection for possible cerebrospinal rhinorrhea is indicated. If there is a question as to whether the clear material obtained is serum, cerebrospinal fluid, or mucus, glucose determinations should be obtained. The glucose level of cerebrospinal fluid is approximately one half that of the serum. Mucin content can also be determined to identify the type of drainage.

In children, minor displacement of nasal bones will result in growth changes and ultimate deformity unless corrected at the time of initial injury.

ROENTGENOGRAPHIC EXAMINATION FOR FACIAL INJURIES

It is unwise to rush the patient to the x-ray department until a possible concomitant major injury (skull or cervical spine), which would make movement of the patient hazardous, has been evaluated. Complete roentgenograms should be obtained, however, when the patient's condition permits. Special views must be obtained for accurate diagnosis of facial bone injury. One must remember that most facial fractures are diagnosed by a careful physical examination, and in spite of proper roentgenograms, fractures of thin bones, such as the maxilla, ethmoid, and nasal bones, may be missed because of superimposition of shadows.

The following roentgenographic views are recommended:

1. Mandible: posteroanterior, lateral, and lateral oblique. A Towne projection of the mandible shows the ascending ramus and condyles. In addition, a Panorex view and dental occlusal views may be advisable for specific injuries.

2. Midface: Water's view with possible stereo views for maxillary and orbital fractures; submento-occipital view to demonstrate the zygomatic arches. Tomography is desirable when clouding of the maxillary antrum prevents definition of the orbital floor.

3. Nasal bones: lateral views taken with soft tissue technique. An anteroposterior view is helpful to evaluate the septum.

REPAIR OF FACIAL INJURIES

Optimal Time for Repair.   When life-threatening and limb-threatening injuries have been thoroughly evaluated and stabilized, soft tissue injuries of the face requiring only local anesthesia can be repaired. Repair of complex injuries listed previously or severe fractures of the facial skeleton should be postponed until the patient's condition is satisfactory for general anesthesia. Perceived urgency for any repair of a facial injury should not override the surgeon's judgment to provide a situation in which a repair with careful technique can be performed. There is a long "period of grace" for facial wounds because of the excellent blood supply and local host defense mechanisms of facial skin secretion and saliva. Therefore, a given inoculum of bacteria in a facial wound multiplies more slowly to greater than the apparently critical 10^5 organisms per gram of tissue. Most soft tissue wounds of the face can be closed safely at 24 hours after injury. If there is a question of safety, quantitative and qualitative bacterial analysis can be performed on a biopsy of tissue from the wound to confirm that the wound is unlikely to become infected despite the delay.

Facial bone fractures should be repaired when the patient's general condition permits. Mandibular fractures that can be reduced and immobilized by the application of dental arch bars and intermaxillary fixation (elastics or wire) can be treated immediately under local anesthesia. If necessary, repair of facial fractures requiring a general anesthetic can safely be delayed up to two weeks following injury. An exception is fine bone of the orbital floor, which becomes difficult to manipulate due to fibrous fixation. A decision to operate in this case should be made within the first week to ten days following injury. Antibiotics should be administered to patients with open fractures, including mandibular and maxillary fractures occurring through a tooth socket and those that involve openings into the maxillary antrum.

ANESTHESIA

In cooperative patients, anesthesia may be administered by regional block, field block, or local infiltration for most facial injuries. Five areas of the face lend themselves to regional nerve blocks: (1) supraorbital, (2) infraorbital, (3) maxillary, (4) mandibular, and (5) nasal. Topical anesthetics may also be used on the nasal mucosa or in the conjunctiva provided proper precautions for sensitivity reactions are observed. General anesthesia is frequently necessary in adults and is essential in children (see Chapter 7).

GENERAL PLAN FOR CARE OF THE WOUND

If local anesthesia is to be administered, the skin should be thoroughly cleansed and prepared with an antiseptic after nerve blocks have been completed. The wound is irrigated with saline, and all dirt, hair, clothing, and other foreign material are removed. Dirt and carbon particles may produce permanent "tattooing" of the skin if they are not completely removed at the initial debridement. Tattooed areas that remain after vigorous mechanical cleansing should be removed with a dermabrasion instrument or a scalpel.

Facial fractures are repositioned and stabilized as necessary with interosseous wires, pins, interdental wiring, or arch bars to provide a stable skeleton for additional repairs.

Fractures of the teeth and alveolar process or dental lamina as well as loose teeth are indications for splinting the area in order to save teeth that might otherwise be lost. Although often necessarily delayed until more urgent repairs are carried out, early realignment of the alveolar process provides the highest probability of dental salvage.

Injuries of specialized structures are repaired, including those to the facial nerve, lacrimal system, parotid gland and duct, and cartilages of the nose and ear. The use of the dissecting microscope will produce superior results when dealing with the fine detail of the facial nerve and lacrimal apparatus.

The remaining soft tissues such as muscle, subcuticular layers, and skin are closed, with emphasis on atraumatic handling of tissues and accurate approximation. Fine suture materials should be used. A properly constructed and well-applied dressing completes the repair.

SPECIFIC SOFT TISSUE INJURIES

Because of the importance of the face for identity and because of its unique blood supply, there are some surgical principles that apply almost solely to the face. Debridement should err on the side of conservatism. This is especially true for the lower eyelid, the alae of the nose, and the corner of the mouth, where overaggressive debridement can lead to severe deformity. Partially avulsed parts with the slightest chance of survival should be meticulously replaced. Apparently avulsed tissue should be searched for locally and if found in a rolled-up flap, should be unrolled and replaced. Important anatomical landmarks such as the vermilion borders, nostril sills, eyebrows, and helical rims should be used to advantage during repair. Therefore, it is obvious that these landmarks should not be removed by shaving or debriding.

ORAL CAVITY, ALVEOLAE, AND TEETH

Injuries to the oral cavity present special problems. Tongue, cheek, palate, and lip mucosa should be sutured. Deep hemostatic sutures prevent delayed bleeding or hematomas or both. Lips should be repaired in layers, including the muscle, and the vermilion border should be meticulously aligned. In addition, the nasal and oral cavities should be isolated from one another by suturing of the nasal mucosa and oral mucosa.

Treatment of a displaced alveolar process consists of manual repositioning, with care being taken to preserve vascularity of the bony fragments carried in the soft tissue attachments. The application of dental splints is usually necessary for immobilization and stability. Displaced or fractured teeth either should be repositioned or should have dental pulp treatment, immediate restorative dentistry, or extraction based on the clinical assessment of tooth vitality.

A displaced tooth (including one totally extracted or traumatically impacted) can be replaced into its alveolus. If the degree of displacement is minor, pulp removal and root canal filling need not be done. If the tooth is obviously devitalized, root canal therapy may be performed prior to replacement. An attempt at "grafting" a traumatically extracted developing tooth in a child is feasible if this can be accomplished shortly after the injury.

The treatment of a fractured tooth depends on the presence or absence of an opening into the dental pulp. If the pulp chamber is exposed in a fracture, local treatment of the pulp wound should be carried out immediately by a dental consultant.

The last modality of treatment is extraction or discarding of the traumatically extracted tooth. This should be done only when all the preceding attempts at salvage have been considered.

NOSE AND EARS

Repair of multiple lacerations both of the nose and of the ear is time-consuming. These wounds generally require a three-layer closure, including a layer of cartilage or perichondrium. In the case of the ear, comparison with the uninjured side is valuable during the anatomical repair. It is helpful to fix the cartilaginous pieces into their proper positions and then proceed with soft tissue repair. The prominence and importance of these features in facial appearance and expression justify all efforts to obtain precise repair. It also seems justified to attempt replacement of amputated parts if the patient is seen within a few hours of injury. Postoperative splinting by wet cotton dressings is helpful in preventing a hematoma of the ear. If such a hematoma occurs, it should be incised and drained and a well-molded dressing applied to prevent a "cauliflower" ear deformity.

PAROTID AND SUBMAXILLARY GLANDS AND DUCTS

Proper repair and management are necessary to prevent the two most common wound complications following these injuries, namely, cyst formation and salivary fistula. The parotid gland is made up of tough glandular material, and extensive debridement is usually not required. The capsule of the gland accepts sutures well. If the parotid is severely contused, drainage of the gland is indicated even when the larger ducts are intact. The parotid duct is repaired most easily over a plastic stent that is brought out intraorally through the orifice of the duct. Sutures should be of chromic catgut; nonabsorbable material could provide a nidus for calculus formation. Sialoadenograms can be carried out by injection of 3 ml of radiopaque material through a polyethylene tube into the parotid duct. This provides useful information regarding the integrity of the duct and the gland.

Lacerations of the ducts of the submaxillary glands are relatively uncommon. They usually do not require formal repair, because the ducts find new openings into the mouth and these injuries cause no further problem.

Eyelids and Lacrimal Apparatus

Repair of the eyelids requires careful approximation of the conjunctiva and tarsus in one layer using absorbable material. Knots should be placed external to the tarsus away from the conjunctival surface to prevent irritation of the globe. Closure of this layer is helped when the surgeon is careful to align the gray line. The skin and subcutaneous layer are then closed without the need for suturing the orbicularis oris muscle. Stepping procedures to interrupt a vertical healing interface can be carried out; however, when moderate tissue loss is present, these procedures have a tendency to use up additional lid tissue. This may be impractical if a lid deficit exists. In horizontal lacerations of the upper eyelid, integrity of the levator palpabrae superioris should be checked. If ptosis due to its division is present, the muscle should be carefully reapproximated.

In general, careful layer repair with 6–0 or 7–0 sutures will suffice for the initial repair. Tarsal repairs after partial lid loss may require closure under some tension, but this is not necessarily incompatible with an acceptable result.

Loss of conjunctiva often can be remedied using flaps from the conjunctival fornices. If full-thickness lid losses occur, an ophthalmological or plastic surgical consultant will be of help. In the case of large upper lid avulsions, lower lid flaps often can be used to correct upper lid defects. The reverse of this, borrowing upper lid tissue to fill in full-thickness lower lid defects, should not be attempted. The lower lid should be reconstructed, using nasal cartilage–mucosa grafts with local skin flaps.

In large defects of the lid, it is necessary to provide a moist, clean environment for the globe in order to prevent desiccation. This can be done with the patient in a steam croup tent or by a cover glass that is taped airtight to the skin of the face around the orbit after ointment has been inserted into the eye.

Lacerations of the medial portions of the eyelids may involve the lacrimal canaliculi leading from the upper and lower lids to the sacculus, or the sacculus itself may be injured. Usually when the sacculus is injured or punctured, the superficial leaf of the medial canthal ligament also has been divided. This structure should be repaired. Injuries to the canaliculus can be repaired by threading a suture of 5–0 nylon through each open end of the canaliculus and bringing it out through the skin medially and laterally to the laceration. The overlying soft tissues are then repaired. One intact canaliculus, superior or inferior, is usually sufficient to prevent epiphora.

Eye Lacerations, Contusions, and Chemical Burns

The immediate treatment of an eye laceration is to immobilize the injured eye as soon as possible. This is best accomplished by patching both eyes and moving the patient by litter. No attempt should be made to remove what appears to be a foreign body or a blood clot because of the danger of injuring intraocular structures. The iris may be indistinguishable from the blood clot and the contents of the eyeball may be inadvertently extracted. Any manipulation of an injured eye causes pain, with resultant squeezing of the lids by the patient and a tendency toward further damage. All lacerations must be regarded as contaminated. Therefore, broad-spectrum antibiotics should be given parenterally as soon as possible after injuries of the globe are sustained. The possibility of an intraocular foreign body should always be considered and its presence excluded by careful examination, including roentgenographic study.

Small corneal or scleral lacerations, with incarceration of ocular contents, may be left unsutured. More extensive lacerations require careful apposition with fine 6–0 or 7–0 silk or 6–0 chromic catgut sutures. If iris or uveal tissue is incarcerated, replacement or excision is indicated prior to suturing. This should be done by an ophthalmological consultant.

Sympathetic ophthalmia is a constant threat following wounds involving the uveal tract. It probably results from an allergic response to uveal pigment in the contralateral eye caused by the disorganization of pigment-containing cells of the injured eye. The only satisfactory treatment is prevention, which is achieved by prompt enucleation when indicated.

An injured eye can be safely observed for two weeks. After that time, if wound healing is delayed because of incarceration of uveal tissue or if an intraocular foreign body is present and irritation continues, enucleation usually should be done. Many considerations are involved, such as residual visual function and the overall condition of the eye. Even eyes with severe lacerations to the ciliary body may survive. Intracranial injury and the presence of a foreign body should always be excluded.

Contusion of the eyeball is a common cause of loss of vision. Blunt injury directly to the eye or transmitted from the impact of a high-velocity fragment can be devastating. Sudden blunt force to the anterior portion of the eyeball results in tears of the iris, ciliary body, or other ocular structures. Occasionally, rupture of the eyeball itself is seen. Vision can be restored in certain cases of blindness following closed blunt trauma to the eye by microscopic surgical decompression of the optic nerve in the optic canal.

Hemorrhage into the anterior chamber, or hyphema, resulting from blunt trauma is serious and quite common. Even a small amount of blood in the anterior chamber immediately after an injury is a grave prognostic sign. Severe bleeding may occur three to five days later, with persistent elevation of intraocular pressure or profound staining of the cornea with blood pigment. Intraocular pressure may be reduced by diuretics and intravenous urea. If the elevated pressure persists, irrigation with fibrin-olysin may be helpful in removing the clot from the anterior chamber.

Hemorrhage into the orbit due to injury to the ophthalmic artery may cause marked proptosis of the globe. Decompression through the lateral orbital septum may be necessary to salvage vision.

Other results of blunt trauma to the eyes include traumatic iridocyclitis, dislocation of the lens or rupture of the lens capsule, tearing of the choroid with choroidal hemorrhage, and retinal detachment.

Chemicals damage the eye by injuring the eyelids, conjunctiva, and cornea. The extent of the damage depends on the nature of the chemical and the length of time the substance is in contact with the ocular tissues. Acids are less damaging to the eye than alkalis, which cause the most serious chemical burns. Alkali appears to combine with the tissues, apparently in an active form, causing progressive damage over a long period of time.

Immediate and copious lavage with nonirritating fluid is of paramount importance. Isotonic saline usually is used in hospital emergency departments. Plain tap water or any nonirritating material should be used immediately after the injury. A rubber-bulb irrigating syringe is ideal for flushing conjunctival cul-de-sacs. Lavage should be continuous for 20 to 30 minutes when the patient is first seen and repeated every half hour. Local and systemic antibiotics should be administered immediately in an effort to avoid secondary infection. Steroid ophthalmic ointment and solutions may help prevent inflammation and secondary scarring. The use of atropine may be indicated. The prognosis is always guarded.

The serious sequela of chemical burns is corneal ulceration accompanied by corneal opacities, necrosis, or perforation. Scarring of the conjunctiva may occur with the development of symblepharon (adhesion of the lids to the eyeball).

BITES (ANIMAL AND HUMAN)

Animal bites and human bites must be considered separately. The bacterial inoculum of most animal bites is small. Infection usually does not ensue unless there was a great degree of crushing of tissues associated with the bite. Therefore, unless there is a large amount of contusion and crush, most animal bites can be debrided, copiously irrigated, and closed. There is not uniform agreement about the need for antibiotic coverage. An exception to this may be severe cat bites. They often are heavily contaminated with *Pasteurella multocida* and require treatment like a human bite.

Human bites, inflicted by someone other than the patient himself, differ from most animal bites. The bacterial count of human saliva is 10^7 to 10^8 bacteria per milliliter and this high degree of inoculum precludes primary closure of these wounds. However, bites of the face should be debrided, irrigated, and dressed until the bacterial level is reduced to a level compatible with successful delayed treatment. The use of systemic penicillin is justified for these wounds.

TREATMENT OF FACIAL BONE FRACTURES

The object of repair of facial fractures is the anatomical reduction and fixation of the displaced fragments. Many fractures need no treatment because of minimal displacement and a stable position. The simplest mechanism available should be used to reduce and stabilize a fracture. Many of the cumbersome indirect methods of the past have been supplanted by simpler, more direct methods. Comminuted fractures such as gunshot fractures are frequently best managed by indirect means such as packing, because direct exposure and wiring often leads to necrosis of the fragments and loss of substance.

FRACTURES OF THE MANDIBLE

Fractures of the mandible occurring in a tooth-bearing region are anatomically reduced by restoring occlusion and holding the patient's mouth in occlusion with arch bars or interdental wires and intermaxillary elastics. The maxillary dentition serves as the landmark to reduce the mandibular fragments. Fractures in the ramus of the mandible may or may not be reduced by restoring the dental occlusion. Fractures in the edentulous mandible can often be managed by securing the dentures to their respective arches and then maintaining occlusion as in the patient with teeth. It is frequently less cumbersome to manage such fractures by a direct reduction and fixation with a small metal plate. All mandibular fractures that cannot be reduced by indirect means should be considered for open reduction and direct wiring or plating at the fracture site.

FRACTURES OF THE MAXILLA

As in the case of fractures of the mandible, reduction of maxillary fractures is accomplished through re-establishment of the occlusion. But unlike the mandible, the maxilla lies free of its superior bony base and therefore the fractured maxilla must be suspended by wires from the superiorly located structure that is stable. In LeFort I and II fractures the zygomatic arches will serve as such a base, and in LeFort III fractures the zygomatic process of the frontal bone is commonly used. The intact mandible is used to establish occlusion prior to the superior suspension. Comminution of the fine interorbital bones is not rare. Indirect management by attachment of the medial canthal ligaments, one to the other with wire suture, and indirect support from external plates of metal or dental compound serve to reduce and immobilize these fragments.

Gunshot wounds of the maxillary antra commonly carry small bony fragments into this space. To avoid chronic sinusitis, it is frequently necessary to debride the involved antrum through a Caldwell-Luc incision in the upper labial gingival sulcus to establish a satisfactory nasoantral drainage. This is best done within the first two weeks after injury to avoid the difficulties encountered with fibrous consolidation of the fragments.

FRACTURES IN AND AROUND THE ORBIT

The zygomatic bone and arch fractures can be elevated and positioned by placement of an elevator under the fragment deep to the temporal fascia either from above (through the eyebrow or sideburn incision) or below (through a buccal sulcus incision). If there is instability after reduction, direct wiring at the lateral and inferior orbital rim may be necessary.

When the inferior rectus muscle has been demonstrated to be incarcerated in fractures of the orbital floor or when significant orbital contents have prolapsed into the maxillary antrum, the reduction of these blowout fractures can be accomplished from below by a Caldwell-Luc transantral approach or directly by exploration of the orbit through the lower eyelid. Many clinically inapparent blowout fractures that demonstrate minimal displacement roentgenographically will not require surgical treatment.

FRACTURES OF THE NOSE

Nasal fractures are usually the result of direct trauma and usually involve more than one fracture within the nasal pyramid. The inability to correct all the nasal deformities at the time of initial injury is sometimes frustrating. The following corrections of nasal fractures can and should be made in the emergency treatment:

1. Elevation of the depressed nasal dorsum with a padded instrument

2. Repositioning of the laterally displaced nose in its proper anatomic position

3. Repair of the badly torn nasal lining

4. Repositioning of the dislocated septum

5. Incision and drainage of septal hematomas

Following these maneuvers, nasal fractures require stabilization by a dressing. This should include a nasal packing of impregnated gauze (unless rhinorrhea is present), and an external splint made of light aluminum, plaster, or plastic held securely to the face with tape. Packing should not be done in the presence of rhinorrhea because this might lead to meningitis.

ANNOTATED BIBLIOGRAPHY

1. Schultz RC: Facial Injuries, 2nd ed. Chicago, Year Book Medical Publishers, Inc., 1977.
   An excellent brief text on the classification, description, and basic management of facial injuries commonly encountered in our society.
2. Thompson RVS: Primary Repair of Soft Tissue Injuries. Carlton, Victoria, Australia, Melbourne University Press, 1969.
   A very readable, well-illustrated manual outlining the repair of soft tissue injuries of the head and extremities.
3. Converse JM, Kazangian VH: Surgical Treatment of Facial Injuries, 3rd ed. Baltimore, Williams and Wilkins Co., 1974.
   The best reference book for definitive treatment of soft tissue and skeletal injuries of the face.
4. Touloukian RJ, Krizek TJ: Diagnoses and Early Management of Trauma Emergencies. Springfield, Charles C Thomas, 1974.
   This abbreviated manual with descriptive figures, tables, and rules is very useful in the emergency department to remind other members of the surgical team of the important features of diagnosis and early care.
5. Dingman RO, Natvig P: Surgery of Facial Fractures. Philadelphia, W.B. Saunders Co., 1964.
   Very well-illustrated text for diagnosis and treatment of facial fractures.
6. Robson MC, Krizek TJ, Heggers JP: The Biology of Surgical Infection. *In* Ravitch MM (ed): Current Problems of Surgery. Chicago, Year Book Medical Publishers, Inc., March, 1973.
   A review of the soft tissue response to bacteria elucidating the principles of quantitative bacteriology and antimicrobial usage.

Chapter

15

Neck

The neck contains many vital structures crowded into a small area; consequently, blunt or penetrating trauma to this region frequently injures one or more components of the vascular, neurological, respiratory, digestive, or skeletal systems. Serious injuries to the neck would be even more common were it not for the protection afforded posteriorly by the cervical spine and thick paracervical muscles and anteriorly by the shoulders and mandible, which shield the flexed neck.

The magnitude of the underlying injury is often obscured by an apparently innocent neck wound. Furthermore, a neck injury may be disregarded because concomitant head or chest trauma divert the examiner's attention. In either instance, failure to appreciate the seriousness of the neck injury may lead to tragic consequences — delayed hemorrhage, airway obstruction, deep neck infection, or cerebral infarction.

INITIAL MANAGEMENT

AIRWAY

The first priority in the management of patients with neck trauma is the establishment of an adequate airway. This may require the clearing of blood, secretions, broken teeth and dentures from the mouth; traction on the tongue; or insertion of an oral airway. In patients who are comatose or likely to aspirate, an endotracheal tube must be inserted. If the patient has sustained severe trauma to the larynx or trachea, an endotracheal tube often cannot be passed and an emergency airway must then be established below the area of injury by means of a tracheostomy or emergency cricothyroidotomy. The hypoxic patient may obtain temporary relief from the percutaneous insertion of a 14 gauge needle or Teflon catheter through the cricothyroid membrane. (See Chapter 1, *Tracheal Catheter.*)

Delayed airway obstruction is occasionally observed several hours after blunt neck trauma and results from the development of edema or an expanding hematoma that causes tracheal compression. Intrinsic laryngeal or tracheal edema may produce airway obstruction as late as 48 hours after injury. Continuous close observation of patients with blunt neck trauma will permit early recognition and treatment of delayed airway obstruction.

Emergency Cricothyroidotomy. If an emergency airway is necessary, suction, light, and a few simple instruments (including a scalpel) should be at hand. The patient's head is slightly extended and held in the midline and the thyroid and cricoid cartilages identified; this brings the cricothyroid membrane into prominence and a quick incision can be made directly into the larynx through the skin, subcutaneous tissue, and membrane (Fig. 15–1). This temporary operation can be done in less than a minute with a minimal loss of blood. As soon as the airway is established the patient is prepared for an elective tracheostomy.

Elective Tracheostomy. This procedure is done best in an operating room with a complete complement of lights, suction, instruments, and operating table. However, in extreme emergencies it can be done at the bedside with the patient's head raised, extended, and fixed and with adequate assistance available. Whenever possible, the patient's airway is controlled by means of a previously inserted endotracheal tube. Following skin preparation and draping, a transverse skin incision is made at the level of the second or third tracheal ring. The fascia and muscles are divided in a longitudinal direction and the thyroid isthmus retracted or divided.

A tracheal hook is extremely useful in grasping the trachea and delivering it into the wound. Many surgeons, particularly those who work with children, prefer to place stay sutures in the trachea and leave them in for 48 hours or longer to give ready control or access to the tracheostomy opening. Small right angle retractors, one for each side of the trachea, are also very useful. Care is taken to carry the dissection directly over the trachea and not to one side, and to identify and preserve or ligate any vascular structures crossing the trachea. After the cervical fascia is divided,

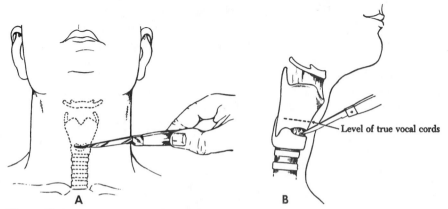

Figure 15–1. Emergency cricothyroidotomy. Site of incision: *A*, Anterior view. *B*, Lateral view.

most of the dissection, to the level of the trachea itself, can be accomplished bluntly. When the trachea is reached, it is firmly grasped with a tracheal hook or by stay sutures before it is opened. Arguments exist as to whether a portion of a tracheal ring should be excised. If a portion of ring is excised there is less possibility of complete obstruction if a tracheostomy tube slips out of the trachea before a fibrous tract is formed. However, loss of a portion of ring may increase the incidence of tracheal scarring and post-tracheostomy narrowing. The tracheal rings are identified and care taken not to place the tracheostomy too high or too low. The most common error, especially in children, is to place the opening too low. If the opening is made between the second and third tracheal rings and the third ring is divided, difficulties with placement are avoided.

The tracheostomy tube should be selected carefully. It should fit the trachea snugly, without unduly compressing the walls, and should be of sufficient length to extend into the trachea to the level of the fifth or sixth ring, but not so long as to pass down a bronchus. Modern tracheostomy tubes are constructed of flexible plastic materials with soft low-pressure balloons to decrease tracheal trauma. To secure the tube in place it is best to affix a strap to the tube externally and pass it completely around the neck, fastening it with a square knot. Some surgeons also prefer to suture the tube to the skin opening. After the tube is in place, light packing is placed around it that can be removed in 24 hours. The tracheostomy tube should not be changed for 48 hours unless it becomes occluded. After 48 hours, a fibrous tract has begun to form so that the tube can be easily replaced.

NECK STABILIZATION

While the primary importance of a patient's airway cannot be overemphasized, protection of the spinal cord must not be overlooked. Patients with head and neck trauma, especially those who are unconscious, should be treated as though their cervical spine were fractured until this possibility can be excluded. The head and neck are continuously supported in a neutral position until anteroposterior and lateral x-rays of the cervical spine are obtained. Hyperextension of the neck in an attempt to visualize the larynx may result in irreparable damage to the cervical spinal cord if cervical fractures are present. When this possibility exists, nasotracheal intubation or a temporary cricothyroidotomy (coniotomy) are safer alternatives (Fig. 15–1).

VENTILATION

Once an adequate airway has been established, proper ventilation must be assured. If necessary, ventilation is supported by whatever means available, e.g., mouth-to-mouth breathing, Ambu bag, or mechanical respirator. The chest is evaluated by physical examination and x-ray to assure that no hemothorax or pneumothorax exists that requires the immediate insertion of a thoracostomy tube.

HEMOSTASIS

In most instances, bleeding from penetrating neck wounds can be controlled with direct pressure. Blind clamping into a neck wound is strictly condemned as this may jeopardize the chances of primary vascular repair or produce permanent nerve damage.

INTRAVENOUS INFUSION

An intravenous line is ordinarily inserted into an upper extremity vein through which blood is drawn for typing, crossmatching, and hematocrit. In patients with injuries that cross the root of the neck, a lower extremity vein should be utilized for intravenous infusions in order to avoid inadvertent loss of fluids through a subclavian or innominate vein injury.

DETECTION OF INJURIES

Once the patient's initial examination and management have been completed, a thorough history and more complete physical examination should be performed. Special attention is directed toward the detection of the following groups of injuries.

VASCULAR

Vascular injuries are suspected if shock, active bleeding, or large, expanding hematomas are present. A potentially serious vascular injury may underlie an apparently small innocent neck wound in a patient who may not show any major clinical signs in the early stage.

Physical examination should include palpation of the carotid, superficial temporal, and upper extremity pulses with comparison of the quality of the pulses and blood pressure on both sides of the body. Diminished or absent pulses are good evidence of a vascular injury, but the pulses may be normal in the presence of a significant injury because: the artery is only partially severed and a good flow of blood continues into the distal vessel; the injured artery has no readily palpable point for evaluating distal pulses, e.g., internal carotid, vertebral, or thyrocervical trunk arteries; the patient is in shock, with all pulse determinations made difficult; or the injury is to the venous system.

Auscultation is an extremely important yet frequently overlooked mode of examination. A systolic bruit is a characteristic finding in patients with a partial arterial injury and a resultant false aneurysm, whereas a continuous bruit suggests the presence of a traumatic arteriovenous fistula.

Vertebral artery injuries are especially elusive but should be suspected whenever: a neurologic deficit develops in the centers supplied by the vertebral-basilar system (brain stem, cerebellum); carotid artery compression fails to slow the bleeding or obliterate a bruit coming from a wound whose apparent trajectory crosses the posterolateral aspect of the neck; or massive bleeding accompanies a cervical transverse process fracture. The fact that the vertebral artery is protected by the bony framework of the cervical transverse processes accounts for the failure of compression to control bleeding from this vessel.

Carotid artery injuries are often suspected in penetrating wounds of the neck but may also result from blunt trauma, and they should be considered in any patient with a hematoma in the upper anterior triangle of the neck, a Horner's syndrome (ptosis, miosis, enophthalmos and loss of sweating on the ipsilateral side of the face), transient ischemic attacks, loss of consciousness following a lucid interval, or the development of hemiplegia. These findings may be absent initially and appear days to weeks later when a slowly developing intramural hematoma obliterates the lumen of the carotid artery.

NEUROLOGICAL

The most important part of the complete neurological examination is the precise determination of the level of consciousness. An accurate and descriptive recording of the patient's initial level of consciousness is essential if subtle changes are to be detected that may suggest an intracranial injury or an expanding intramural hematoma of the extracranial carotid artery.

The most serious neurological effect of neck injury is quadriplegia, which results from severing the cervical spinal cord. Trauma to the root of the neck may produce brachial plexus damage, usually in association with a vascular injury.

The vagus, recurrent laryngeal, spinal accessory, hypoglossal, phrenic, and cervical sympathetic nerves are also subject to injury from neck trauma. These injuries are easily overlooked unless a detailed neurological examination is performed. Vagus and recurrent laryngeal nerve injuries usually produce hoarseness and are confirmed by observing an immobile vocal cord on direct or indirect laryngoscopy. The spinal accessory and hypoglossal nerves are assessed by noting the motor function of the trapezius and tongue muscles respectively. A cervical sympathetic nerve injury is recognized by the presence of an ipsilateral Horner's syndrome.

Trachea and Larynx

Injuries to the trachea and larynx are suspected in patients with dyspnea, hoarseness, stridor, or subcutaneous emphysema (Fig. 15–2). These injuries are seen most frequently in patients who have sustained blunt neck trauma as occurs in automobile accidents in which the neck abuts against a steering wheel or dashboard. Fractures of the larynx or trachea can often be palpated through the overlying intact skin.

Pharynx and Esophagus

Severe pain and dysphagia are characteristic symptoms of a perforation of the pharynx or esophagus. Physical examination should include digital palpation of the oropharynx and hypopharynx, as well as careful palpation of the neck in an attempt to feel subcutaneous crepitation.

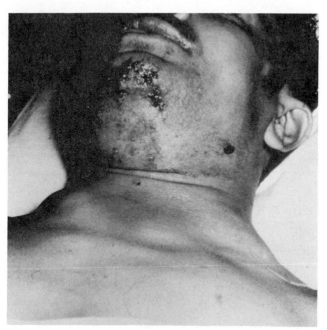

Figure 15–2. Patient who sustained a fractured larynx in an automobile accident. Note the visible neck swelling which represents subcutaneous emphysema.

INTRATHORACIC

An intrathoracic injury should always be suspected in patients with penetrating wounds of the neck. The path of a knife blade may be difficult to determine, and stab wounds, as well as gunshot wounds, of the neck can produce hemothorax, pneumothorax, and occasionally cardiac tamponade.

Initial physical examination and chest x-ray may be normal. However, if positive pressure breathing is instituted, a small previously unrecognized injury to the lung parenchyma may allow for the development of a life-threatening tension pneumothorax. A high index of suspicion, repeat physical examination, chest x-ray, and occasionally diagnostic thoracocentesis are warranted if the patient's condition deteriorates rapidly.

DIAGNOSTIC PROCEDURES

After the physical examination has been completed, the following diagnostic procedures should be performed unless immediate surgical intervention becomes necessary.

NECK X-RAYS

Anteroposterior and lateral films of the neck help to detect displacement of the trachea, narrowing of the airway, subcutaneous emphysema, cervical fractures, and retained missile fragments (Fig. 15–3).

CHEST X-RAYS

Posteroanterior and lateral chest films may reveal widening of the superior mediastinum, pneumomediastinum, pneumothorax, or hemothorax (Fig. 15–4).

ESOPHAGRAM

A barium esophagram is informative if extravasation is noted; however, a normal study does not exclude esophageal injury (Fig. 15–5).

ENDOSCOPY

Direct laryngoscopy, tracheoscopy, and esophagoscopy are extremely helpful in locating injuries to the larynx, trachea and esophagus. Whenever

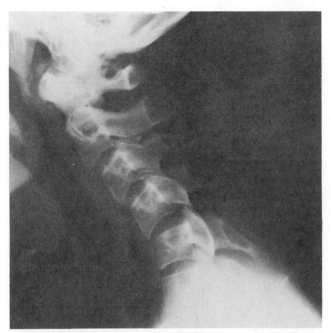

Figure 15–3. Lateral x-ray of the neck in patient who sustained blunt trauma. Note the subluxation of C4 over C5, the fractured hyoid bone and the retrotracheal air collection.

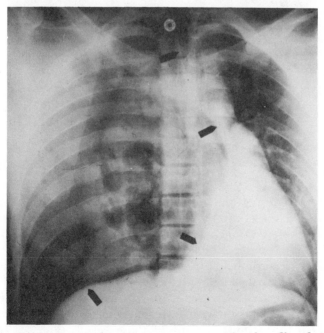

Figure 15–4. Tension pneumothorax seen on posteroanterior chest film of a patient who sustained a stab wound of the right neck. Note marked shift of the mediastinum to the left.

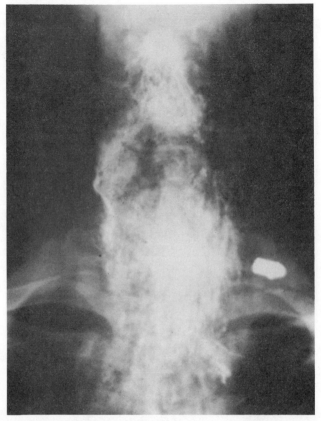

Figure 15–5. Barium esophagram showing extravasation of contrast material from a gunshot wound of the cervical esophagus.

possible, these procedures should be performed in the operating room immediately prior to neck exploration.

ARTERIOGRAPHY

When considering the need for arteriography, neck injuries are categorized into one of three zones (Zone I, below the sternal notch; Zone II, between the sternal notch and the angle of the mandible; and Zone III, above the angle of the mandible) (Fig. 15–6).

Injuries extending below the sternal notch (Zone I) should be evaluated with a preoperative retrograde femoral aortic archogram. This allows good visualization of the innominate, common carotid, subclavian, and vertebral arteries and is invaluable in determining the appropriate operative approach to an injury of any of these vessels (Fig. 15–7). Injuries confined to Zone II are easily exposed and repaired and therefore

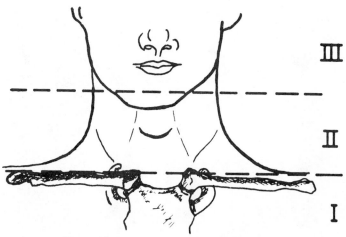

Figure 15–6. Zones of injury in neck trauma.

arteriography is not essential for their evaluation. Injuries extending into Zone III should be evaluated with a carotid arteriogram, preferably performed in selective fashion through the retrograde femoral route. This gives specific information about the status of the internal carotid artery and the intracerebral circulation, and helps to determine the feasibility of repair as well as the possible consequences of ligation (Fig. 15–8).

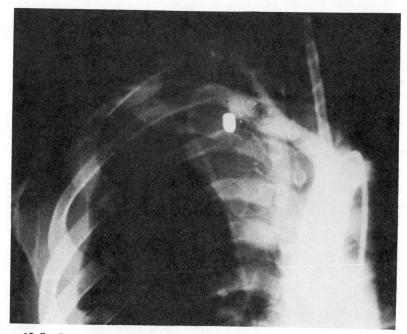

Figure 15–7. Retrograde femoral aortogram demonstrating transection of the proximal right subclavian artery in a patient who sustained a gunshot wound of the right neck.

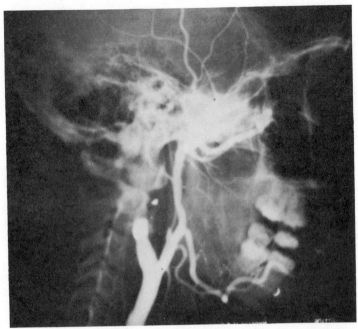

Figure 15-8. Carotid arteriogram from a patient who sustained a gunshot wound to Zone III. Note complete thrombosis of internal carotid artery.

SURGICAL EXPLORATION

Surgical exploration of the neck is imperative in all patients whose neck wound penetrates the platysma muscle layer. If the depth of the wound is uncertain, it should be assumed that the platysma muscle has been penetrated. Probing of neck wounds is never justified. Routine exploration of penetrating neck wounds has decreased mortality figures by eliminating the late complications of hemorrhage, airway obstruction, and neck abscess. A nasogastric tube inserted while the patient is in the operating room prevents gastric dilatation and aspiration, and aids in identifying the esophagus during the operation. The operative field is widely prepared and draped to provide exposure of the entire anterior chest and neck. General anesthesia is employed in all instances.

INCISIONS

An incision from the angle of the mandible to the sternoclavicular joint, paralleling the anterior border of the sternocleidomastoid muscle, provides excellent exposure to the important ipsilateral structures of the midneck. This incision is extended down through the midline of the sternum if the preoperative arteriogram has demonstrated an injury to the intrathoracic portion of the innominate, right subclavian, or left common carotid artery. The intrathoracic portion of the left subclavian artery is approached through an anterior thoracotomy in the left third intercostal space. The vertebral arteries and the extrathoracic portion of the subclavian arteries are approached through a supraclavicular incision combined with resection of the medial half of the clavicle if necessary. Injuries that traverse both sides of the neck are explored through a transverse or "collar" incision.

MANAGEMENT OF SPECIFIC NECK INJURIES

VASCULAR

Injuries to the innominate, common carotid, subclavian, vertebral, and internal carotid arteries are repaired by either lateral arteriorrhaphy, resection and end-to-end anastomosis, saphenous vein patch, or bypass. Synthetic grafts are avoided because of their increased potential for infection in the presence of a contaminated wound. Injuries to the internal carotid artery near the base of the skull pose a difficult problem in repair, and occasionally ligation of the proximal artery and packing the distal stump with muscle is required. In patients with evidence of cerebral infarction associated with a carotid injury, repair of the injured vessel is probably not advisable because of the likelihood of converting an ischemic cerebral infarction to a hemorrhagic one with progressive neurological deterioration. All other carotid injuries are repaired utilizing (when necessary) an internal shunt for cerebral protection. The remaining arteries and veins in the neck may be safely ligated, although repair is frequently performed if it can be accomplished without difficulty. Pressure should be immediately applied to all venous injuries in order to avoid air embolism.

NEUROLOGICAL

Injuries to any of the important nerves of the neck are easily overlooked unless they have been suspected prior to operation. Once recognized, these injuries are carefully debrided and the nerve repaired with fine synthetic sutures approximating the perineurium. Fracture dislocations are ordinarily reduced with traction; however, operative reduction may be necessary. Laminectomy is reserved for patients with deteriorating neurological findings, usually with x-ray evidence of bony fragments or missiles within the spinal canal.

TRACHEA AND LARYNX

Laryngeal and tracheal injuries must be primarily repaired, otherwise strictures and stenoses will develop. Minor hematomas, lacerations, and undisplaced fractures of the larynx, resulting from blunt trauma, may require only close observation, broad-spectrum antibiotics, and high humidity. More serious lacerations or contusions of the larynx that result in the loss of mucosa must be treated with split thickness skin grafts held in place by an internal stent for two to three weeks. Severely displaced fractures of the larynx require open reduction, mucosal repair, or grafting, and internal stenting for six to nine months. Large avulsion injuries of the trachea may require replacement with Marlex mesh.

PHARYNX AND ESOPHAGUS

Injuries to the pharynx and esophagus are debrided and closed in two layers. Broad-spectrum antibiotics are administered and the wound is drained for three or four days. Large defects in the cervical esophagus may be impossible to repair primarily, and in this situation both ends of the esophagus are brought out of the wound as cutaneous esophagostomies. Staged reconstruction of the cervical esophagus is subsequently accomplished.

Small defects in the esophagus may be difficult to visualize. An overlooked esophageal injury will invariably lead to the development of deep neck infections and mediastinitis. In order to avoid missing these injuries, the neck wound should be filled with saline, and positive pressure breathing per mask should be administered prior to completing the neck exploration. Escaping air bubbles seen in the saline can be traced to the site of esophageal injury.

MISCELLANEOUS

Injuries to the thyroid and salivary glands are treated by debridement, thorough hemostasis, and neck drainage. Thoracic duct injuries are suspected when a milky fluid accumulates in the operative field. The duct is carefully searched for and ligated.

Chapter

16

Blood Vessels

Advances in vascular surgery have changed our attitude toward injuries of the blood vessels. The time-honored procedures of ligation of major vessels or amputation of a limb, based on the concept of saving life, are infrequently indicated. The modern techniques of direct operative repair and early restoration of blood flow have immensely extended the surgeon's opportunities — and his responsibilities. The techniques of arterial reconstruction should be familiar to every surgeon who may be called upon to deal with major trauma.

URGENCY OF TREATMENT

The time lag from injury to operation has therefore taken on new meaning. Prompt treatment is essential not only to prevent death from exsanguination but also to improve the chances for successful restoration of arterial blood flow. There is no precise time in which the anoxic damage to tissues that are deprived of blood supply becomes irreversible. Furthermore, each case varies according to the site of injury and adequacy of collateral flow. Experience has shown, however, that the best results are obtained when vascular repair is accomplished within eight hours after injury. Adequate assistance during operation and the facilities of a well-equipped operating room are essential for success.

CARE IN TRANSIT

The most crucial factor from the time of injury until arrival in the hospital is intervention in life-threatening problems, namely, maintenance of airway and treatment of shock. Treatment of shock includes control of external bleeding. Continued bleeding through a dressing may be controlled by use of a blood pressure cuff placed proximally and inflated above systolic pressure. Patients with potential vascular injuries associated with obvious fractures of long bones should have the injured limb splinted prior to transit to prevent further injury to the neurovascular structures. Attempts at restoration of blood volume before and during transit may be valuable if the patient will be in transit for more than 30 minutes to an appropriate trauma facility.

EMERGENCY DEPARTMENT RESUSCITATION

Continued external bleeding upon arrival at the emergency department is also best controlled by a pressure dressing or, if that fails, by a proximal sphygmomanometer tourniquet inflated above systolic pressure. One should avoid harried, rapid attempts at "clamping" the injured artery in the emergency facility setting. This is fraught with the risk of failure and frequently leads to irreparable damage to the involved artery. Likewise, local explorations without proper lighting and assistance should be discouraged. Some patients have absent distal pulses in association with dislocations or fractures. Dislocations require immediate reduction to relieve arterial kinking, compression, or entrapment. Examples of such dislocations include 90-degree eversion dislocations of the ankle, anterior dislocations of the shoulder, and posterior knee dislocations. Return of pulse following dislocation eliminates the threat of early limb loss, but one should obtain an arteriogram to rule out arterial injury.

DIAGNOSIS

The classic signs of arterial injury include external bleeding, large or enlarging hematoma, absent or decreased pulse, absent or decreased motor and sensory function, swelling, pain at the site of injury, distal pain caused by ischemia, pallor, coldness, and thrill and bruit if an arteriovenous fistula is present. If one or more of these signs or symptoms are present, the diagnosis of arterial injury should be assumed and subsequently checked by either emergency arteriography or exploration of the involved artery. Absence of all of these signs or symptoms, however, is still compatible with arterial injury. Because of this, all patients with a penetrating wound in proximity to a major artery should have arteriography, if available, to rule out a vascular injury. The urgency to diagnose and repair an injured artery immediately after injury is obviously not as critical in patients without positive signs or symptoms, but patients with poor distal flow and ischemia require early operative repair.

All patients with long bone fractures and decreased pulse should be suspected of having an arterial injury. Spasm should never be diagnosed without arteriographic or operative confirmation. In the unusual instance when spasm is confirmed by arteriography, intra-arterial injection of vasodilators such as papaverine may be beneficial.

PRINCIPLES OF OPERATIVE TREATMENT

Hemostasis is the first priority. Control of external bleeding through most penetrating limb wounds is best achieved in the operating room by digital pressure directly over the perforated artery. Surgical prep and surgical incision are then performed around the occluding finger. Occasionally, this technique is unsuccessful and a proximal tourniquet must be placed.

Proximal and Distal Control

All incisions should be made along the pathway of the involved vessel and should be kept between the natural anatomical planes to avoid unnecessary injury to associated muscles, nerves, and smaller vessels. During operation, both proximal and distal control should be obtained before dissection of the injured segment. When the injury is at the interface of two anatomical compartments, proximal control should be achieved in the proximal anatomical compartment. This objective is achieved by a suprainguinal incision and a retroperitoneal isolation of the external iliac artery for common femoral artery injuries, a supraclavicular incision and isolation of the subclavian artery for distal subclavian or axillary injuries, and median sternotomy and isolation of the appropriate aortic vessels for innominate, proximal subclavian, or common carotid arterial injuries. A left thoracotomy and clamping of the descending aorta immediately above the diaphragm provides excellent proximal control in those patients with suspected abdominal aorta injuries, severe shock that is unresponsive to fluid administration, and significant abdominal distention.

Vascular Repair

When the care of severe associated injuries will delay vascular repair, a temporary shunt, such as the Javid shunt, provides good distal perfusion prior to vascular reconstruction. Once the repair is begun, the injured artery is dissected free and the adventitia should be removed from the media 3 to 5 mm proximal and distal to the site of subsequent repair. A Fogarty balloon catheter should then be passed distally to extract possible clots, after which 15 to 25 ml of heparin solution (100 u/ml) should be instilled in the distal artery through a Fogarty irrigating catheter. Passage of the Fogarty balloon catheter proximally is usually not necessary but the proximal instillation of 3 to 5 ml of heparin solution (100 u/ml) is recommended.

The suture used for arterial repair should be monofilament polyethylene suture; size varies from 3–0 for the abdominal aorta to 7–0 for vessels in the forearm or calf. The technique of vascular repair varies with the type and severity of the injury.

Simple closure or lateral suture is indicated for clean, partial circumferential knife wounds. The end-to-end anastomosis is indicated for most knife wounds, gunshot wounds, and lacerations caused by bone fragments. Contusions to the wall of arteries are best treated by resection of the contused segment and an end-to-end anastomosis; there is no other way to rule out significant intimal damage. The artery resected should extend approximately 1 mm beyond the site of gross injury. The surgeon must carefully rule out unobtrusive injury to the intima prior to arterial reconstruction.

Arterial segments up to 3 cm may be resected prior to a safe, tension-free, end-to-end anastomosis. The end-to-end anastomosis is most easily accomplished by placing and tying two lateral sutures 180 degrees apart. The assistant holding the atraumatic vascular clamps must keep tension off these sutures while they are being tied and throughout the subsequent repair. Each corner suture is then used to approximate the anterior and posterior walls respectively using the continuous technique, placing each subsequent bite approximately 0.5 mm from the previous bite and 0.5 to 1 mm from the anastomosis line. Just before completion of the anastomosis, the distal clamp is removed, allowing a small amount of air and some blood to escape, and the proximal clamp is then released. Any oozing through needle holes or between sutures is readily controlled by gentle finger pressure for five minutes. Occasionally an additional interrupted suture is needed; this suture must be carefully placed so as not to narrow the lumen. The "splay" technique, in which both ends to be approximated are cut at an angle, is useful for repairing small arteries.

More extensive injuries require resection of a longer segment of artery, and therefore need arterial replacement. Such injuries are usually seen with shotgun wounds, rifle wounds, or blunt injuries with long bone fractures. Arterial replacement is best achieved with a saphenous vein taken from the uninjured limb. Patients with injury to larger vessels such as the abdominal aorta or patients without available saphenous veins may require prosthetic replacement of the injured artery. Following reconstruction, operative arteriography should be employed if there is any question concerning the adequacy of patency or distal flow. Drainage of the wound is optional, but when it is used, soft rubber Penrose drains for 24 to 48 hours are preferred.

COVERAGE OF VASCULAR REPAIR

Following vascular reconstruction, the repaired vessel should be covered by adjacent soft tissues. This is usually no problem, because the vessel ordinarily lies in its normal anatomical plane surrounded by muscle and subcutaneous tissue. Occasionally, however, associated large soft tissue defects preclude both coverage of the vessel and primary wound closure. In most such instances, protection of the vascular repair can be achieved by placing a long saphenous graft through an uninvolved extra-anatomical plane and well away from the area of the large soft tissue defect. For example, an ileopopliteal bypass graft through the obturator foramen provides vein graft protection in patients with massive shotgun wounds to the anterior and medial thigh.

Occasionally, patients with massive soft tissue defects and arterial injury do not have an uninvolved extra-anatomical plane, thereby precluding coverage of the vascular repair. Although in the past this has been considered as indication for amputation, some success has been achieved by placing a long saphenous vein graft on a healthy viable muscle. This graft is then covered by split-thickness porcine skin grafts that are changed every 48 hours for a period of four to six weeks. At the end of this period the completely granulated wound is covered by a split-thickness autogenous skin graft.

The associated massive soft tissue injury from either a shotgun wound, rifle wound, or occasionally a shearing pedestrian injury should be treated by thorough debridement and dressed open. Primary closure of these wounds increases the incidence of infection and results in further necrosis of soft tissues. The adequacy of debridement in such wounds is often questionable, so that a "second look" under general anesthesia at 24 to 48 hours is helpful.

ASSOCIATED LONG BONE FRACTURES

Patients with closed wounds and transverse midshaft long bone fractures are best treated by combined intermedullary rodding and vascular reconstruction. Patients with open comminuted fractures are best treated by balanced skeletal traction, care being taken to interpose healthy muscle between the vein graft and the bony fragment to prevent subsequent injury in the postoperative period.

FASCIOTOMY

Long medial and lateral fasciotomies through the skin, subcutaneous tissues, and muscle fasciae are indicated in those patients with moderate to severe problems of ischemia before surgery as reflected by minimal changes in motor or sensory function or a moderate degree of calf or compartment swelling, tightness, or changing calf contour. In patients who have substantial loss of motor or sensory function preoperatively, massive soft tissue defects with interruption of deep and superficial venous system, or a prolonged interval before an operation that includes venous ligation, a complete fasciotomy using the fibulectomy-fasciotomy technique should be seriously considered. This fasciotomy provides decompression of all four compartments. If there is some question concerning the extent of fasciotomy needed at the time of surgery, measurement of the tissue pressure in the calf muscles will be helpful. Whenever tissue pressure is greater than 45 cm of water, a fibulectomy-fasciotomy should be performed. Following fasciotomy, the underlying muscles bulge through the fasciotomy incisions until the edema subsides, after which they are covered by split-thickness skin grafts.

POSTOPERATIVE CARE

The most important priority postoperatively is to maintain the vascular volume and blood pressure so as to keep the vascular repair open. The addition of heparin, other anticoagulants, or low molecular weight dextran is no substitute for good operative technique. Absence or disappearance of pulse in the immediate postoperative period is an indication for immediate arteriography and subsequent operative re-exploration if correctable mechanical problems exist.

Splinting of the involved limb in the early postoperative period prevents sudden movement and damage to the repaired artery, particularly in those patients with associated fractures. When swelling is present in the postoperative period, it is best to keep the patient at bed rest until the swelling or edema has subsided. If no swelling is present, early ambulation is most beneficial.

VENOUS INJURIES

A venous injury should be suspected in any patient with significant swelling or edema in whom an arteriogram shows no arterial damage. Such patients are candidates for venography in order to confirm the venous injury and to provide a road map for subsequent exploration when the hematoma is evacuated and an attempt is made to repair the venous injury.

The operative approach for venous injuries is the same as for arterial injuries. The type of repair for venous injuries varies with the extent of injury but in most instances a simple lateral repair can be accomplished. This repair may produce some narrowing, but the narrowing is usually insignificant in the postoperative period. Small injuries, which cannot be repaired by a lateral repair, are best treated by end-to-end anastomosis. Larger injuries, particularly in those patients with significant soft tissue injuries, are best treated by venous ligation. Interposition of a saphenous vein for a large venous injury is seldom indicated and should be reserved for those patients without other major injuries in whom prolongation of the operative time will not seriously increase operative risk. Synthetic graft interposition for large venous injuries needs further clinical evaluation. Most patients with venous ligation do well if the involved limb is kept elevated following operation.

Patients with massive soft tissue injuries resulting in ligation of both the deep and superficial venous systems should have fibulectomy-fasciotomy with decompression of all four muscle compartments. The legs of such patients must be kept elevated for a period of four to six weeks until the limb edema has completely subsided. If edema recurs when the patient begins to walk again, elevation should be reinstituted until all edema has subsided. Almost all patients will develop adequate collateral circulation if the limb is kept elevated long enough.

PRIMARY AMPUTATION

Primary amputation may be the better part of valor when other life-threatening injuries take priority. When the surgeon is faced with life-threatening hemorrhage elsewhere that requires his primary and prolonged attention, amputation may be the most effective way to control severe bleeding from a gravely damaged limb. Furthermore, primary amputation may be indicated in aged patients who have little likelihood of good functional return because of major injury to associated nerves and soft tissues. Finally, primary amputation is indicated in patients with complete neurovascular severance and massive soft tissue loss when primary repair carries too high a risk of infection and lethal bleeding from an exposed anastomosis. Amputation is indicated also when there is the possibility of a functional return that, if successful, would be marginal.

17

Peripheral Nerves

Loss of peripheral nerve function can result from contusion, stretch, traumatic devascularization, or transection. In contusion, stretch, or traumatic devascularization:

1. The nerve sheath is intact.
2. The loss of function may be physiological and not anatomical.
3. Function may return through the natural healing process.
4. Early attempts at surgical "repair" are not indicated.
5. The injury should be identified and its location noted.

In cases of transection:

1. Surgical repair is indicated primarily or secondarily (see below).
2. Axonal regrowth starts a few millimeters proximal to the point of injury and takes place at a rate of about 1.5 mm per day.
3. Exact anatomical alignment of nerve ends promotes regeneration.
4. Malalignment of nerve ends may impede or prevent axonal regeneration.
5. Tissue between the nerve ends prevents axonal regeneration.

Loss of function from paralyzed muscles should be treated, when indicated, by appropriate static and dynamic splints and passive range of motion exercises. The patient should be instructed concerning the problem of decreased sensibility in both the upper and lower extremities.

DIAGNOSIS

Peripheral nerve injury should be suspected and carefully searched for during examination of an injured extremity. Injury to specific nerves can be identified by evidence of the loss of specific sensory and motor functions distal to the level of injury.

Upper Extremity

1. Median Nerve

a. *Sensory* — loss of sensibility over the palmar aspect of the thumb, the index and long fingers, and radial half of the ring finger (Fig. 17–1).

b. *Motor* — loss of ability to rotate the thumb to a position of grasp. (Such loss is present in approximately one third of patients with median nerve injury.)

c. *Median injury above the elbow* — inability to flex the thumb and index phalanges. Inability to forcefully flex the wrist or pronate the forearm.

2. Radial Nerve

a. *Sensory* — decreased sensibility over the radiodorsal aspect of the forearm and the dorsum of the thumb, the index and long fingers, and part of the ring finger (Fig. 17–1).

b. *Motor* — inability to extend the wrist and the fingers at the metacarpophalangeal joint and the thumb at all joints.

3. Ulnar Nerve

a. *Sensory* — decreased sensibility, both dorsal and palmar, over the little finger and ulnar half of the ring finger (Fig. 17–1).

b. *Motor* — inability to spread and close the fingers or achieve flexion of the metacarpophalangeal joints without interphalangeal flexion. Weak thumb pinch. Hyperextension of the metacarpophalangeal joint and flexion of the interphalangeal. Clawing of ulnar two digits is present in most patients.

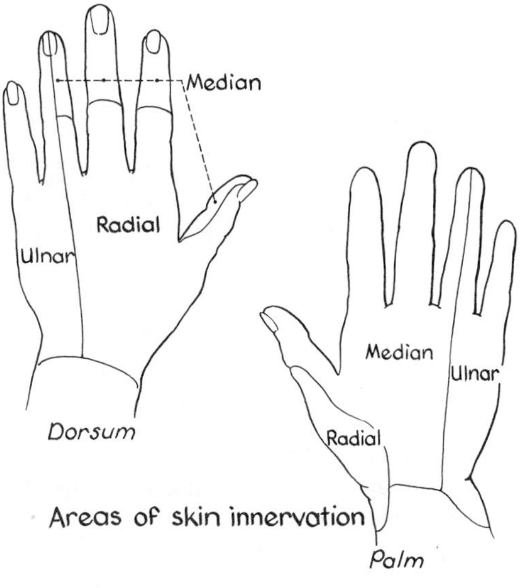

Figure 17–1. Sensory distribution in the left hand for the radial, ulnar, and median nerves.

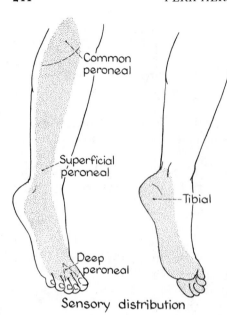

Figure 17–2. Sensory distribution in the lower extremity for the peroneal and tibial nerves.

4. Brachial Plexus

    a. *Sensory* — mixed area losses, depending on the location of the lesion in plexus.

    b. *Motor* — no clear peripheral nerve distribution, but mixed weakness of the arm, forearm, and hand musculature, depending on the location of the injury in plexus.

LOWER EXTREMITY

1. Peroneal Nerve

    a. *Superficial branch*

        (1) *Sensory* — decreased sensibility over dorsum of the foot and toes (Fig. 17–2).

        (2) *Motor* — loss of ability to evert foot (paralysis of peronerus longus and brevis).

    b. *Deep branch*

        (1) *Sensory* — decreased sensibility in first web space between the great and second toe (Fig. 17–2).

        (2) *Motor* — inability to dorsiflex the ankle or extend the toes.

2. Tibial Nerve

    a. *Sensory* — decreased sensibility over the plantar aspect of the foot (Fig. 17–2).

    b. *Motor* — loss of plantar flexion of the ankle and toes.

3. Sciatic Nerve

Combination of the motor and sensory losses for tibial and peroneal nerves. If the injury is in proximal thigh, motor loss may include weakness of knee flexion.

TREATMENT

When it is clear that a peripheral nerve has been transected, a decision must be made whether repair should be undertaken primarily or secondarily. Immediate suture saves time in regeneration and may reduce scar formation at the site of the nerve injury. With it another operation may be avoided. However, it is time consuming, requires accurate identification of "normal" nerve ends, and demands meticulous operative technique. Late repair does not jeopardize the final result of nerve suture if performed within three to six months.

EARLY REPAIR

The indications for early repair are as follows:

1. A clean wound.
2. Availability of soft tissue for coverage of nerve repair.
3. Nerve suture without tension.
4. Ideal patient condition for operative procedure.
5. Familiarity of the surgeon with nerve suture technique.

Contraindications to early repair are:

1. Gross contamination.
2. Established infection.
3. Extensive contusion, in addition to laceration of the nerve.
4. Inadequate soft tissue coverage for the sutured nerve.
5. Significant segmental loss of nerve tissue.
6. Other injuries requiring life-saving attention.

The technique of early repair consists of:

1. Careful debridement (see Chapter 18).

2. Adequate identification of the nerve. The cut ends of the nerve and tendons are occasionally confused, particularly in the hand, with the result that one may be sutured to the other. Identification can be readily made according to the criteria in Table 17–1. The use of magnification to aid in identification and precise repair is highly recommended.

3. Debridement of the uncontused nerve proximally and distally with a sharp blade.

TABLE 17–1. CRITERIA FOR NERVE IDENTIFICATION

Nerve	*Tendon*
A. Soft	A. Firm
B. Friable, capable of stretch	B. Inelastic and tough
C. Off-white or light ivory color	C. White, often "glistening"
D. Branches present	D. No branches
E. No true attachments	E. Attached to bone and muscle
F. Longitudinal fascicular arrangement	F. No longitudinal cords seen

4. Gentle approximation. The nerve ends must come together in a clean bed without tension. If necessary, the extremity may be flexed to accomplish this. If flexion of adjacent joints does not allow for a tension-free repair, a nerve graft reconstruction is indicated. Do not pinch the nerve; only the sheath should be handled with fine instruments.

5. Precise alignment
   a. Identify position of major fasciculi and consider epineural suture (Fig. 17–3) or modified fascicular repair (Fig. 17–4).
   b. Note the alignment of the epineural blood vessels proximally and distally.
   c. Place one coaptation suture at an identifiable point.

6. "Atraumatic" suture technique
   a. Use 8–0, 9–0, or 10–0 nonabsorbable suture depending on size of nerve.
   b. Pass the suture only through the nerve sheath.
   c. Preserve the alignment of the fascicular nerve ends.

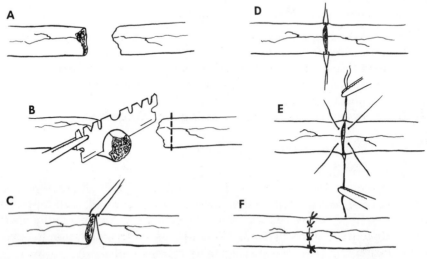

Figure 17–3. Technique for epineural nerve repair. *A* and *B*, Recut ragged nerve ends. *C*, After lubrication of suture materials in local fat, place primary suture with surface vessels properly aligned. *D*, *E*, and *F*, Sutures in nerve sheath only.

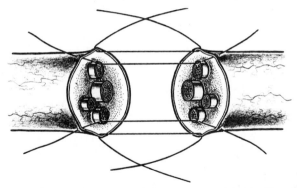

Figure 17–4. Modified fascicular nerve repair. (From Boswick JA: Neural Microsurgery in Reconstructive Microsurgery. *In* Reconstructive Microsurgery. R. K. Daniel and J. K. Terzis. Little, Brown and Co., Boston, 1977.)

    d. Four to six stitches are usually sufficient for epineural suture (Fig. 17–3).

Immobilization can be established as follows:

1. Place the limb in a position that will relax the sutured nerve.
2. Apply a well-padded splint.
3. Keep the part immobilized for three weeks.
4. If necessary, extend the limb gradually to avoid early tension on the repair by reapplying splints with the limb in appropriate position.

POSTOPERATIVE CARE

Postoperatively, treatment is as follows:

1. Avoid injury to the areas with loss of sensibility. The lack of protective sensibility sets the stage for a patient to sustain inadvertent, unrecognized injury.

2. After a period of immobilization, it is essential to provide splinting and passive motion to prevent postparalytic contracture.

3. Electrical stimulation of paralyzed muscles may minimize denervation atrophy in the period before reinnervation and return of voluntary motor function. However, dynamic splinting with carefully balanced traction that functions continuously is effective in maintaining function.

4. Tinel's sign: About five weeks after suture, gently percuss the skin over the course of the severed nerve. Begin distally and proceed proximally until the patient reports an "electric shock" sensation in the sensory distribution of the nerve. This is the point to which regeneration has progressed distally from the suture line. Regeneration over a distance of about two inches should be apparent five weeks after operation.

Chapter

18

The Hand

The basic principles of early care of acute hand injuries are the prevention of further damage and the earliest possible restoration of maximal function. These objectives are best achieved by the careful handling and splinting of damaged parts, early reduction of fractures and dislocations, repair of tendons and nerves at an optimal time, and care of the wound so as to minimize contamination and infection. If these principles are followed, healing will occur without iatrogenic delay and rehabilitation can begin soon after the injury.

EVALUATION AND PLANNING

In making the initial evaluation and planning treatment, one should proceed as follows:

1. Assess the total patient for associated injuries, complicating medical conditions, and factors that would increase the risk of anesthesia.

2. Obtain a detailed history of the mechanism of injury in order to determine its severity and extent, to plan for the initial operation, and to assess the prognosis for eventual function.

3. Systematically evaluate all injured tissues before an anesthetic is given. This examination and evaluation should be done under sterile conditions, and a mask and gloves should be worn. Probing of the wound gives little information on the degree of damage to the deep parts; it adds to the risk of infection and may cause further injury.

4. Evaluate the injured parts of the hand in the following order:

Skin.   Estimate the established skin loss and any added loss anticipated from excision of the wound. Plan the methods and timing of closure.

Nerves.   Examine the hand for sensory and motor loss (see Chapter 17).

Bones and Joints.   Review multiple roentgenographic views in preference to unnecessary painful manipulation of injured tissues. Use the uninjured hand for comparison.

248

Tendons. Specifically test function of individual extensor and flexor tendons to demonstrate tendon or muscle disruption.

Blood Supply. Note the color of the hand and test for capillary return by digital pressure.

After evaluation, the priorities for immediate repair of the parts of the hand should be determined. The condition of the wound may preclude immediate repair of one or more of the parts. As a rule, each successive step depends on the preceding step.

Skin. If appropriate, close the wound to restore coverage to the hand in order to promote early healing.

Nerves. The decision as to whether damaged nerves are repaired at this point depends on a number of features (see Chapter 17).

Bones and Joints. Unless the hand has rigid members with good hinges, the repair of tendons is futile.

Tendons. Repair tendons if conditions are acceptable and if the foregoing prerequisites are favorable; otherwise plan a delayed repair.

OPERATION

OPERATING ROOM

The sterile techniques, equipment, and assistance available only in an operating room contribute to the quality of the final result. Only simple lacerations of the skin without damage to the other tissues should be repaired in an emergency department setting.

ANESTHESIA

General anesthesia or axillary block of the entire arm is preferred. The choice of type of anesthesia is based on the patient's age, recent food intake, associated injuries, and overall status, as well as the physician's familiarity with the various techniques.

TOURNIQUET

Work only in a bloodless field. Inflate a tourniquet on the upper arm to 250 to 300 mm Hg after the hand and forearm are emptied of blood by wrapping or by elevation. If the operation is prolonged, deflate the tourniquet for five to ten minutes at 90-minute intervals. Control bleeding and empty the arm of blood before inflating the tourniquet again. Before closing the wound, evaluate the circulation of the skin by releasing the tourniquet and noting the flush of postischemic vasodilation.

REPAIR OF THE PARTS OF THE HAND

Cleanse the wound gently but thoroughly with soap or detergent and water. Inspect the depths of the wound carefully. With meticulous care, excise all devitalized tissue and remove all foreign material. Enlarge the wound to allow cleansing and identification and repair of the injured parts. Avoid crossing flexion creases at right angles, "T" incisions, and the eminences of the hand.

Skin. If possible, close the wound to promote early wound healing. Accurately approximate sharply incised or carefully debrided skin edges to obtain prompt healing. This should be done only if the skin edges are viable and if they can be approximated without tension. Unfavorable conditions for closure include extensive contusion, contamination, presence of dirt or other foreign material that cannot be completely removed, and excessive length of time since injury. Under such circumstances, closure should be delayed. As to sutures, if in doubt, leave them out!

Use split-thickness skin as a permanent graft or as a dressing graft to close defects. A convenient donor site is the proximal volar surface of the forearm. Use direct pedicle flaps over avascular tissues or over moving parts, but only if conditions are ideal. Local pedicle flaps can be rotated up to 45 degrees to cover exposed bones, joints, or tendons. Base such a flap proximally and preserve the vascularity of the distal tip of the flap by careful incision and undermining. A digit with severe, irreversible damage that requires amputation may provide an excellent local pedicle flap after removal of bone and tendon.

Distant pedicle flaps from the abdomen or chest are rarely necessary. Such flaps are reserved for coverage of essential deep structures that cannot be covered by split-thickness grafts or local pedicle flaps.

Nerves. Primary nerve repair is often possible. Contraindications to primary repair include loss of substance, severe stretching or crushing of the nerves, and extensive mutilation and contamination.

Accurately align and meticulously but loosely approximate the freshened nerve ends with a few fine (8–0) sutures of nylon or polyethylene through the nerve sheath only, or with 10–0 sutures, repairing the individual fascicules. Nerves may be repaired to the level of the distal interphalangeal joint.

Bones and Joints. Accurate reduction of displaced bones and joints is necessary for optimal function of the moving structures of the hand. In a closed wound, if the reduction cannot be achieved easily by manipulation, open reduction and internal fixation may be necessary. Immobilize the hand with the fracture in a position of function. The major complication of fractures of the hand is stiffness; nonunion and osteomyelitis are rare. In most cases of fractures, the patient may begin active motion three to four weeks after injury.

In an open fracture, internal fixation may be necessary to maintain the

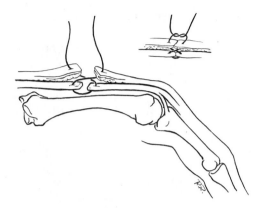

Figure 18–1. Use a simple figure-of-eight suture brought out through the skin to approximate the ends of a divided extensor tendon. Relieve tension by splinting, and resting the wrist and metacarpophalangeal joints in extension.

reduction. Loose closure of the subcutaneous tissue with skin edges left open is usually indicated.

Tendons.   Repair tendons unless there is a contraindication. Repair extensor tendons using a simple figure-of-eight wire suture brought out through the skin (Fig. 18–1) or use a horizontal crisscross suture (Fig. 18–2) or one or more simple horizontal mattress sutures. Relieve tension by extension of the wrist and metacarpophalangeal joints for three to five weeks.

Primary repair of flexor tendons should be performed when experienced personnel are available, unless the wound is grossly contaminated or the tissue is crushed or torn and primary healing is unlikely. Accurate approximation by a horizontal crisscross suture of 5–0 nylon, wire, or polyethylene (Fig. 18–2) is suitable for flexor tendons. Relieve tension by

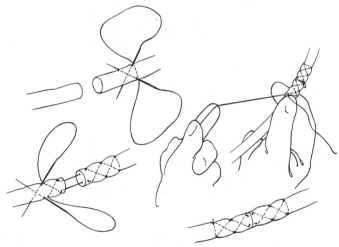

Figure 18–2. Use a horizontal crisscross suture to approximate the ends of a divided flexor tendon. Relieve tension by splinting the wrist in flexion with the fingers in a position of function.

splinting the wrist in 20 degrees of flexion with the fingers in a position of function for three weeks.

In the finger, repair one or both tendons. If the profundus tendon is severed at the level of the midportion of the middle or distal phalanx, repair by advancement; excise the distal portion and suture the proximal end into a short stump of the distal end. This places the repair distal to where the tendon glides (Fig. 18–3). For injuries in the fingers, dynamic

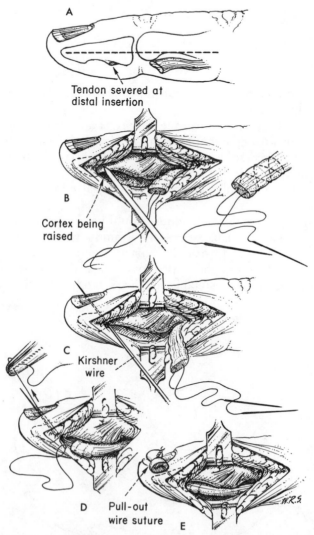

Figure 18–3. Flexor profundus advancement to tendon stump. *A,* Adequate tendon stump for tendon suture; *B,* tendon stump split; wire suture placed in proximal end of tendon; *C,* proximal end advanced to distal stump with pull-out wire through fingertip; *D,* tendon suture complete and pull-out wire tied over rubber catheter. (From Nora, PF: Operative Surgery, 2nd Ed. Lea & Febiger, Philadelphia, 1980.)

traction is indicated starting the day of surgery or one to two days postoperatively.

In the palm or thumb, a lacerated tendon can usually be repaired without jeopardizing motion of the uninjured tendons.

In the forearm, all tendons should be repaired for optimal balance of the hand, but adherence to other tendons may occur. Therefore, some loss of individual agility of the digits may be anticipated.

DRESSING

A bulky pressure dressing, usually with a plaster or metal splint, is useful for *compression* to minimize edema; for *immobilization* to decrease pain and aid in the healing of bones, joints, and soft tissues; and for *maintenance of position.*

1. Place nonadherent gauze in a single layer over the wounds.
2. Place gauze pads between the fingers.
3. Place the hand in a position of function, as reaching for a glass, with the wrist extended 20 degrees, the thumb in line with the radius, and the fingers slightly flexed with the tips equidistant from the tip of the thumb.
4. Keep in mind that the nature of the injury or repair may necessitate flexion or extension of the wrist or fingers.

AFTERCARE

The hand should be elevated on pillows or suspended while the patient is in bed. The hand and arm should be elevated when the patient is up. Undue pain may indicate tightness of the dressing. After one or two days, gentle, frequent, active motion should be encouraged in parts not requiring immobilization.

SPECIAL INJURIES

GREASE GUN INJURIES

These injuries result in the intrusion of grease through planes, spaces, and tendon sheaths. The grease causes an intense chemical reaction and subsequent fibrosis. Infection may add to the tissue destruction. Early decompression of all involved spaces and planes, plus removal of as much of the grease as possible, is indicated. Leave all spaces open to reduce the chance of infection. The same principles apply to injuries from paint guns and other high-pressure injection injuries.

Amputation of a Finger

1. Identify nerves, put them on a stretch, and divide them proximally so that they will retract as far as possible.
2. Preserve all possible length of bone; consider removal of articular cartilage if the amputation is through a joint.
3. Close the skin with a split-thickness skin graft to preserve length when indicated.
4. If bone is exposed, consider a pedicle flap.

Wringer Injuries

These injuries may result in ischemia, necrosis, and damage to the skin, tendon, muscle, and bone.

1. Gently clean the skin.
2. Apply a sterile bulky pressure dressing with the hand in the position of function.
3. Elevate the hand.
4. Change the dressing each day or as indicated.
5. Evacuate fluid, incise the fascia, and debride any necrotic tissue.

Crush (Corn Picker) Injuries

These and similar injuries crush, tear, and avulse skin, nerves, and tendons and cause multiple fractures.

1. Meticulously clean the wound, remove all foreign material, and excise all nonviable tissue, including skin, muscle, tendon, and bone.
2. Mold the fragments into position or pin large bone fragments when possible.
3. Delayed wound closure is usually indicated.

FRACTURES AND DISLOCATIONS IN THE HAND

These types of fractures and dislocations and their sites are listed in Table 18–1.

The basic objectives of management of these injuries are the *maintenance* of function of uninjured parts and the *maximum return* of function of fractured or dislocated parts. The principles by which these injuries should be treated call for the injured parts to be restored promptly to as near their normal relationships as is possible. Overzealous efforts to salvage badly injured digits must not be allowed to prejudice eventual function of those digits that were not injured.

TABLE 18–1. TYPES OF FRACTURES AND DISLOCATIONS
IN THE HAND

Fractures and Dislocations of the Thumb including the Metacarpal
Fractures of the base of the thumb metacarpal
Bennett's fractures
Fractures of the shaft of the thumb metacarpal
Fractures of the phalanges of the thumb
Dislocations of the metacarpophalangeal joint

Fractures of the Finger Metacarpals
Fractures of the shafts
Fractures of the necks of metacarpals

Fractures and Dislocations of the Phalanges of the Fingers
Fractures of the proximal phalanx
Fractures of the middle phalanx
Fractures of the distal phalanx
Mallet or baseball finger (or fracture)
Chip fractures
Dislocations of the metacarpophalangeal joints
Dislocations of the proximal interphalangeal joint

Splinting of the entire hand or parts of it in the position of function
often starts with immobilization of the wrist in slight dorsal flexion. The
finger or fingers are held in moderate flexion at each joint and the thumb is
held in slight rotation.

Only injured digits or, at times, uninjured contiguous digits should be
splinted. Uninjured digits usually should remain unsplinted to permit
active motion. Splints for fractures or dislocations of the hand should be
discontinued at the earliest practical time, which will vary according to the
specific injury or injuries.

FRACTURES AND DISLOCATION OF THE THUMB INCLUDING THE METACARPAL

Injuries to the thumb usually occur as a result of a fall or a blow on the
tip, although trauma at any point on the thumb that forces any part beyond
its normal range of movement may result in a fracture or dislocation or
both.

Fracture of the Base of the Thumb Metacarpal. Undisplaced
fractures require approximately four weeks in a plaster cast in which is
incorporated the entire thumb, the base of the hand, and the forearm.
Displaced fractures require accurate reduction. This often can be achieved
by manipulation under local or general anesthesia and maintained by a
cast.

Bennett's fracture is a fracture, partial dislocation, or subluxation of
the base of the thumb metacarpal, requiring precise reduction for an
optimal result. At times Bennett's fracture can be reduced adequately by

closed manipulation and held in plaster. Many of these injuries, however, require internal fixation for stabilization. Internal fixation with small pins may be accomplished at an open operation or by percutaneous pinning, while the fracture is held reduced by an assistant (Fig. 18–4). With open reduction and internal fixation, the pins are cut short to remain permanently. With percutaneous pinning, the pins project through the skin. They are protected with a sterile dressing and removed after sufficient healing of the fracture has occurred.

Fractures to the Shaft of the Thumb Metacarpal. Undisplaced fractures and those that can be reduced by manipulation under local or general anesthesia require only a plaster cast comparable to that used for fractures of the base of the metacarpal. About four weeks of immobilization will usually suffice for healing.

Dislocations of the Metacarpophalangeal Joints. The metacarpophalangeal joint differs from the interphalangeal joint not only in size but also in the manner in which the tough palmar ligament is incorporated into the volar capsule. Dislocation is usually produced by hyperextension, which may cause the proximal end of the phalanx to displace onto the dorsum of the metacarpal. Reduction is achieved by pressure on the base of the displaced phalanx; this is pushed into place (Fig. 18–5B). Traction is contraindicated because a tongue of volar plate may be dragged into the joint and become interposed between the phalanx and the metacarpal, necessitating open reduction (Fig. 18–5C).

A complex dislocation occurs when the head of the first metacarpal is buttonholed through a tear in the capsule and is entrapped by the "noose" of joint capsule, short thenar muscles, and the interposed volar plate. Attempts at reduction by traction merely tighten the "noose." Under these circumstances, the thumb is usually found parallel to the metacarpal rather than hyperextended on it (Figs. 18–5C and 18–5D). When reduction is not

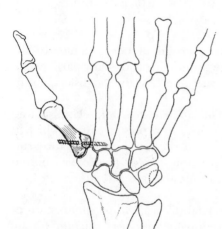

Figure 18–4. Percutaneous (or open) pinning to stabilize a Bennett's fracture in good reduction. (From DePalma AF: The Management of Fractures and Dislocations: An Atlas, Vol. 2. Philadelphia, W. B. Saunders Co., 1970.)

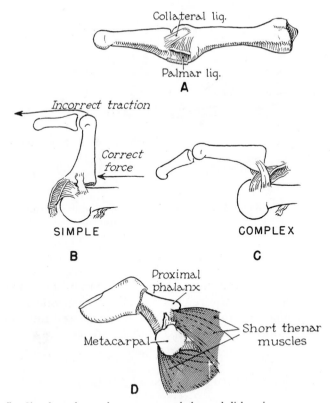

Figure 18–5. Simple and complex metacarpophalangeal dislocation.

A, The volar aspect of a metacarpophalangeal joint capsule is reinforced with a palmar ligament or fibrocartilage.

B, In a simple dislocation the phalanx is hyperextended and the palmar ligament hangs like a curtain over the metacarpal head. Traction may pivot the phalanx on the intact collateral ligaments and interpose the palmar ligament between the bone. The phalanx should be pushed into place.

C, The finger is not hyperextended on, but more nearly parallel to, the metacarpal in a complex dislocation. The volar joint plate and palmar ligament are interposed, and usually prevent reduction by manipulation.

D, In the metacarpophalangeal joint of the thumb the short thenar muscles augment the pivot force predisposing to complex dislocation. (From McLaughlin HL: Trauma. Philadelphia, W. B. Saunders Co., 1959.)

achieved by hyperextending the thumb and pushing on the base of the phalanx, open reduction is necessary.

Following closed or open reduction, a plaster cast as described for fractures of the first metacarpal is indicated for 10 to 14 days. Thereafter, the thumb should be protected from reinjury for several weeks.

Fractures of the Phalanges of the Thumb. Undisplaced fractures of the proximal phalanx require the use of splints or a cast for three or four weeks. Displaced fractures can usually be reduced by manipulation, although internal fixation is occasionally required.

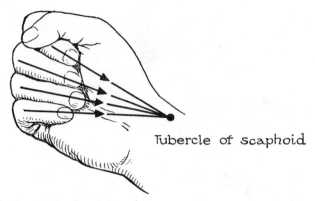

Tubercle of scaphoid

Figure 18–6. Axes of the flexed fingers do not correspond to those of the metacarpal or forearm bones but converge on the tubercle of the scaphoid. Finger splinting in flexion should be in this direction. (From McLaughlin HL: Trauma. Philadelphia, W. B. Saunders Co., 1959.)

Fracture injuries of the distal phalanx are painful but usually inconsequential. The majority require only a dressing for protection, although occasionally the amount of displacement warrants closed reduction, which is maintained by a protective splint.

FRACTURES OF THE FINGER METACARPALS

Fractures of the Shafts. Fractures of the metacarpal shafts in adequate apposition and good alignment and those that can be reduced by manipulation need to be immobilized for approximately four weeks. Rotational deformity must be avoided, because it may result in finger overlap when the digit is flexed. Proper rotation may be assessed by a simple guideline (Fig. 18–6). When each digit is flexed so as to make a fist,

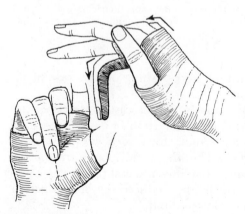

Figure 18–7. Metal splint incorporated in cast to support flexed finger that is contiguous to a fractured metacarpal shaft. (From McLaughlin HL: Trauma. Philadelphia, W. B. Saunders Co., 1959.)

the tip of each finger should point toward the tuberosity of the carpal navicular. Although restoration of normal length is desirable, efforts to achieve full length should not be allowed to prejudice function of contiguous fingers.

A plaster cast over the forearm and the hand, extending just proximal to the metacarpophalangeal joints, provides adequate immobilization for many metacarpal fractures. For others, the finger or fingers contiguous to the digit with the fracture must be splinted on a metal splint incorporated in the cast (Fig. 18–7). When fingers are splinted there should always be moderate flexion at each joint. Two or three weeks of immobilization will usually suffice.

In certain injuries, open reduction and pinning of metacarpal fractures (Fig. 18–8) may be indicated to assure precise reduction and to maintain optimal alignment. Open reduction and internal fixation, however, should be reserved for those fractures in which operation may be expected to give a better functional result than would be obtained by nonoperative methods.

Fractures of the Necks of Metacarpals. These fractures may occur on any of the metacarpals, but the little finger is the most frequently involved. They frequently occur during fist fights and are sometimes called boxer's fractures. They may occur any time a finger forcibly strikes a solid object when the fingers are tightly flexed.

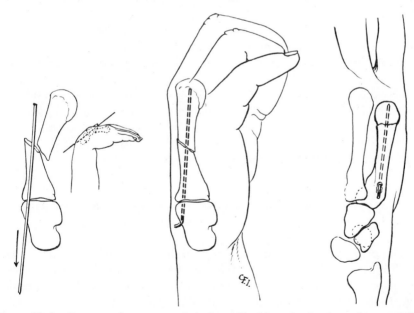

Figure 18–8. Fracture of a metacarpal shaft stabilized in reduction by an intramedullary pin. (From Milford, Lee: The hand. *In* Crenshaw, AH (ed.): Campbell's Operative Orthopaedics, 5th ed. St. Louis, C. V. Mosby Company, 1971. Reprinted by permission.)

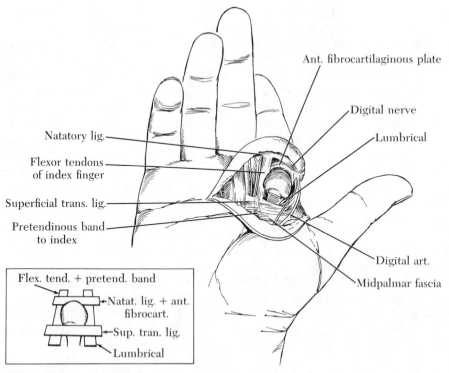

Figure 18–9. Entrapped dislocated index metacarpal head. (From Kaplan EB: J. Bone Joint Surg. *39A*:1081, 1957.)

Many fractures of the neck of metacarpals are impacted tightly. When fragments are impacted in up to 50 degrees of angulation, the position is usually acceptable. Only a compression dressing is needed for a few days. Active exercises of the joints of the contiguous finger should be initiated promptly. Fractures impacted in 75 degrees of angulation and angulated unimpacted fractures require reduction. Under local or general anesthesia, the fracture is reduced by manipulation and held by splinting the injured finger with all joints slightly flexed for two to three weeks.

FRACTURES AND DISLOCATIONS OF THE PHALANGES OF THE FINGERS

Dislocations of the Metacarpophalangeal Joints. In most cases, reduction is not difficult and often may be achieved without anesthesia. The proximal end of the displaced phalanx should be pushed into position (Fig. 18–5). Redislocation is very unlikely to occur; therefore, simple splinting or a compression dressing for 12 to 16 days will suffice.

Occasionally an anteriorly displaced head of the metacarpal will be trapped by the joint capsule or the flexor tendon (Fig. 18–9). Manipulative reduction in this situation may be unsuccessful. If so, open operation is necessary to free the metacarpal head from entrapment. After operation, splinting of the finger in moderate flexion for two to three weeks is advisable.

Dislocations of the Proximal Interphalangeal Joint. Chip fractures of various sizes may be associated with these injuries. Dislocations uncomplicated by fractures usually can be reduced easily by strong manual traction, often without anesthesia. The finger should be splinted with each joint in 15 to 20 degrees of flexion for two weeks.

A dislocation complicated by a fracture may present a very complex problem. When the fracture is of insufficient size to make the joint unstable and does not lead to subluxation, the fracture may not require treatment. If the fracture involves a significant part of the articular surface, open reduction and pinning with small wires is indicated.

FRACTURES OF THE PHALANGES

Fractures of the Proximal Phalanx. These fractures may lead to considerable loss of motion in the interphalangeal joints, particularly in the proximal interphalangeal joint.

Undisplaced fractures of the proximal phalanx require about three weeks of splinting.

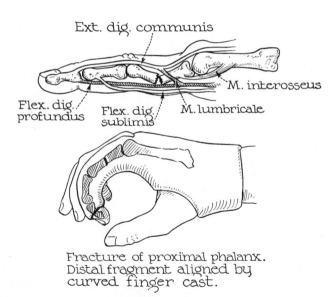

Ext. dig. communis

M. interosseus

Flex. dig. profundus

Flex. dig. sublimis

M. lumbricale

Fracture of proximal phalanx. Distal fragment aligned by curved finger cast.

Figure 18–10. Fracture of proximal phalanx of the index finger with palmar angulation; reduction and plaster cast immobilization. (Reproduced with permission from Compere EL, Banks SW, Compere CL: Pictorial Handbook of Fracture Treatment, 2nd ed. Copyright © 1947 by Year Book Medical Publishers, Inc., Chicago.)

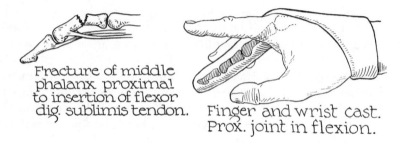

Fracture of middle phalanx proximal to insertion of flexor dig. sublimis tendon.

Finger and wrist cast. Prox. joint in flexion.

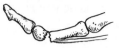
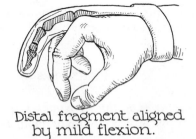

Fracture of middle phalanx distal to insertion of flexor dig. sublimis tendon.

Distal fragment aligned by mild flexion.

Figure 18–11. Fracture of middle phalanx of long finger with dorsal angulation, and another with palmar angulation; reduction and plaster splinting for each. (Reproduced with permission from Compere EL, Banks SW, Compere CL: Pictorial Handbook of Fracture Treatment, 2nd ed. Copyright © 1947 by Year Book Medical Publishers, Inc., Chicago.)

Displaced fractures of the proximal phalanx are usually angulated anteriorly (Fig. 18–10). In most cases, reduction can be accomplished by manipulation with local anesthesia. The entire finger should be immobilized in 15 to 20 degrees of flexion, especially the middle joint. Special precaution is necessary to ensure that the tip of the flexed finger points toward the carpal navicular as a safeguard against malrotation and finger overlap (see Fig. 18–6).

A plaster cast holding the wrist in slight dorsal flexion and incorporating a metal splint for the injured finger provides excellent immobilization. The finger portion of the cast may be constructed with plaster of Paris (Fig. 18–10). Three weeks of immobilization will allow enough union of the fracture to permit active motion. The patient should protect the finger from reinjury for five to six weeks.

Fractures of the Middle Phalanx. Fractures in this portion of the finger, especially those close to the middle joint, often cause permanent loss of motion in that joint. In many instances loss of flexion in the distal joint occurs because of tendon fixation at the fracture site.

Undisplaced fractures of the middle phalanx require about three weeks of simple splinting that holds the middle and distal joints in 15 to 20 degrees of flexion. Immobilization of the metacarpophalangeal joint is unnecessary.

Displaced fractures should be reduced into adequate apposition and alignment without rotational deformity. Fractures in the middle phalanx may be angulated dorsally or toward the palm (Fig. 18–11). Correction of the angulation in either direction by manipulation usually is not difficult. Precautions against malrotation are necessary. Splinting should immobilize the three joints of the injured finger in 15 to 20 degrees of flexion. These fractures usually unite within three to five weeks.

Fractures of the Distal Phalanx. Fractures in this portion of the finger usually remain in adequate reduction even though they are severely comminuted. Angulation can be corrected easily by manipulation under digital block anesthesia. There are no tendon attachments to displace the fragments and splinting is not necessary. These are painful injuries, and some splinting to protect the end of the finger from bumps and pressures contributes significantly to the patient's comfort. A splint applied to the finger for fractures of the distal phalanx should extend only to the midportion of the middle phalanx to allow active motion of the proximal and middle joints.

Mallet Finger or Baseball Finger (or Fracture). This injury is caused by a sharp blow on the end of the finger such as that sustained when the finger is struck by a baseball, hence the name by which it is often called. At times the injury is an avulsion of the extensor tendon from the distal phalanx. In other instances, a small fragment of the dorsal proximal portion of the distal phalanx, including some of the articular surface, is broken (Fig. 18–12).

Either a tendon avulsion or a fracture causes considerable pain and tenderness over the dorsum of the distal joint and the loss of the ability to extend the distal phalanx completely. The distal phalanx remains in a "dropped" position, hence the term mallet finger.

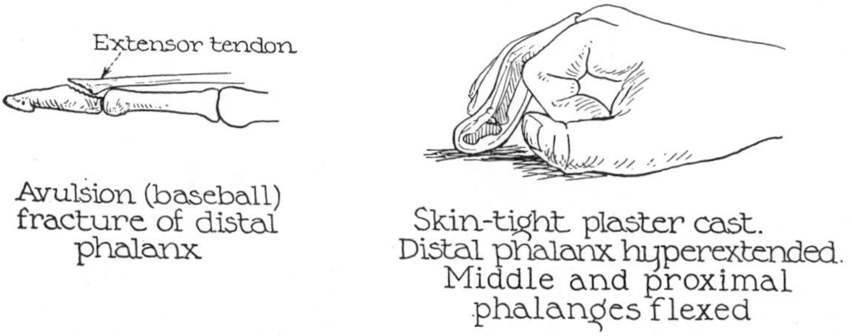

Extensor tendon

Avulsion (baseball) fracture of distal phalanx

Skin-tight plaster cast. Distal phalanx hyperextended. Middle and proximal phalanges flexed

Figure 18–12. Baseball or mallet finger treated by plaster immobilization holding the middle joint in almost 45 degrees of flexion and the distal phalanx in hyperextension. (Reproduced with permission from Compere EL, Banks SW, Compere CL: Pictorial Handbook of Fracture Treatment, 2nd ed. Copyright © 1947 by Year Book Medical Publishers, Inc., Chicago.)

Simple splinting consists of a short splint that does not immobilize the middle joint but holds the distal phalanx in extension. Splinting should be maintained for five or six weeks, and thereafter use of the short splint at night for several weeks may contribute to a more satisfactory result. If there is a fragment of bone greater than one third of the articular surface and separated by more than 1 mm, a more satisfactory result will be achieved by open reduction with pinning or wiring the fragment in place.

19

Traumatic Amputations and Replantation of Amputated Parts in the Extremities

TRAUMATIC AMPUTATIONS

COMPLETE AMPUTATIONS

Complete traumatic amputations of extremities occur from time to time as a result of various kinds of trauma, such as railroad or other vehicular accidents, entanglements in farm or industrial machinery, or crushes caused by collapsing buildings or falling heavy objects. These same kinds of trauma may lead to partial but almost complete amputations in which an extensive comminuted open fracture, a severed major artery, and severe muscle damage are present, yet some continuity of muscle, fascia, and skin remains.

PARTIAL BUT ALMOST COMPLETE AMPUTATIONS

Many severely damaged limbs that may be considered to have been almost completely amputated have been salvaged during the past two decades largely as a result of widespread surgical knowledge and skills regarding vascular repair, including the use of vein grafts. The required surgical judgment and techniques are not unlike those necessary for replantation (see page 270). While restoration of arterial and venous circulation is crucial in order to avoid amputation in many extensively damaged extremities, other precise surgical procedures are also of great importance. Thorough cleansing of the open wound and debridement of devitalized tissues, particularly muscle, must be carried out to minimize the chances of sepsis. If present, sepsis will jeopardize the vascular repair, may lead to amputation at a higher level, and even risk the life of the patient. The surgeon must be familiar with the techniques required to achieve adequate soft part coverage of the sites of vascular repair and with the principles of staged wound closure. Complete primary wound closure seldom, if ever, should be used in such severely injured extremities,

265

particularly in lower extremities. Fractures must be treated so as to favor union in satisfactory alignment, yet the method of fracture management must not prejudice vascular repairs and wound healing or predispose to wound sepsis.

Overzealous efforts to save a "near amputation" must not jeopardize the life of the patient. Moreover, the anticipated function of the salvaged limb must justify not only the risk to the patient but also the prolonged hospitalization, expense, and period of temporary disability that will be necessary. For example, efforts to save a lower extremity would hardly be justified if the injury included a severed femoral artery, a severely comminuted fracture of the femur, and a crushed and severed sciatic nerve that defies repair. In fact, an irreparably severed sciatic nerve in combination with only one of the other two injuries may be sufficient indication to complete the amputation. The burden of proof rests on the surgeon who undertakes to salvage a limb, particularly a lower extremity, that has sustained severe damage to essential soft tissue components and bone, especially in view of the risk involved and the current status of lower extremity prostheses fitting and effectiveness.

Alternative Procedures for Amputation

Assuming that it is not tenable to attempt to save an extremity with a partial but almost complete amputation, the amputation must be completed. The alternative procedures are identical with those for complete traumatic amputations and are in accordance with several well-established surgical principles.

Preoperative Control of Hemorrhage

Hemorrhage must be controlled as an emergency measure. Fortunately, exsanguinating life-endangering hemorrhage usually does not occur, because the severed blood vessels retract promptly into the muscle mass of the stump and because the normal clotting mechanism goes into effect. Even so, significant shock-producing hemorrhage must be stopped and shock countermeasures instituted by blood-volume replacement using balanced salt solutions and whole blood transfusions (see Chapter 2).

In the usual case, a firm compression dressing over the stump will adequately control continuing hemorrhage. Briskly bleeding arteries may be clamped prior to application of a compression dressing. As a last resort, a tourniquet may be applied just proximal to the amputation site, but in such instances the tourniquet should be removed as soon as surgical facilities and personnel can be made available for control of hemorrhage, but not until intravenous fluids and blood transfusions have been provided to control shock.

Debridement of Stump

Following prompt adequate resuscitation and with the patient under general or, rarely, spinal anesthesia (the latter alternative is only for lower extremities), adequate surgery on the open stump must be carried out. All devitalized tissue, particularly muscle, must be excised, and severed major blood vessels must be ligated. Nerve trunks must be identified, pulled downward, cut short with a sharp instrument, and allowed to retract into living muscle.

Bone

The level at which the bone is finally severed identifies the level of amputation. In many instances, projecting bone must be sawed off. In determining the saw line, so-called sites of election for definitive amputations usually should be ignored in traumatic amputations and the bone shortened merely to the level just proximal to the remaining viable muscle mass. The same precautions used in elective amputation should be followed to ensure a smooth bony stump without projecting jagged bony spicules. Excess periosteum should be excised, and in some instances a cuff of periosteum may be excised so as to leave the distal one fourth inch of bone devoid of periosteal covering to minimize the hazard of painful spur formation.

Skin

Handling of skin is a problem requiring precise surgical judgment. A time-honored guideline, particularly in military surgery, has placed the level of primary amputations resulting from trauma at the lowest level of viable tissue. A companion guideline has called for open circular amputations in such injuries. In a way the two guidelines may be paradoxical. In traumatic amputations, a long flap of healthy viable skin may extend distal to the bone end, particularly after it has been sawed at the level of the remaining viable muscle. If the flap of skin is cut away in order to carry out an open circular amputation, obviously the amputation has not been at the lowest level of viable skin.

TYPES OF AMPUTATION

The surgeon has the choice of performing an open amputation (either open circular or with an open flap or flaps) or a closed amputation with sutured skin flaps. The latter usually is to be avoided in traumatic amputations. Ordinarily, some form of open amputation is preferable in that it runs less risk of sepsis in the stump because of the open drainage it provides; moreover, it furnishes a "second look" at the stump at the optimal time to verify that stump debridement was adequate. In very few traumatic amputations — and practically all of these involve the arm or forearm — is the surgeon justified in primarily closing fashioned flaps of the stump. Even in these, an open amputation has many advantages and provides less risk.

Open Circular Amputation

In traumatic amputations in which the skin has been severed near the level of the postdebridement stump, the open circular amputation is usually indicated. Often called a guillotine amputation — erroneously, because it is not a "meat cleaver" procedure — the technique calls for the muscle to be severed at the level to which the circular cut skin retracts, and the saw line of the bone to be at the level to which the muscle retracts. The result is a short inverted cone.

Following an open circular amputation, continuous traction on the skin is mandatory. Following application of a dressing that is limited to the

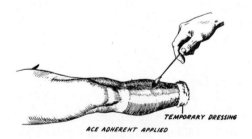

ACE ADHERENT APPLIED

TEMPORARY DRESSING

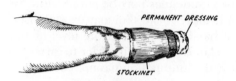

PERMANENT DRESSING

STOCKINET

Figure 19–1. Steps in application of skin traction following amputation in the middle third of the leg. Tincture of benzoin may be used instead of ace adherent. While the sagittal section shows arrangement for continuous traction in a banjo cast, traction may be provided over a pulley at the foot of the bed. (From Hampton, O. P. Jr.: *Wounds of Extremities in Military Surgery.* St. Louis, C. V. Mosby Co., 1951. Reprinted by permission.)

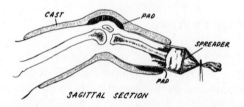

CAST   PAD

SPREADER

PAD

SAGITTAL SECTION

open wound, a few pounds of skin traction may be provided with adhesive strips as in ordinary Buck's traction or as shown in Figure 19–1. The illustrated technique may be used for continuous traction over the foot or side (for upper extremities) of the bed or in a "banjo" cast that permits the patient to turn and be out of bed in a chair. The spreader as shown in Figure 19–1 should be utilized in all forms of skin traction to avoid excessive pressure on the skin against the bone end.

Skin traction must be maintained until the skin has become fixed by healing processes. As edema in the stump decreases and atrophy of the muscle occurs, skin margins often tend to fold over the raw stump, thereby reducing the size of the open wound. Complete healing by scar formation may take place. Regardless, skin traction is required for at least three weeks and often one or two more. Ordinarily, skin traction may provide adequate immobilization in the desirable position of the joint above the amputation. At times, however, that joint should be held by a rigid splint.

Open circular amputations usually, but not always, require revision that may include shortening of the bone before fitting of a prosthesis. Reference is made to standard texts and the surgical literature regarding the indications for stump revision following open circular amputations, preferable levels for definitive amputations, and the selection and fitting of prostheses.

Open Flap Amputation

A modified open flap procedure may be indicated following traumatic amputations. Just as in open circular amputations, thorough debridement of the stump, adequate hemostasis, shortening of visible nerve trunks, and perhaps shortening of a projecting bone end are carried out before considerations of flap design. Seldom if ever should bone be shortened to permit flaps to be fashioned. Rather a flap or flaps may be created only from healthy viable skin extending distal to the stump after debridement and shortening of the bone if necessary. Under this concept, standard anterior and posterior flaps are unlikely to be feasible; therefore, a flap or flaps may be asymmetrical and based at unusual places. In summary, a flap or flaps come from remaining available healthy viable skin.

Open flap amputations require careful dressing. Precautions are necessary to avoid torsion of flaps and excessive pressure on them, either of which might jeopardize their viability. Even so, a reasonably snug compression dressing is indicated to minimize edema of the stump. Rigid splinting of the joint above the amputation usually is indicated. The splint should extend a short distance beyond the stump to protect it.

The optimal time for closure of open flap amputations is three to five days after the initial surgery. Preferably, the dressing applied in the operating room at the end of that surgery remains undisturbed until the patient again is in the operating room and under anesthesia. Only signs and symptoms of infection in the stump justify an earlier dressing. Even under these circumstances, the first dressing is preferably carried out under anesthesia in the operating room, which is set up for any indicated surgery on the wound. Infection in the stump usually demands further debridement. Conversion of the open flap to an open circular amputation may be indicated. If not, after adequate redebridement, the wound is dressed again with the flap or flaps protected.

If the amputation stump is clinically clean when it is exposed in the operating room, the flap or flaps may be sutured so as to close the stump. Drainage with a Penrose drain or drains is usually advisable. A compression dressing and a protective splint complete the reparative surgical procedures.

SUMMARY — TRAUMATIC AMPUTATIONS

In traumatic amputations, resuscitation and other life-saving measures take first priority but, after appropriate resuscitation, some surgery on the stump is usually indicated (particularly to minimize the chances of life-threatening sepsis). Following adequate debridement of the stump and control of hemorrhage, the surgeon must choose between open circular, open flap, and closed flap techniques. As a rule, the latter should be reserved for selected traumatic amputations of the upper extremity. Open circular or open flap amputations are usually indicated in the lower extremity. As a rule, bone should not be shortened at the first surgery merely to permit flaps to be fashioned. The need for a later amputation at a higher level under optimal conditions is a small price to pay for improving the chance of achieving a healthy, well-healed stump.

REPLANTATION

ROLE OF THE EMERGENCY DEPARTMENT

In the emergency department critical and life-endangering injuries should not be overlooked in the enthusiasm of the primary care physician to transport the patient to a replantation center. A two-team approach is advisable with one physician ministering to the patient while another contacts the regional replantation center and appropriately prepares the amputated part. The final decision regarding feasibility of replantation should be the responsibility of the replantation specialist.

Prior to transport, intravenous fluids, antibiotics, and appropriate tetanus prophylaxis are administered. Adequate blood volume and blood pressure should be assured. Following saline lavage, a stump dressing should be carefully applied. The arrest of hemorrhage can usually be achieved through such a pressure dressing. The amputated part requires little treatment. Foreign material may be washed off with lactated Ringer's solution, but lengthy irrigation of the exposed tissues should be avoided, because it may make identification of structures more difficult. The amputated part should be placed dry in a dry polyethylene bag and the bag placed in regular ice (Fig. 19–2).

TRANSPORTATION

If the condition of the patient and amputated part are satisfactory for transfer, the replantation surgeon must give precise instructions regarding transportation:

1. Standard precautions for evacuation of any injured patient are necessary, including providing analgesia, arresting hemorrhage, and restoring adequate blood volume.

2. Transportation must be as rapid as possible, especially for cases of major limb replantation, but there is no need for panicky haste.

3. Air transport is preferable for journeys beyond four hours by ambulance.

4. Qualified personnel are mandatory when parenteral fluid or systemic support is required.

5. Incompletely amputated digits or limbs should be splinted to minimize further vascular injury.

ROLE OF THE REPLANTATION CENTER

When patient arrives at the replantation center, the following procedures are done:

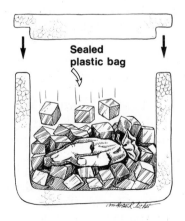

Sealed
plastic bag

Figure 19–2. The amputated part transported in a dry polyethylene bag placed in regular ice. (From Kleinert, H. E., and Jupiter, J. B.: Replantation—An Overview. Clinical Trends in Orthopedics, Thieme-Stratton, Inc. New York. In press.)

1. The patient's overall condition and associated injuries, if any, are re-evaluated, and history of any pre-existing illness is noted.

2. Detailed medical and social histories (to include mechanism of injury, handling of the part, and normothermia time) are obtained.

3. A complete blood count, coagulation studies, urinalysis, routine chemistry studies, blood type and crossmatch, and roentgenograms of the stump and amputated part are ordered. Arterial blood gas with pH measurement is obtained if major limb replantation is expected.

4. If not already administered, tetanus prophylaxis and intravenous antibiotics are begun.

5. A preoperative anesthesia evaluation is made.

6. The part and the stump are inspected without debridement or dissection, and then the part is returned to ice.

7. A detailed explanation of the proposed procedure, the possibility of further surgical procedures, the financial cost, and long period of rehabilitation is presented to the patient and available relatives.

SELECTION FOR REPLANTATION

The initial aim in replantation is the re-establishment of vascular continuity. The ultimate goal, however, is a functional restoration greater than that provided by a prosthesis. With appropriate patient selection, modern equipment, and well-trained personnel, a survival rate of 95 percent of replanted parts in ideal situations and 40 percent in salvage cases can be expected.

CONTRAINDICATIONS TO REPLANTATION

The following conditions present contraindications (either absolute or relative) to replantation:

Absolute

1. Severe crush or avulsion injuries with extensive vascular or segmental damage to either affected limb or amputated part. Roentgenograms may reveal multiple fractures and vascular damage indicated by red line or ribbon signs.

2. Significant associated injuries.

3. Frozen parts or those preserved in nonphysiological solutions.

4. Chronic illness — for example, cardiac disease sufficient to make transportation or prolonged surgery hazardous.

Relative

1. Single-digit amputations. An index finger replantation unless the digit can function almost normally may not be performed. In a more distal amputation, however, replantation is justified.
2. Patient over 50 years of age.
3. Extensive avulsion injuries.
4. Lengthy warm ischemia time (in excess of six hours), especially with skeletal muscle involvement.
5. Previous injury or surgery to the amputated part or limb.
6. Psychological. Those patients insufficiently motivated or unwilling to accept a prolonged period of convalescence.

SALVAGE REPLANTATION

In certain circumstances, relative contraindications may be disregarded:

1. The patient is a child. Replantation should be attempted in most instances, because the results of primary repair in children are superior.
2. There is multiple digital loss. Available intact parts can be utilized to restore some function to the hand.
3. The amputated part is the thumb. Of foremost importance, the thumb will function well even if motion is only in the basal joint if sensibility can be restored.
4. Situations of injured dominant hand, bilateral injuries, or associated disabilities such as contralateral paralysis or blindness.

THE REPLANTATION PROCEDURE

General Equipment

Standard equipment necessary for performing replantation includes a stable hand table, a lead hand to help immobilize the stump and severed part, a bipolar coagulation unit, and microvascular surgical instruments such as jeweler's forceps, atraumatic microvascular clamps, and special needle holders. An operating microscope with two binocular operating positions and foot pedal control is essential.

Personnel

It is desirable to have a team of surgical nurses and technicians well versed in microvascular and replantation surgery. In the ward, nurses experienced in evaluation of the circulation are essential.

Solutions

Appropriate irrigation solution prepared prior to replantation includes (1) Xylocaine 1 percent, 2 ml/100 ml Ringer's; (2) heparin 200 units/100 ml Ringer's. An antibiotic solution is used for general irrigation.

Anesthesia

The majority of upper extremity replantations are performed under axillary block using a long-acting agent. Should general anesthesia be necessary, halothane is to be avoided because of the associated shaking phenomenon at the termination of anesthesia. Continuous patient monitoring includes pulse and electrocardiography, urinary catheterization with hourly volume readings, and a rectal temperature probe. More proximal amputations or those involving significant metabolic or volume problems require monitoring of the central venous pressure, blood gases, and electrolytes. Intravenous therapy with antibiotics as well as blood transfusions with replacement of volume for volume is indicated.

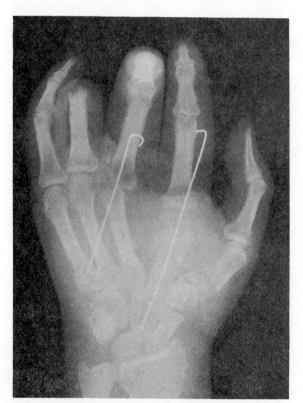

Figure 19–3. The principle of bony shortening and internal fixation at the site of replantation.

Methods

Skeletal Management.   Adequate shortening permits tension-free neurovascular and soft tissue approximation. The degree of shortening depends upon the extent of debridement and adequacy of skin cover. Fixation can be achieved with compression plates for long bones and crossed Kirschner wire or interosseous wires for metacarpals or phalanges (Figs. 19–3 and 19–4). Primary arthrodesis or silastic arthroplasty may be required where the amputation passes through a joint.

Tendons.   In hand or digital amputations, the extensor and flexor tendons should be repaired primarily with an atraumatic technique, along with repair of the digital flexor sheath.

Arteries.   At all levels, repair of all major arteries (radial and ulnar at the wrist and both digital arteries in the fingers) is recommended. Adequate proximal flow should be confirmed prior to repair in instances in which more proximal section of the vessel and interposition vein grafts are required.

Nerves.   Nerves are repaired with careful fascicular alignment with fine monofilament suture of 9–0 or 10–0 nylon. Primary tension-free repair obviates secondary procedures and results in improved functional results.

Veins.   Sufficient venous repairs are necessary for successful replantation. The more veins repaired, the greater is the chance of survival.

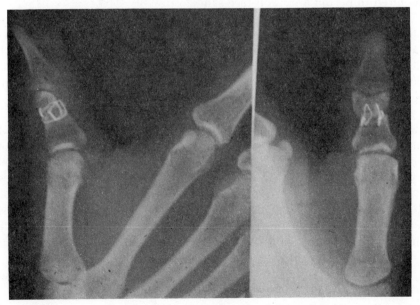

Figure 19–4. The principle of skeletal shortening and internal fixation at the site of replantation.

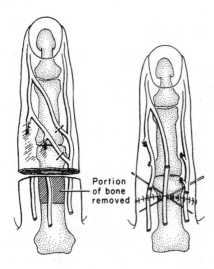

Portion
of bone
removed

Figure 19–5. Technique of increasing the available number of veins for anastomosis. The distal veins are traced to their confluence and divided. The absolute number of veins available is increased.

Localization of dorsal digital veins may be aided by longitudinal incisions (Fig. 19–5).

Skin. The skin would be closed loosely with a few interrupted sutures to avoid any compression. Hemostasis must be absolute, because free blood can act as a potent thrombogenic agent. Z-plasties are advised for circular wounds. Fasciotomy is routinely considered in crushing injuries or when edema is a concern. Split-thickness skin grafts may also be required to permit a tension-free skin closure.

Dressing. The dressing should be bulky and supportive without obstructing venous drainage. Circular dressings should be avoided, because they may have a tourniquet effect after becoming blood-soaked. The hand should be splinted in a functional position with the fingers and nail beds adequately exposed to allow postoperative assessment of the vascular repair. Circulation and digital temperatures are to be checked hourly.

Medications. Aspirin (10 grains) is administered rectally prior to vascular anastomosis to inhibit platelet aggregation and continued every 12 hours postoperatively. Low molecular weight dextran may be used postoperatively in a dose of 5 to 7 mg/kg/24 hours in a continuous infusion to help expand blood volume, prevent sludging, and inhibit platelet adhesiveness. Parenteral heparin is still used on occasion when extensive crushing exists: 10,000 units is given in an intravenous bolus just prior to vessel anastomosis and continued in an intravenous drip titrated to keep the activated partial thromboplastin time 1½ to 2 times control. Heparin and dextran should not be used together, because they may produce a bleeding diathesis.

A broad-spectrum antibiotic, usually a cephalosporin, is continued parenterally for 48 to 72 hours postoperatively.

General Considerations of Fracture Treatment

Diagnosis of the nature and the extent of injuries depends upon synthesis of information derived from the history, the physical examination, the x-rays, and laboratory data. All the data obtained should be evaluated in relation to the patient's clinical presentation. Any inconsistencies suggest unusual or overlooked conditions and must be investigated. This synthesis of information into an early, accurate diagnosis is simplified by the process of pattern recognition.

HISTORY

It is essential to obtain as much information as possible on the details and mechanism of the accident. This is of value in the diagnosis, because injuries consistently occur in patterns and knowing the mechanism of injury may lead to a correct diagnosis. Treatment is also dependent on the history; the fracture fragment displaced by one mechanism of injury can often be reduced by reversing the process; i.e., external rotation fractures of the ankle are reduced by internal rotation. The patient should be questioned specifically as to how the injury occurred. Examples of questions are: "How far did you fall? Was your seatbelt fastened? Where were you sitting in the car? Did you hear something snap?" When the patient, because of the nature and severity of the injury, cannot provide information, it should be sought from companions, emergency medical personnel, and traffic officers: "What types of vehicles were involved? What was the extent of the damage? What was the estimated velocity of the vehicle?" The severity of the injury is related directly to the amount of force expended upon the bone and soft tissue, or $F = Mv^2$. This is reflected in the increased comminution or shattering of bone and the greater displacement of fracture fragments in injuries caused by high-velocity motor vehicle accidents. Accompanying such injuries is an increased incidence of damage to nerves, vessels, and other soft tissue structures such as ligaments.

Many fractures occur consecutively. The patient twists and breaks an ankle and then may fall on an outstretched hand, which in turn is fractured. A pedestrian is struck by a car, suffering a fracture of a tibia and fibula. The impact throws him over a guard rail and he rolls down an embankment. The sharp fracture fragment further lacerates the skin and soft tissues, complicating what was initially a more simple injury. The history of tumbling following the initial impact raises the possibility of such consecutive injuries. Care should be taken to avoid additional injuries to the patient during extraction from wrecked vehicles and buildings and in the emergency department during examination as splints are removed, x-rays are taken, and the patient is transferred from one stretcher to another.

Occasionally a patient with a fracture will be encountered who relates only a minimal injury, such as rolling over in bed or making a false step. This situation should alert the physician to the possibility of a pathological fracture, defined as a fracture through an area of bone weakened by pre-existing disease. Hip fractures in the elderly are associated with osteopenia. Patients with fractures through areas of metastatic disease may give a history of previous treatment for a tumor. In such fractures the amount of force expended is usually very small. As a result, the displacement of the fracture fragments is minimal.

The general medical history should not be overlooked. While there are few, if any, diseases that will interfere directly with fracture healing, there are many that can complicate treatment. Pre-existing cardiopulmonary disease may affect the choice of anesthesia. Neurological disease such as hemiparesis or Parkinson's can influence the indications for operative treatment. The history of an active focus of infection externally (such as acne or furunculosis) or internally (such as pyuria or middle ear infection) may also affect indications for treatment. An inquiry must be made regarding medications that the patient is currently taking for the treatment of diabetes, hypertension, heart disease, and other chronic conditions. A history of allergies, drug sensitivities, medications, and excessive consumption of alcohol and use of addictive drugs should be recorded.

PHYSICAL EXAMINATION

The physical examination should be complete, careful, and gentle. The findings should be recorded in the chart immediately. If indicated, the examination should be repeated at appropriate intervals to ensure that no injuries or complications are overlooked. The most painful areas should be examined last. Failure to do this will lead to imprecision because of muscle spasm and poor pain localization.

Particular attention should be given to the condition of the dressings and splints applied by the emergency medical personnel. The splints should be checked to ensure that they are functioning properly without producing areas of constriction or excessive pressure.

Aphorism: To minimize soft tissue damage and to avoid conversion of a closed to an open fracture, "splint 'em where they lie" on first contact.

Air splints present a specific hazard, because these can become tighter as the patient is moved from winter cold into a warmer hospital atmosphere. The limbs should be protected by proper splinting during the evaluation in the emergency department and in the x-ray department. Splints should be removed only at the time definitive treatment is begun. Wounds should be inspected and carefully re-covered with sterile dressings.

The cardinal signs and symptoms of fractures or dislocations are pain, deformity, unnatural motion, and swelling. The pain of musculoskeletal injuries varies widely with the patient and with the circumstances. It is not uncommon for a patient with a fracture to continue to use the injured extremity for several days before progressive swelling, loss of function, and pain cause him to seek medical help.

Aphorism: Treat every case of injury as a fracture until it is proved to be otherwise.

Aphorism: Do not be deceived by the absence of deformity and disability; in many cases of fracture, some ability to use the limb persists.

The loss of pain sensation in patients with head injuries and patients with paraplegia, acute or of long standing, may delay the diagnosis of injury. Pain patterns may be confusing. Pain may be referred, usually distal to the site of the injury. This is particularly true with injuries to the spine and the hip. The pain threshold of the patient who is taking drugs or is intoxicated may be altered.

Reduction and immobilization of a fractured or dislocated extremity should be followed by substantial pain relief. Failure of treatment to relieve pain promptly should suggest strongly that either the reduction is not satisfactory or that there may be an unrecognized injury or complication.

Aphorism: Continued severe pain usually indicates circulatory constriction and requires immediate attention, day or night.

Pain is particularly severe when caused by ischemia. Pain recurring or increasing after initial relief following reduction and immobilization of fractures is an important danger signal. Plaster dressings should be bivalved and split to the skin for their full length. Compression dressings should be released and the limb closely inspected.

Aphorism: In splitting a plaster cast, divide the plaster and the underlying padding to the last thread.

Compartment syndromes such as Volkmann's ischemic contracture and anterior compartment syndrome are characterized by severe deep boring pain. This pain is aggravated by movement of the fingers and toes in such a way as to put tension upon the affected muscles.

Deformity is the distortion of the body beyond the limits of normal variation. The deformity may be minimal or gross, subtle or self-evident, and is best evaluated by comparing the injured limb with the opposite normal uninjured limb. This comparison is done automatically by most examiners and is taken for granted. How much we depend upon such comparisons is not appreciated until we are faced with the evaluation of an injured limb in a patient whose opposite limb has been injured or previously amputated. Many deformities associated with fractures and dislocations are classical and consistent. Their recognition should establish the diagnosis quickly. Some of these are the dinner fork deformity of Colles' fractures; the shortening and external rotation of the leg accompanying hip fractures; and the flexion, adduction, and internal rotation of the femur associated with posterior dislocations of the hip. Any deformity, even when not classical, should suggest the presence and location of the injury.

When the bone or the soft tissues or both are completely disrupted, abnormal motion occurs at the site of injury. Such is the case with ligamentous injuries of the knee when varus or valgus stress applied to the extended knee allows medial or lateral movement at the joint. It is also seen in long bone fractures that may be angulated but that can be straightened during the application of traction or a splint. Movement of the fracture fragments may produce crepitus, the grating sensation occurring as the broken ends rub together. This is not to be deliberately produced during the clinical examination, since such manipulation produces pain and muscle spasm and may cause further soft tissue injury.

Swelling that occurs rapidly after injury may obscure deformities and interfere with clinical examination.

Aphorism: Reduce the fracture with as little delay as possible. Do not wait for the swelling to subside.

Massive swelling limits the effectiveness of plaster and other dressings and splints used to immobilize the injured limb. Swelling that persists into the healing period promotes stiffness of the joints, particularly in the fingers, and limits the excursion of the tendons in their sheaths. Soon after injury, swelling is due almost entirely to the extravasation of blood into the damaged area. Consequently, the amount of swelling may be a useful guide for estimating the amount of local blood loss. This can be quantified to a degree by measurement and comparison of the injured and uninjured sides using the formula

$$V = \frac{L \times C^2}{4\pi}$$

where volume (V) is determined by calculation after measuring length (L) and circumference (C). An increase in circumference is particularly important because this factor is squared in the formula, while differences in length are of relatively little significance. Rapid swelling in an extremity suggests arterial bleeding from vessels of considerable size.

Every effort should be made to limit swelling following injury. This can be accomplished by the application of cold, proper splinting, elevation of the injured part, and careful application of compression dressings. These dressings should always include the distal portion of the limb and extend proximally to well above the area of injury. Proximal constriction must be avoided.

In an awake, conscious patient, sensation and motor function should be tested grossly to determine whether or not spinal cord trauma has occurred. Sensory loss due to peripheral nerve injury requires more detailed examination. Spotty, atypical loss of sensation in an extremity suggests vascular insufficiency, usually from arterial injury. Motor function of specific muscle groups can be inhibited by pain and deformity. In many patients with head injuries the cooperation required for an accurate sensory-motor examination cannot be obtained. Anxiety, severe pain, prior receipt of analgesics including alcohol, and a language barrier can interfere with an examination. Sensation and motor function must be tested repeatedly before, during, and after treatment to ensure that changes are not overlooked.

Aphorism: Examine the injured part for signs of vascular and nerve injuries and record your findings.

Lack of adequate perfusion in the extremities may be due to hypovolemic shock, in which case all extremities are involved, or to arterial or venous constriction or injury in a particular limb. A pale, cool hand or foot with collapsed veins is more commonly seen with arterial insufficiency, while a cyanotic cool hand or foot with prominent veins suggests venous insufficiency. Arterial pulses should be palpated in every patient but may be difficult to evaluate in a hypotensive patient. Local swelling at the site may also interfere. Splints and dressings can usually be displaced sufficiently to permit palpation of the pulses. If a deformity is present, straightening of the limb or reduction of the dislocation may be followed immediately by improved pulsation and perfusion. Release of a constricting dressing or cast may produce a similar improvement. Doppler measurements are of some use as an objective sequential measurement.

Aphorism: Make certain the obvious fracture is the only injury.

The general physical examination must not be neglected. Every patient should be turned to permit examination of the back. A rectal examination and a pelvic examination should be carried out in all seriously injured patients. Scars from previous operations suggest the possibility of pathological fracture, and abdominal scars may prove to be contraindications to peritoneal taps or lavage. Abrasions, lacerations, and contusions should be noted, because the location of these may be of diagnostic importance or may affect the subsequent choice of surgical approaches, and also may have important potential medicolegal implications.

Aphorism: The saving of life comes first. Treat impending asphyxia, hemorrhage, shock, and other life-endangering conditions before treating the fracture.

ROENTGENOGRAPHIC EXAMINATIONS

Roentgenographic examinations should not be ordered until after the patient has been carefully examined. Ideally, the roentgenographic examinations should be used to confirm the initial diagnosis and to define further the nature of the injury. A "skeletal survey" should not be used as a substitute for a careful examination. A useful practice is to take large films and to read the corners of the films for unexpected bits of information.

Aphorism: Obtain roentgenograms in at least two planes and examine them yourself.

All diagnostic roentgenograms should be taken during one visit to the x-ray department. In many urgent situations, the requirements of the surgeon and the radiologist may be different. For the surgeon, it may be sufficient only to know that a fracture is present. For this a formal series of films may not be necessary. For the radiologist, a standard set of films, plus some special procedures, may be necessary to reveal every detail of the injury. The patient's condition may dictate some compromise. In the emergency department, a cross-table lateral of the cervical spine may be adequate to rule out a fracture dislocation. Multiple views of the cervical spine may be taken later under more optimal conditions if they are required. In certain seriously injured patients who need immediate operation or resuscitation, the time lost taking large numbers of roentgenograms cannot be spared without adding substantial risk. In such situations the surgeon must rely upon the clinical findings, augmented by large scout films, and occasionally may have to operate without any preliminary roentgenograms. A more thorough roentgenographic evaluation may be obtained later as the patient's condition permits.

In less urgent situations a complete roentgenographic examination should be made (Table 20–1). In some situations, special views, comparison views, planigrams, and CT scans may be required to assess the nature and location of the total injury. Fractures are characterized by their appearance on the roentgenogram (Fig. 20–1). Four types of displacement may occur: shortening, lengthening, angulation, and rotation. The description of epiphyseal injuries devised by Salter and Harris (1963) is widely used and has prognostic and therapeutic value (Fig. 20–2). All seriously ill patients should be accompanied to x-ray by knowledgeable individuals capable of helping to prevent pulmonary aspiration, shock, or arrhythmia and capable of recognizing and treating these complications if they develop.

HYPOVOLEMIC SHOCK

Since the classical experiments carried out by Blalock in the 1930s, it has been known that the slow silent sequestration of blood into an injured limb or limbs is difficult to appreciate because there may be no visible signs

TABLE 20-1.   GUIDELINES FOR AN ADEQUATE
X-RAY EXAMINATION

Technical Considerations
A small focal spot should be used.
Collimation of x-ray beam enhances detail and decreases exposure.
The central ray should be centered over the site of fracture.
Intensifying screens should be used.
Technique should provide information about the soft tissue as well as bone.

Diagnostic Considerations
An adequate number of views should be obtained: "one view is no view, but
two may not be enough."
The joints above and below the fracture must be seen, ideally on the same films.
In children, comparison views of the opposite uninjured extremity should be used
to evaluate epiphyseal configuration.
The pelvis should always be x-rayed in the presence of major lower limb injuries.

Professional Considerations
Communication between the physician and the radiologist is essential, particularly regarding
1. The seriousness of the patient's condition
2. The history of the injury
3. The clinical diagnosis
4. Any contraindications to routine roentgenographic positioning or maneuvers
5. An informed professional should accompany seriously injured patients to the x-ray
   department and assist the technician in positioning the patient.
Consultation between the physician and the radiologist concerning the need and indications
for special procedures such as special views, tomography, computerized axial
tomography, etc.

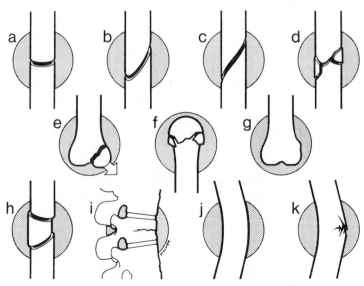

Figure 20-1.   The semantics of fractures. *a*, transverse; *b*, oblique; *c*, spiral; *d*, comminuted; *e*, avulsion; *f*, impacted; *g*, torus; *h*, segmented; *i*, compression; *j*, bending; *k*, greenstick.

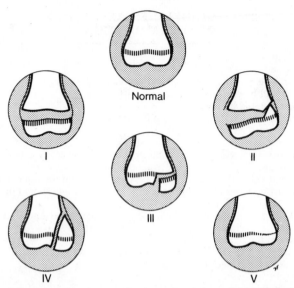

Figure 20–2. The Salter-Harris classification of epiphyseal injuries. (From Salter RB, Harris WR. Injuries involving the epiphyseal plate. J. Bone Joint Surg. 45A:587–622, 1963.)

except for the local swelling. This sequence occurs most frequently with injuries about the shoulder and pelvic girdles, in the thigh, and in cases of multiple extremity injuries. The estimated average blood loss in patients with fractures is commonly greater than anticipated (Table 20–2). This is due to the fact that bleeding continues for 24 to 48 hours after the fracture, during which time blood forms the major component of soft tissue swelling. It is essential that surgeons understand the importance of silent bleeding in the production of hypovolemia and hypovolemic shock in patients with fractures and that they take this into consideration in the resuscitative treatment with fluid and blood.

Bleeding into the soft tissues around the fractures can be limited by gentle handling and prompt application of splints and dressings. Early reduction of fractures with restoration of limb length by traction or by immobilization in plaster casts helps limit bleeding.

TABLE 20–2.   ESTIMATED LOCAL BLOOD LOSS IN FRACTURES (IN LITERS)

Humerus	1.0–2.0
Elbow	0.5–1.5
Forearm	0.5–1.0
Pelvis	1.5–4.5
Hip	1.5–2.5
Femur	1.0–2.0
Knee	1.0–1.5
Tibia	0.5–1.5
Ankle	0.5–1.5

FAT EMBOLISM

Fat embolism occurs most frequently in patients with multiple long bone fractures, fractures of the pelvis, and crush injuries. The most important manifestation of this phenomenon is inapparent hypoxemia, that is, the presence of significant hypoxemia that cannot be recognized on clinical examination. This hypoxia is often present when the patient arrives in the emergency department and should be treated by administration of oxygen while the patient is being evaluated and treated. Measurement of the arterial blood gases on admission and at appropriate intervals thereafter is helpful to ensure that serious inapparent hypoxemia is not overlooked. Early adequate oxygenation is the best method of preventing more serious problems with fat embolism.

The full-blown picture of fat embolism appears after 24 to 72 hours and is characterized by dyspnea, tachypnea, profuse tracheobronchial secretion, petechial hemorrhages, and changes in the sensorium ranging from apprehension and agitation to coma. Petechial hemorrhages, best seen on the sclera, conjunctiva, chest wall, and axillae, may appear as early as 12 hours or as late as 72 hours after injury. Their presence establishes the diagnosis of fat embolism. The neurological findings are characteristically diffuse and nonlocalizing. In addition to a decrease in the PaO_2, an associated thrombocytopenia of less than 150,000 platelets/mm^3 is often present. An electrocardiogram may show right heart strain. The chest roentgenograms are occasionally helpful and may show diffuse microatelectasis evenly distributed throughout both lung fields.

The treatment of fat embolism consists of maintaining adequate tissue oxygenation using an endotracheal tube and a volume-controlled respirator as needed. In severe cases, massive doses of corticosteroid hormones may be helpful. The disease is self-limited, and the patient will recover completely if he can be maintained through the critical period.

OPEN FRACTURES

Open fractures and dislocations are injuries in which the fracture site or joint is in direct communication with the external environment through a wound in the skin or mucous membranes. An operation for the open reduction of a fracture or dislocation produces the same situation. Inherent in such open injuries is the possibility of infection. Prior to the development of antiseptic and aseptic surgical techniques, the mortality rate for open fractures was high and the treatment of choice was often immediate amputation before infection became established. Even today the mortality rate for open fractures of the pelvis is 50 percent. Despite our current methods of treatment there is a continuing toll of infected nonunited fractures, chronic draining sinuses, bone necrosis, osteomyelitis, soft tissue abscesses, and late amputations. An open fracture or dislocation demands early effective treatment to prevent infection.

Open injuries occur as a result of three mechanisms: (1) the rupture of the skin and soft tissues due to the explosive effects of the deforming force, (2) the puncture or laceration of the integument by the sharp bony fragments of the fracture, and (3) wounds of the skin and soft tissues from external objects that also produce a fracture.

Although soft tissue wounds may appear to be quite insignificant and even at some distance from the fracture, they must be carefully examined prior to closure to be certain that they do not communicate with the fracture site. Seen on x-ray, the presence of gas (air) in the tissue planes in the fractured limb immediately following injury suggests the presence of an open fracture through which the air has been aspirated at the time of fracture. Occasionally the patient may have a portion of the fractured bone protruding through the wound or easily visible in its depth. There may be extensive injury of the skin and soft tissues as well as of the bone. Three factors affect the incidence of infection in such open fractures: (1) the nature of the wound, (2) the type of contamination, and (3) the initial treatment. Tidy wounds, which are defined as bursting or incised wounds in which the skin edges are sharply defined and soft tissues are divided cleanly, contain very little dead or questionably viable tissue. Untidy wounds are the result of tearing and crushing forces that leave skin edges ragged and abraded, fatty layers disrupted, and muscles crushed to a pulp and shredded. These wounds contain a good deal of dead and severely compromised tissues. Untidy wounds provide an excellent medium for the growth of bacteria, particularly when an element of ischemia is present because of interference with the local circulation by injury, swelling, or constriction, or all three.

Bacteria and debris such as dirt, gravel, shotgun pellets, and metal fragments may be present in wounds associated with open fractures. Bacterial contamination depends in part upon the environment in which the injury was incurred. Open fractures sustained in fields contaminated by human and animal feces are more apt to contain spores of tetanus and gas gangrene bacilli. Bacteria can be introduced into the wound at any time following injury. This emphasizes the importance of immediate application of an occlusive dressing over the wound to prevent further contamination and aseptic management thereafter to reduce the incidence of nosocomial infection.

Initial treatment should be directed toward changing an untidy wound into a tidy wound. This is accomplished by removing all dead and questionably viable soft tissue and ensuring an adequate blood supply to the remaining tissue by the process of debridement. (The unnecessary sacrifice of skin, soft tissues, and bone fragments is to be avoided.) The wound should be extended longitudinally so that the fracture fragments can be examined. Tight fascial sheaths should be opened in the same manner to provide decompression, prevent constriction, and allow room for swelling. Dead muscle can be recognized by its appearance and the fact that it does not contract when stimulated by grasping with a thumb forceps. In this way the media upon which bacteria can grow is removed from the wound.

At the same time, contaminating debris is removed mechanically and by copious irrigation. While loose bone fragments may be discarded, every effort should be made to preserve large fragments, particularly if they remain viable because of periosteal and soft tissue attachments. Dirt that has been ground into the end of a fracture fragment can be removed with a curette or rongeur. In shotgun wounds, loose pellets are easily removed and the wadding from the shell should be carefully looked for and extracted. Widely dispersed pellets should be left alone, because the damage caused by searching for and removing them may be greater than the damage resulting from leaving them in situ.

Bacterial contamination should be reduced by removing the foreign material to which the bacteria may be attached and by diluting their number by copious irrigation. The use of a Water Pik is favored by some. Further growth of the bacteria in the wound may be suppressed by appropriate prophylactic use of antibiotics. This consists of the early intravenous administration of broad-spectrum antibiotics. To be most effective this should be begun as soon as the presence of an open fracture is recognized and before definitive debridement is begun. All patients with open fractures should receive appropriate prophylaxis against tetanus.

After debridement, the fracture must be reduced and immobilized. External skeletal fixation by the Roger Anderson or Hoffmann technique is a useful option, especially when there is extensive loss of skin and soft tissue. It is essential to secure satisfactory reduction and immobilization of the fracture fragments, because this in itself will help to prevent infection by limiting swelling and promoting good circulation to the injured area.

The closure of the wound often constitutes a problem. Primary closure should be done only when (1) contamination is small, (2) the wound is tidy without extensive soft tissue injury, (3) the wound can be readily closed without tension, and (4) the fracture can be reduced and maintained in position easily. When these criteria cannot be met, the wound should be left open, carefully dressed with sterile fine mesh gauze (roller bandage) and closed four or five days later (delayed primary closure). Split-thickness skin grafts may be used to carry out primary or delayed primary closure. When primary or delayed primary closure cannot be accomplished, secondary closure should be done as early in the course of treatment as possible.

GAS GANGRENE

Gas gangrene is one of the most dreaded complications of open fractures and occurs most frequently in fractures associated with substantial soft tissue injury to muscles and in which circulation to the injured area is impaired because of vascular injury or constriction. The clinical picture is characterized by a short prodromal period followed by the onset of a severe dull boring pain and tachycardia. There is usually only a low-grade fever. Examination of the wound reveals a characteristic mousy smell and a thin serosanguinous exudate. Such wounds should be widely opened immediately with further debridement and excision of affected muscle. Everything possible should be done to ensure that circulation in the remaining tissue is not impaired. In fulminating cases, guillotine amputation may be necessary.

INDICATIONS FOR AMPUTATION

Occasionally a patient will be seen whose extremity is so badly damaged that amputation is the treatment of choice. The decision to proceed with amputation should be made only after consultation with another surgeon, whenever possible. The taking of appropriate photographs of the limb to document its condition is recommended. In many situations, when the mangled limb has multiple fractures, extensive soft tissue damage, and gross contamination, the decision is an easy one. In other cases, the decision may not be as clear. The indications for amputation can be appraised systematically by considering the condition of five components: skin, muscle and tendon, bone, nerves, and blood vessels. After initial evaluation, one must ask oneself the questions: Can early or late skin coverage be obtained? Can loss of muscle and tendon be compensated for? Can bone loss be restored by later grafting? What is the prognosis for nerve regeneration after nerve suture or grafting? Can circulation be restored by suture or grafting?

When there is irreparable loss or damage to three or more component systems, amputation is usually indicated. The most critical component is the blood supply, because intact circulation is essential for limb survival. When amputation is carried out under these circumstances, as much limb length as possible should be preserved. Primary closure should not be attempted. A guillotine amputation with skin traction applied to the stump will usually suffice. The decision regarding delayed closure or revision of the stump can then be delayed safely for several days.

INDICATIONS FOR REPLANTATION

There has been sufficient experience with the replantation of amputated limbs to derive some general principles regarding its application. Replantation should not be considered in patients who have other major injuries, are over 50 years of age, or who have untidy avulsion or amputations with crushed tissues. Replantation of the lower limb is rarely if ever justified. The condition of the opposite limb should be considered.

Time is of the essence because the amputated part, if not cooled, remains viable for only four to six hours, but with cooling, it remains viable for up to about 18 hours. The best results are obtained with finger replantation (60 to 80 percent success rate). A skilled surgical team is required. The initial treatment of the amputated part is very simple. It should be placed in a plastic bag, without any additional fluid, and transported in a container with ice. At the time of replantation the tissue should be thoroughly cleaned and debrided.

METHODS OF TREATING FRACTURES

Fractures may be treated by a variety of methods, each of which has its particular advantages and disadvantages and associated complications. The selection of an appropriate method of treatment depends upon the type of injury, the presence of other associated injuries, the condition of the patient, the facilities available, and the capabilities of the physician.

PARTIAL IMMOBILIZATION

Many fractures about the shoulder can be treated simply with a sling, a sling and swathe, or a figure-of-eight bandage. Some fractures of the foot and ankle can be treated with adhesive tape strapping. Crutches to limit weight bearing on the leg may be all that is required. Partial immobilization promotes early function and simplifies patient care but may not be effective in relieving pain. The cooperation of the patient and family is essential, because with this treatment immobilization is not complete and further displacement of the fracture fragments can occur.

IMMOBILIZATION

Many undisplaced fractures require only immobilization in a splint or a plaster cast. Splints must be carefully adjusted to fit the individual patient. Plaster of Paris is an ideal material because it is readily available, conforms easily to the part, and is absorbent and inexpensive. Plaster casts deteriorate with abuse and exposure to water. Complications associated with plaster casts include pressure sores, nerve palsies, and displacement of fracture fragments because of loosening.

CLOSED REDUCTION AND IMMOBILIZATION

When there is a dislocation or a displaced fracture, the initial step in treatment is to reduce the dislocation or to obtain a satisfactory position of the fracture fragments. When this is done without an open operation by traction or manipulation or both, it is called a closed reduction.

Some form of anesthesia is almost always required for such a closed reduction. An intravenous injection of diazepam or morphine sulfate may be sufficient. Sometimes a local anesthetic agent may be injected directly into the joint or into the fracture-hematoma. On occasion, a nerve block or Bier block may be used (see Chapter 7). In many cases, however, spinal or general anesthesia is required. The choice of the anesthetic method to be used depends upon the injury, the presence of associated injuries, the condition of the patient, and the facilities available.

While many dislocations and fractures can be reduced satisfactorily by closed manipulation, this technique will fail (1) when soft tissues such as muscle, tendon, or joint capsule are interposed between the fragments; (2) if fragments of bone are either caught in the joint or distracted from the site of fracture by muscular contraction; or (3) when the reduction is intrinsically unstable, as is the case in most fracture-dislocations. It is usually possible to judge initially the cases in which a closed reduction cannot be successful so that an alternate method of treatment may be chosen. In cases of doubt, a closed reduction should first be attempted, but if reduction is not satisfactory, an alternate method should be pursued.

The criteria used to decide if a reduction is satisfactory vary widely with the different bones and the location of the fracture in the individual bone. In general, fractures involving articular surfaces of joints must be reduced and the anatomical contours accurately restored, because any residual incongruity of the joint surface can lead to late traumatic arthritis. In many other areas, the reduction need not be anatomical as long as length, alignment, and rotation are preserved and as long as the final position does not impair function significantly.

Following reduction, the injured part may be partially immobilized, e.g., in a sling and swathe following dislocation of the shoulder, or immobilized in a plaster cast or dressing. Closed reduction and immobilization of fractures is usually simple and can be carried out with a low morbidity and few complications. Since no incision is made, the risk of infection of the fracture site is avoided.

Open Reduction and Internal Fixation

When a satisfactory reduction cannot be obtained or has not been obtained by closed methods, open reduction should be done by means of an operation to visualize the fracture site followed by internal fixation with screws, plates, pins, and so forth. Open reduction is the primary method of choice when (1) soft tissue or bone interposition between the fracture fragments prevents the reduction of the fracture, (2) the fracture cannot be held in anatomical position, or (3) the fracture dislocation is intrinsically unstable. In many cases, internal fixation may be so firm that no other immobilization is required. In other cases, the additional support of plaster casts and dressings may be needed.

Open reduction and internal fixation requires a high degree of technical skill and is associated with technical complications such as the loosening or breaking of screws, pins, plates, and other components. Since a closed fracture is converted into an open fracture by the operation, there is increased hazard of infection. Open reduction enables the surgeon to remove any obstacle to an accurate anatomical reduction. Internal fixation may also allow early function of the injured part and minimize the amount of external immobilization required. This is particularly valuable in the patient with multiple fractures who requires special pulmonary care.

EXTERNAL SKELETAL FIXATION

This method of treatment is a form of fixation or immobilization of the fracture fragments by the use of pins drilled into the bone fragments and left protruding through the skin. The protruding ends of the pins are then rigidly fixed to provide immobilization. The simplest form of this technique is called "pins in plaster." In this method, the pins are incorporated in the plaster dressing or cast enveloping the limb. The pins can also be attached to one another by articulated bars in the more elaborate systems popularized by Roger Anderson and Hoffmann. When pins are used, there is always the risk of pin track infection and the technical problems of loosening. The more sophisticated equipment is expensive and may not be readily available. External pin fixation is most useful in immobilizing fractures of the pelvis and in fractures of the extremities associated with extensive skin and soft tissue injury.

TRACTION

Traction is employed most frequently in patients with fractures of the hip and femur, less frequently in fractures of the upper extremities.

Skin traction is effected by adhesive or adherent strips attached to the skin and held in place by a circular bandage. The area (cm^2) of skin to which the strips are applied determines the amount of traction that can be applied. The strips should therefore extend proximally on the limb as far as possible. Even with strips attached from toes to groin in an adult, the upper limit of traction that can be applied safely is about 5 kg. Skin traction is applied easily and can be used for definitive treatment or for postoperative stabilization. The complications of skin traction are blisters and skin irritation from the strips, nerve palsies, circulatory impairment, and pressure sores from the circular bandage. Skin traction cannot be applied over wounds, abrasion, or areas of chronic skin disease.

Skeletal traction is effected by the insertion of pins or wires through the bone. Appropriate bails are attached to the pins and rope is then attached to the bail. Insertion of pins and wires requires local anesthesia and introduces the hazard of infection along the pin track. The advantage provided, however, is that as much traction as desired can be applied. Skeletal traction can be used as either a definitive or a temporary form of treatment. The pins can be incorporated in a plaster cast dressing when desired. Removal of the pins is easy and does not require anesthesia.

FRACTURES IN CHILDREN

It has often been said that fractures in children are different. In reality, it is the children who are different. The diagnosis, complications, and indications for treatment in children's fractures are the same as those in adults. Children differ from adults in that their bony skeleton is immature and undergoing continuing growth. This growth takes place at the epiphyses at the ends of the long bone. These areas are not as strong anatomically as the adjacent bones and ligaments so that epiphyseal separations or fractures occur frequently. Damage to the epiphysis may result in failure of continued normal growth with a resulting shortening or deformity or both. The degree of shortening or deformity or both depends upon the amount of growth potential remaining in the epiphysis and is, of course, much greater in the young child than in the adolescent, whose epiphyseal line is about to close spontaneously. The likelihood of a growth disturbance is related to the type of injury. Here the classification of Salter and Harris (see Fig. 20–2) is particularly useful. When the epiphysis is displaced but not broken (Types I and II), a subsequent growth disturbance is infrequent. When the epiphysis is fractured (Types III and IV) or crushed (Type V), the prognosis is much worse. In injuries involving the epiphyseal areas in children, x-rays of the uninjured opposite side are of great value in helping to compare and determine the presence and nature of any epiphyseal difference.

The growth of bone in a child is accomplished by continuous remodeling as new bone is laid down and old bone is resorbed. This process leads to some improvement in angular deformities in healed long bone fractures in children. The amount of remodeling to be anticipated depends upon the amount of bone growth that can be expected. There is no bone growth compensation for displacements in rotation. Anticipation of future remodeling should not lead the surgeon to accept a poor reduction of a fracture in a child.

MULTIPLE INJURIES

With the exception of dislocations, the treatment of extremity injuries has a lower priority than the treatment of life-threatening injuries in the cranial, thoracic, and abdominal cavities. The reduction of a dislocation of the hip, shoulder, knee, elbow, etc., should not be postponed. These injuries can usually be reduced expeditiously immediately following induction of anesthesia while the patient is being prepared for other operative procedures. At this time, gross displacements of fractures that threaten the integrity of the skin or circulation should also be corrected. Great care should be taken to protect the injured limb during operations on other parts of the body. Proper splinting should always be employed and any focal pressure that might cause necrosis or constriction of neural or vascular structures must be avoided.

Multiple fractures and other injuries can occur in one extremity or may involve all four extremities and the trunk. As the number of such injuries increases, so does the number of complications arising in their treatment. The presence of other fractures influences the indications for the treatment of individual fractures. For instance, most fractures of the shaft of the humerus are treated without operation, utilizing a hanging plaster technique. This requires the patient to be ambulating or only semirecumbent. If he must be recumbent because of other injuries, this technique is unsatisfactory and another method must be employed. In patients with multiple fractures there are strong indications for an aggressive program of early open reduction and internal fixation of many, if not all, of the fractures.

FRACTURE HEALING

Fracture healing is a local phenomenon that is rarely affected by systemic illness and disease. The local factors of greatest importance are (1) the blood supply to the fracture fragments, (2) soft tissue interposition, and (3) the amount of motion at the fracture site.

The cancellous bone of the metaphysis generally has a rich blood supply. Fractures through areas of cancellous bone heal rapidly and delayed union or nonunion is unusual. In contrast, the blood supply to the hard cortical bone of the diaphyseal tubes of the long bones is more critical. This is especially true when there are segmental fractures or comminuted fractures. Occasionally, as a result of the injury or dissection of the fracture fragments at operation, a large fragment may be separated from its periosteal and soft tissue attachments with complete loss of its blood supply. Such a fragment then becomes, to all intents and purposes, an autogenous bone graft. Fractures of this type have a high incidence of delayed union and nonunion because of their poor blood supply.

Soft tissue interposition between the fracture fragments occurs at the time of injury when the maximum degree of displacement of bone fragments and soft tissues occurs. The entrapment of muscle, tendon, or joint capsule commonly acts as an impediment to a closed reduction. The presence of soft tissue interposition is an indication for open reduction at which time these obstacles to reduction and to fracture healing are dealt with.

The amount of immobilization required for satisfactory fracture healing varies with the location and type of fracture. Fractures of the clavicle and the shaft of the humerus heal well with a minimal degree of immobilization. The wide use of cast braces and early ambulation in the treatment of fractures of the shaft of the femur and tibia would indicate that these fractures also do not require rigid immobilization to achieve union. On the other hand, fractures of the carpal navicular and the neck of the femur require rigid fixation. In general, fractures whose fragments have an excellent blood supply from periosteal and muscle attachments require less rigid fixation than fractures whose fragments have a poor blood supply.

The healing reaction around fragments not rigidly immobilized is much greater than that around fragments rigidly immobilized. Swelling, thickening, and the components of callus formation can be palpated. New bone formation around the fractures can be seen on x-rays. A large amount of healing reaction and callus formation does not guarantee solid union. Conversely, the absence of a visible healing reaction in a rigidly immobilized fracture does not mean that solid union is not progressing. Fractures of the phalanges, metacarpals, and metatarsals may progress to

TABLE 20–3. **AVERAGE HEALING TIME FOR COMMON FRACTURES (IN WEEKS)**

Upper Extremity	
Clavicle	6
Humerus	
Neck	6
Shaft	12
Forearm	
Both bones	12
Distal radius	6
Ulna	6
Carpal navicular	10
Metacarpal	6
Phalanx	3
Lower Extremity	
Hip	12
Femoral shaft	16–24
Tibia	
Plateau	8
Shaft	16–32
Ankle	8–12
Fibula	
Shaft	8
Ankle	8
Os calcis	8–12
Metatarsal	8

union with minimal signs of a local healing reaction. Surprisingly, many pathological fractures through tumor metastases will heal, particularly if the tumor is sensitive to irradiation and if local irradiation is administered.

At the time of the fracture the patient, his family, or his employer will want to know how long the injury will take to heal. The average healing times for some common fractures are shown in Table 20–3. Fractures in adolescents require much the same time to heal as do those in adults. In children, healing occurs more rapidly.

Fracture healing is assessed most accurately by a careful clinical evaluation. Has a sufficient time elapsed for healing to occur? Is there local tenderness on palpation over the fracture site? Is there false motion or a "give" at the fracture site when it is stressed? What is the condition of the adjacent soft tissues? What is the range of motion of adjacent joints? The roentgenographic examination will show the position of the fracture fragments, the amount of new bone formation, the degree of osteopenia related to immobilization and disuse, and the condition of any devices used for internal fixation. Broken plates, pins, or screws, and evidence of loosening or movement of such devices strongly suggest that solid healing has not occurred.

Delayed union of a fracture is a condition in which prolongation of fracture healing is occurring, but in which healing will eventually occur. Nonunion is a condition in which healing of the fracture will never occur without some intervention, usually in the form of a bone graft.

Chapter

21

Injuries of the Upper Extremity

FRACTURES AND DISLOCATIONS OF THE SHOULDER REGION

Fractures and dislocations about the shoulder are seen in all age groups. They are caused by falls on the outstretched arm or the point of the shoulder, and by the direct impact of objects on the shoulder. While single injuries are the rule, a complex of multiple injuries can occur. An example of this is the patient struck on the shoulder from behind who sustains an acromioclavicular separation, a comminuted fracture of the scapula, multiple rib fractures in the area where the scapula is driven into the chest wall, and a pulmonary contusion. Stretch injuries of the brachial plexus can accompany violent injuries of the shoulder. Fragments of a broken clavicle rarely damage the brachial plexus or subclavian vessel.

Emergency treatment for injuries of the shoulder consists of an arm sling to support the weight of the arm, and a bandage or swathe to bind the arm against the chest wall (Fig. 21–1).

THE CLAVICLE

The clavicle can be dislocated from either its medial (sternoclavicular) or lateral (acromioclavicular) articulations. These joints are shallow, contain fibrocartilaginous menisci, and are strengthened by strong external ligaments. The main attachments of the clavicle to the scapula are the coracoclavicular ligaments that pass from the coracoid process to the junction of the middle and lateral third of the clavicle. The acromioclavicular joint is much more vulnerable to injury than the sternoclavicular joint.

Since the clavicle is palpable subcutaneously throughout its length, fractures or dislocations or both can be diagnosed by a careful physical examination. The roentgenographic diagnosis of injuries of the clavicle may be difficult, particularly at the medial end because of the superimposition of shadows from the ribs, spine, and mediastinum. It is helpful in assessing the degree of separation of the acromioclavicular joint to obtain a

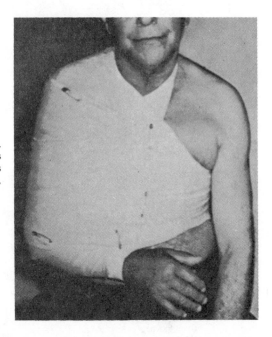

Figure 21-1. Sling and swathe. (From Rhoads JE, Allen JG, Harkins HN, Moyer CA: Surgery, Principles and Practice, 4th ed. Philadelphia, J. B. Lippincott Co., 1970.)

"weighted view." This consists of an anteroposterior view of the shoulder, taken with the patient standing and holding a 5 to 10 pound weight in his hand. Such a pull tends to distract the clavicle from the joint and to reveal the extent of the disruption. An oblique view may help in visualizing this joint. Comparison views of the opposite uninjured acromioclavicular joint are essential.

Dislocation of the sternoclavicular joint usually occurs anteriorly, the proximal end of the clavicle riding over the front of the manubrium and producing an abnormal prominence. When the clavicle dislocates posteriorly above and behind the manubrium, respiration can be impaired by direct pressure on the trachea and major vessels may be injured. The maneuver that produces reduction of both dislocations consists of direct pressure while both shoulders are pulled backward. A figure-of-eight bandage and an arm sling are used for support and stabilization. When recurrent dislocation occurs, consideration must be given to reconstruction of the ligaments or excision of the medial end of the clavicle.

Subluxation or dislocation of the acromioclavicular joint (the "knocked-down shoulder" of the football player) is a common injury. In addition to disruption of the acromioclavicular ligaments, partial or total disruption of the coracoclavicular ligaments always occurs. The diagnosis is made by localizing the pain to the acromioclavicular joint and palpating the deformity. It may be possible to reduce the dislocation by pushing down on the end of the clavicle and upward on the arm. The immediate treatment consists of supporting the weight of the arm with an arm sling. Subsequent

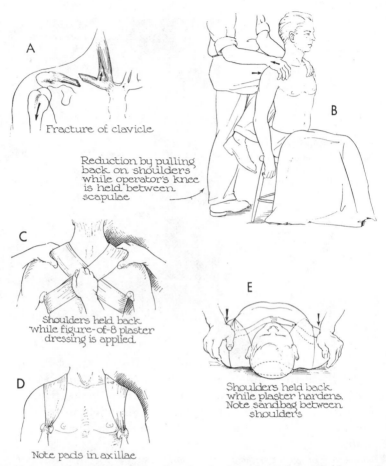

Figure 21-2. Method of hyperextending the shoulders in applying the figure of eight bandage. (Reproduced with permission from Compere EL, Banks SW, Compere CL: Pictorial Handbook of Fracture Treatment, 5th ed. Copyright © 1963 by Year Book Medical Publishers, Inc., Chicago.)

treatment should consist of either an early program of exercises to promote normal shoulder motion or an operation consisting of excision of the lateral end of the clavicle and repair of the coracoclavicular ligaments. Complicated systems of adhesive strapping or splinting or both are not effective. The choice of treatment is related to age, sex, dominant arm, and level of activity. In a young athlete, operation is usually the treatment of choice. In patients treated without an operation, late symptoms associated with traumatic arthritis of the acromioclavicular joint can be relieved by simple excision of the distal end of the clavicle.

Fractures of the clavicle are divided into two groups determined by the insertion of the coracoclavicular ligaments. Fragments of the medial two thirds of the clavicle are unstable. The weight of the arm displaces the scapula downward and forward; the pull of the sternocleidomastoid muscle displaces the medial fragment upward. These fractures are aligned by pulling the shoulder backward and upward (Fig. 21–2). Position is maintained by a figure of eight bandage and an arm sling (Fig. 21–3). Open reduction and internal fixation of fractures of the clavicle is rarely if ever indicated and is the most frequent cause of nonunited fractures of the clavicle.

Fractures of the lateral third of the clavicle are stable, since the major ligaments binding the clavicle to the scapula are intact. These fractures can be treated simply in an arm sling.

DISLOCATIONS OF THE SHOULDER

Dislocations of the shoulder or glenohumeral joint are almost always anterior; posterior dislocations make up only 2 percent of all dislocations. Anterior dislocations are the result of forced abduction and external rotation of the humerus. In young adults, associated fractures of the greater tuberosity of the humerus are unusual, but with advancing age they become quite frequent. Such fractures rarely interfere with reduction of the dislocations and usually require no special treatment. The axillary

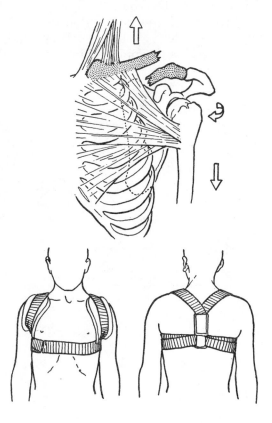

Figure 21–3. Fracture of the clavicle. Top, The shoulder drops forward, inward, and downward, resulting in over-riding of the fragments. Bottom, Immobilization by the standard clavicular strap that tends to hold the shoulder upward, backward, and outward. An arm sling to support the weight of the arm is always used in addition to the figure of eight bandage. (From Rhoads JE, Allen JG, Harkins HN, Moyer CA: Surgery, Principles and Practice, 4th ed. Philadelphia, J. B. Lippincott Co., 1970.)

nerve, which is closely applied to the posterior and lateral aspect of the neck of the humerus, supplies motor fibers to the deltoid muscle and sensory fibers to the lateral aspect of the shoulder, the "shoulder patch area." Injuries of the axillary nerve can occur in association with dislocations of the shoulder and other injuries in this area and must be anticipated.

A patient with an *anterior dislocation of the shoulder* presents with the arm held in abduction and external rotation. He cannot bring his elbow down to the chest wall nor touch his opposite ear with his hand. Palpation over the deltoid muscle reveals that the head of the humerus no longer lies beneath it. Further palpation may find the head of the humerus anterior and below, or lateral to the coracoid process. The sensation on the lateral aspect of the shoulder and the contractility of the deltoid muscle should be checked to determine if injury to the axillary nerve has occurred. An anteroposterior roentgenogram of the shoulder will establish the diagnosis and indicate whether or not there is an associated fracture of the humerus.

Dislocations of the shoulder should be reduced promptly, without delay. Reduction can be accomplished in many patients using an intravenous analgesic drug, reinforced occasionally by injection of a local anesthetic agent into the joint. In some large, muscular patients, a general anesthetic may be required.

The most frequently used method of reducing an anterior dislocation of the shoulder is called the Hippocratic method (Fig. 21–4). In this method, traction is applied to the arm with the foot of the operator against

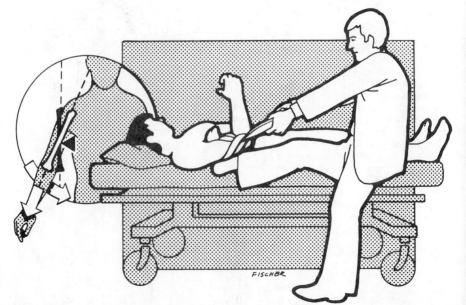

Figure 21-4. The Hippocratic method of reducing an anterior dislocation of the shoulder.

the chest wall for countertraction and to act as a fulcrum against which the humeral shaft can be applied as a lever. A convenient method of applying traction is by means of a skein of yarn, formed into a loose loop about 36 inches in circumference. This is applied to the arm above the elbow. Traction can then be made with the elbow flexed to 90 degrees, weakening the resistance of the biceps and coracobrachialis muscles. The substance of the yarn also allows a firmer grasp than the wrist of the patient. Firm continuous traction is then applied to relax opposing muscles. Jerky rapid movements stimulate the opposing muscles to contract. When the muscles have relaxed, the arm is adducted and brought down to the chest wall. The upper portion of the shaft of the humerus is pressed against the fulcrum of the foot and the head is levered laterally, where it becomes reduced into the glenoid cavity. After reduction, the arm is placed in a sling and swathe, and roentgenograms are taken to confirm the fact that reduction has, indeed, occurred. The function of the axillary nerve is also reassessed.

In an intoxicated combative patient the method of Milch is useful (Fig. 21–5). The patient is placed on a litter in the prone position with the arm hanging over the edge. A weight (5 to 8 kg) is attached to the arm using the skein of yarn. Traction is applied for 5 to 10 minutes, at which time it will be found that the dislocation may be reduced in many cases. If it has not reduced spontaneously, gentle circumduction of the arm will accomplish this. Subsequent treatment is the same.

The reduction of an anterior dislocation of the shoulder by the Kocher maneuver (Fig. 21–6) should not be attempted in primary dislocations, in muscular young adults, or in older patients. It is most useful in patients with recurrent dislocations. In this maneuver, traction is applied to the

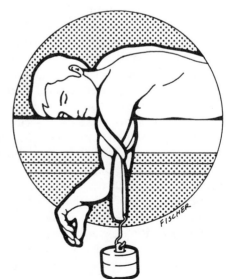

Figure 21–5. The Milch method of reducing an anterior dislocation of the shoulder.

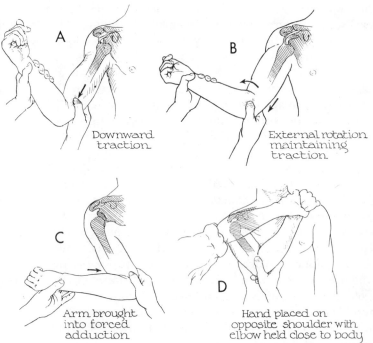

Figure 21–6. Kocher's maneuvers for reduction of an anterior (subcoracoid or subglenoid) dislocation of the shoulder. (Reproduced with permission from Compere EL, Banks SW, Compere CL: Pictorial Handbook of Fracture Treatment, 5th ed. Copyright © 1963 by Year Book Medical Publishers, Inc., Chicago.)

humerus to relax the muscles, the arm is adducted to and then across the chest to move the head laterally, and then the arm is internally rotated to reduce the dislocation. If this is done forcefully, spiral fractures of the humerus can occur because of the torque on the shaft.

Posterior dislocations of the shoulder are rare injuries. While a strong blow in the front of the shoulder can cause posterior dislocation, the great majority of these injuries result from violent uncoordinated contractions of muscles of the shoulder occurring during convulsions or seizures. In fact, a history of a seizure or convulsion followed by persistent shoulder pain should give rise to a strong suspicion that such a dislocation has occurred. The patient will present with his arm held stiffly at his side in marked internal rotation. He will be unable to externally rotate the humerus. The roentgenographic diagnosis of a posterior dislocation of the shoulder is difficult, and anteroposterior, axillary, and lateral views of the gleno-humeral area are essential. Confusion results because little change in the relationship of the head of the humerus to the glenoid will be seen in the anteroposterior view and the details of the relationship on the lateral view are obscured by overlapping shadows. When the head of the humerus on the anteroposterior views appears to be symmetrical (the "light bulb sign") because of marked internal rotation, posterior dislocation is almost always present. Because the diagnosis is difficult, posterior dislocations of the shoulder may be overlooked. A diagnosis of "frozen shoulder" is then incorrectly made, and the patient receives extensive physical therapy without benefit.

The reduction of a posterior dislocation of the shoulder is accomplished by applying traction to the humerus. When sufficient muscle relaxation has occurred, the head of the humerus is pushed forward by direct pressure from behind and seated in the glenoid cavity by externally rotating the humerus. Aftercare is the same as for an anterior dislocation, unless the dislocation recurs with internal rotation of the arm. In such a case, immobilization in a shoulder spica with the arm in external rotation is required.

Fractures of the scapula result from direct blows on the posterior aspect of the shoulder. Since the scapula is contained in a thick muscular envelope, displacement of the fractures is usually small. Palpation along the spine of the scapula may reveal some irregularity. Anteroposterior and tangential views of the scapula are essential for roentgenographic diagnosis. Treatment is directed toward the early restoration of normal motion. This is especially important when the underlying chest wall has also been injured, since loss of scapulothoracic motion — that is, the gliding of the scapula on the chest wall — will result in significant loss of shoulder motion.

FRACTURES AND DISLOCATIONS OF THE ARM

FRACTURES OF THE UPPER END OF THE HUMERUS

Fractures of the tuberosities of the humerus occur most frequently in association with dislocations of the shoulder. They do not present obstacles to closed reduction and usually fall into good position following reduction of the dislocation. Rarely the tuberosity fractures when a portion is avulsed by the strong contraction of the rotator cuff during abduction against resistance. In such a case the fragment may remain displaced. Treatment consists of abducting the humerus to bring the head up to the avulsed fragment and maintaining the position of abduction in a shoulder spica for four to six weeks. Alternatively, the fracture can be exposed surgically and the rotator cuff and the avulsed bony fragment fixed in place. Following this, only an arm sling is required for several weeks.

Fractures of the anatomical neck of the humerus are intra-articular fractures. The fragment of the head of the humerus has no blood supply, resulting in aseptic necrosis and delay of fracture healing. These fractures are usually the result of violent injury with dislocation of the shoulder and can be an obstacle to closed reduction. Successful management usually

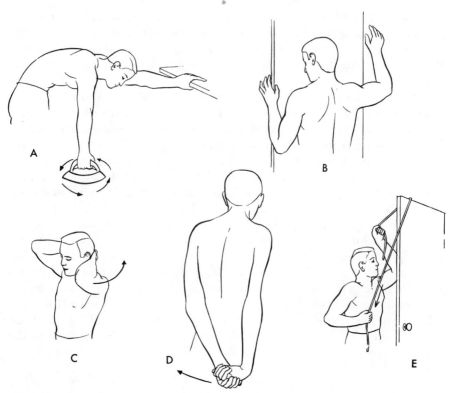

Figure 21-7. Mobilization of injured and painful shoulder. *A,* Gravity-free pendulum exercises are more comfortable and efficient with a weight in the hand. *B,* Crawling up the wall, assisted elevation; a strip of adhesive is placed on the wall to be marked in pencil as a record of the elevation attained each day. *C,* Exercise for restoration of external rotation. *D,* Exercise for restoration of internal rotation. *E,* The normal extremity assists in elevation of the injured member. (From McLaughlin HL; Trauma. Philadelphia, W. B. Saunders Co., 1959.)

requires open operation with removal of the fragment of the head. Occasionally a humeral head prosthesis may be used to improve the functional result.

Fractures of the surgical neck of the humerus, occurring frequently in the elderly, are accompanied by substantial blood loss into the area around the shoulder. As the large hematoma resolves, ecchymosis is seen on the chest wall and breast, extending down the arm even to the palm of the hand. Bleeding is greater in those patients who are on anticoagulants. Because of local hemorrhage following fractures of the surgical neck of the humerus, blood transfusion may be required. Treatment of the fractures can be accomplished easily with a sling and swathe. Emphasis should be placed on early motion by means of pendulum exercises to avoid late stiffness of the shoulder (Fig. 21–7).

Some high humeral fractures in young adults may be displaced by the violence of the injury. Closed reduction may be impossible because of soft tissue interposition, which commonly traps the tendon of the long head of the biceps between the fracture fragments. In such cases, open reduction and internal fixation with screws or intramedullary pins is indicated.

Separation of the proximal humeral epiphysis is uncommon and is almost always of the Salter Type II configuration. With minimal displacement, only a sling and a swathe is required for treatment. Reduction of greater degrees of displacement can usually be obtained by closed manipulation under anesthesia, bringing the humerus into full abduction and external rotation. External fixation in a shoulder spica in this position for three or four weeks is usually sufficient. A badly displaced separation of the proximal humeral epiphysis caused by violent trauma may because of soft tissue interposition require open reduction and internal fixation to obtain a satisfactory reduction.

FRACTURES OF THE SHAFT OF THE HUMERUS

Fractures of the shaft of the humerus are caused by direct blows and by rotation or twisting (torque) on the humerus. Wide displacement may result in soft tissue interposition or injury to the radial nerve (or both). Injury to the radial nerve occurs most frequently in association with fractures of the lower third of the shaft of the humerus. Function of the radial nerve should be tested and the findings recorded regularly and frequently in all patients with fractures of the shaft of the humerus. Treatment of these fractures is usually accomplished by closed methods such as the hanging cast (Fig. 21–8), the sugar tong splint or coaptation splints (Fig. 21–9), and an arm sling. A common error is to make the dressing or cast too heavy; this results in distraction of the fracture site and interferes with normal healing. All of these methods require that the patient be ambulatory and sleep partially sitting up to maintain the effect of gravity.

In patients confined to bed with other injuries, skin traction or skeletal traction through the olecranon may be employed as the initial treatment. Open reduction and internal fixation may be indicated in patients with soft tissue interposition, injury to the radial nerve, or multiple fractures of the same or other extremities.

THE ELBOW REGION

Fractures of the distal end of the humerus include those fractures in the supracondylar region, fractures of the capitellum, and fractures of the epicondyles. These fractures occur frequently in both children and adults and present difficult therapeutic problems. Initially, they are best treated by placing the arm in an arm sling.

Supracondylar fractures in children usually result from falls on the outstretched arm and are accompanied by rapid swelling and occasionally

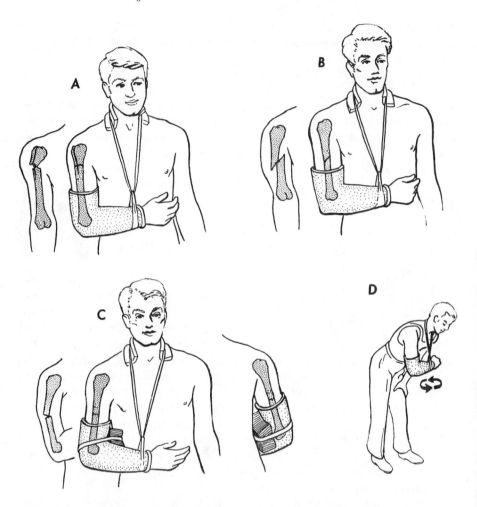

Figure 21-8. Treatment of fractures of the shaft of the humerus with a hanging cast. *A,* An angulated fracture of the proximal portion of the shaft which is corrected by the traction provided by a hanging cast. *B,* Oblique fracture of the middle third of the shaft with considerable displacement which is corrected by the traction provided by a hanging cast. *C,* Fracture of the middle third of the shaft of the humerus in a hanging cast. Lateral angulation is corrected by large pad placed on the inner side of the cast at the elbow. *D,* Circumduction exercises of the shoulder should be carried out diligently to avoid restriction of motion in that joint. (From Rhoads JE, Allen JG, Harkins HN, Moyer CA: Surgery, Principles and Practice, 4th ed. Philadelphia, J. B. Lippincott Co., 1970.)

by nerve and vascular injuries. These fractures deserve a very high priority and, if displaced, will require an axillary block or a general anesthesia for reduction. Gentle closed reduction can be accomplished by traction, realignment, and flexion of the elbow to 90 degrees or more. The arm is then immobilized in a dressing that does not constrict the antecubital space.

Closed reduction should not be attempted if, on initial examination, there is considerable swelling. Attempts at closed reduction should not be repeated more than twice. If there is considerable swelling and/or if initial attempts at closed reduction have been unsuccessful, the treatment of choice is traction, either by skin traction (Dunlop's) ·(Fig. 21–10) or by skeletal traction (Fig. 21–11) by means of a Kirschner wire through the olecranon. Satisfactory position can usually be obtained by traction. After seven to ten days the traction can be removed and a suitable dressing applied. Occasionally, following reduction, fixation of the fracture may be obtained by the percutaneous insertion of one or more Kirschner wires through the fragments.

The major complication associated with supracondylar fractures is

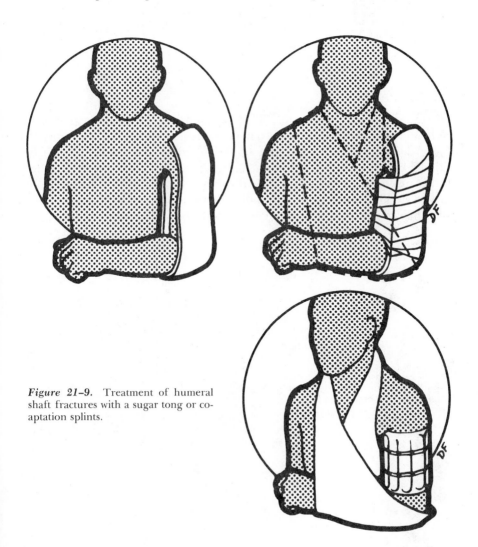

Figure 21-9. Treatment of humeral shaft fractures with a sugar tong or coaptation splints.

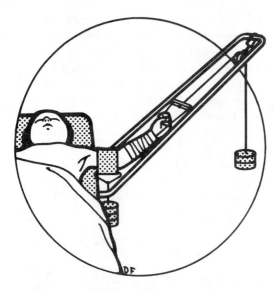

Figure 21–10. Dunlop's traction for the treatment of supracondylar fractures of the humerus.

Volkmann's ischemic contracture. This is a variety of the compartment syndrome and involves the vessels, nerves (median and ulnar), and muscles of the deep flexor compartment of the forearm. The ischemia can be initiated by direct injury to the brachial artery as it is kinked over the edge of the proximal fragment of the displaced supracondylar fracture, by massive swelling about the elbow and forearm associated with the fracture, or by the rigid compression of an external dressing applied to maintain the

Figure 21–11. Skeletal traction for the treatment of supracondylar fractures of the humerus. Note the splint to support the wrist to prevent wrist drop.

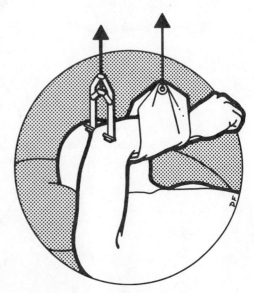

reduction of the fracture. Progression of the process results in necrosis of portions of the median and ulnar nerves and necrosis of the bodies of the deep flexor muscles of the forearm. Late scar formation and contraction of the scar produce the typical rigid claw hand deformity for which little can be done.

This disastrous result often can be prevented by early recognition of the premonitory symptoms and signs and the restoration of adequate circulation to the affected areas before irreversible changes have occurred. Volkmann's ischemic contracture can be anticipated in patients with supracondylar fractures of the humerus as well as occasionally in patients with fractures of the bones of the forearm. The circulation and sensory and motor function in patients with these injuries should be carefully evaluated before instituting treatment, during the maneuvers of closed reduction, and at regular close intervals during the immediate postreduction period. Any dressings used to maintain reduction must be applied without constricting the limb at any level.

The outstanding symptoms of impending Volkmann's ischemic contracture are *paresthesias* in the distribution of the median and ulnar nerves in the hand, *paralysis* of the deep flexor muscles to the fingers, and *pulselessness* in the radial artery at the wrist. *Pallor* and cyanosis of the hand and nail beds are difficult to evaluate clinically and may be misleading. The fingers are held in a flexed position. An attempt to extend the fingers passively increases the pain.

As soon as the complication is suspected, all constricting dressings should be released and the elbow extended until a radial pulse can be palpated. Failure of this maneuver to relieve the signs and symptoms promptly is an indication for immediate operation. Because of the urgency of the situation and the disastrous consequences of delay, procedures such as cervical sympathetic blocks, arteriography, measurement of intracompartmental pressures, and use of Doppler flow meters should not interfere with the rapid transporting of the patient to the operating room. The operation should consist of a long skin incision, a generous fasciotomy, epimysiotomy, neurolysis of the median and ulnar nerves, and vascular repair if indicated. An intraoperative arteriogram may be invaluable in demonstrating the site and extent of arterial injury. The wound should be left open for delayed primary or secondary closure. In such a case fixation of the fracture with Kirschner wires is indicated when possible.

Fractures of the medial and lateral epicondyles of the humerus are due to muscular violence, the strong contraction of the flexor or extensor muscle groups of the forearm against forces moving in the opposite direction. They occur frequently in children. All of the flexor muscles of the hand and wrist have their origin at the medial epicondyle of the humerus. Subliminal repetitive stress in the origin of the flexor muscle mass as in pitching gives rise to Little Leaguer's elbow, or medial epicondylitis. Occasionally the stress of one tremendous throwing effort may avulse the epicondyle. In such a case treatment will depend upon the degree of displacement. If displacement is significant, open reduction and pinning of the fragment is indicated. For lesser degrees of displacement, immobilization of the arm in a plaster dressing with the elbow at 90 degrees and the wrist in slight flexion is adequate. Because of its close proximity, the ulnar nerve may be compressed by local swelling or, in cases of severe displacement, may be displaced forward between the fracture fragments.

Subliminal repeated stress in the extensor origin on the lateral epicondyle gives rise to tennis elbow or lateral epicondylitis. Avulsions of the lateral epicondyle may include the adjacent capitellum, which becomes displaced. These fractures cannot be reduced and maintained in position by closed methods. Open reduction and pinning is necessary if progressive deformity and tardy ulnar palsy is to be avoided.

Isolated fractures of the capitellum occur in adults as a result of falls on the outstretched hand, the impact of the radial head shearing off the capitellum. These injuries require open reduction. When the fragment of the capitellum is floating freely in the joint as a loose body, it should be removed. If the fragment has soft tissue attachments that guarantee its viability, it should be replaced and fixed with a pin.

Dislocations of the elbow occur as a result of falls and hyperextension of the elbow and are frequently seen in athletes. The dislocations are either directly posterior or posterior with medial or lateral displacement. The roentgenograms may reveal associated bony fragments from the epicondyles of the humerus or the coronoid process of the ulna. Dislocations of the elbow may be complicated by injuries of the median and ulnar nerves as well as the brachial artery. It is essential to examine the patient carefully before and after reduction to establish the presence or absence of such complicating injuries. Like other dislocations, early reduction is essential and should have a high priority in a patient with multiple injuries.

While heavy intravenous sedation coupled with the injection of a local anesthetic agent into the joint may provide sufficient analgesia to permit closed reduction, a general anesthesia providing good muscular relaxation is usually required in the well-conditioned athlete.

Closed reduction is accomplished by applying traction on the forearm against countertraction on the arm or against the axilla (Fig. 21–12). Before traction is applied, any medial or lateral displacement must be corrected and the arm aligned in such a way that the complicated articulation of the elbow will mesh properly as the forearm is drawn forward. Failure to do this will make reduction difficult or impossible. With the application of traction, the articular processes are engaged and the reduction is completed by flexing the elbow to 90 degrees. Ordinarily, small bony fragments do not interfere with closed reduction. Rarely, closed reduction is impossible because of interposition of a bony fragment or a soft tissue. In such a case, an immediate open reduction should be carried out.

Following reduction the arm should be immobilized in an above-elbow plaster dressing with the elbow at 90 degrees and the forearm in neutral

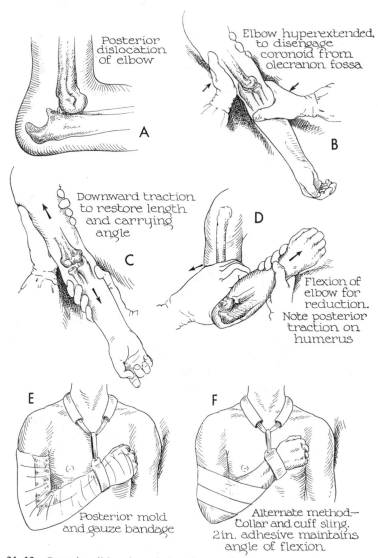

Figure 21-12. Posterior dislocation of the elbow and the maneuvers for reduction and immobilization. (Reproduced with permission from Compere EL, Banks SW, Compere CL: Pictorial Handbook of Fracture Treatment, 5th ed. Copyright © 1963 by Year Book Medical Publishers, Inc., Chicago.)

position—that is, midway between full pronation and full supination. Immobilization should be maintained for about 10 to 21 days and the arm should then be supported in an arm sling for one or two weeks while motion is regained. During this convalescent period, formal physical therapy should be avoided, because heat and passive stretching of any kind may promote the formation of *myositis ossificans* or the formation of heterotopic bone in the damaged brachialis muscle. Only active motion carried out by the patient should be permitted.

Dislocations of the head of the radius occur very rarely as isolated injuries. They are usually seen in association with dislocations of the elbow and angulated fractures of the ulna (Monteggia fractures). Isolated dislocations of the head of the radius do occur in children and are frequently overlooked initially, presenting weeks and months later. This makes their treatment quite difficult without an open reduction. When recognized immediately, they can be reduced by closed manipulation utilizing direct pressure over the head of the radius coupled with pronation and supination of the elbow. Care must be taken not to produce a separation of the proximal radial epiphysis.

A special form of subluxation of the head of the radius does occur frequently in small children and is referred to as "nursemaid's elbow" or "pulled elbow" because of the mechanism. The history is typical: A child of two or three is being swung by his hands or is picked up by his hand to lift him up a curb or high step. The child cries out, complains of pain in his arm, and will not use it. The forearm is held in full pronation and attempts to supinate it are painful. What has happened is that the base of the head of the radius has been subluxed distally by the longitudinal traction and is impacted in the orbicular ligament, producing locking. Reduction is accomplished by flexing the elbow to 90 degrees and supinating the forearm. This will give instant relief of pain and restoration of function. Roentgenograms of the elbow are normal, and it is not unusual for the reduction to occur in the radiology department as the arm is positioned for the various x-rays. No follow-up care is required.

Fractures of the head of the radius are the result of falls on the outstretched arm (Fig. 21–13). As the force is transmitted up the shaft of the radius, the head is compressed against the capitellum of the humerus. As a result, fractures of the radial head are almost always accompanied by damage to the articular cartilage of the capitellum. Fractures of the head of the radius range in severity from those producing small pie-shaped fragments to comminuted fractures involving the entire head. Rarely the radius fractures through the neck or the proximal radial epiphysis. These fractures may be undisplaced, angulated, or completely displaced into the joint. Fractures of the head and neck of the radius can also occur as components of more severe and complicated fractures and fracture-dislocations about the elbow.

The diagnosis of a fracture of the head of the radius may be suspected by a history of a fall on the outstretched arm followed by localized pain on the lateral (radial) side of the elbow. With the elbow flexed to 90 degrees pronation and supination may be limited by pain and this may be accentuated by pressure over the head of the radius.

Roentgenograms of the elbow in several planes may be necessary to define the nature and the extent of the fracture. Careful observation of the position of the normal fat pads in front of and behind the distal humerus (the fat pad sign) may indicate an associated hemarthrosis.

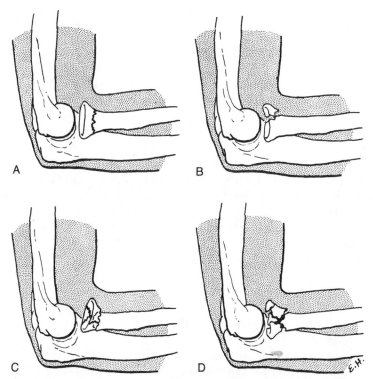

Figure 21–13. Varieties of fractures of the head of the radius. *A,* Undisplaced fracture that should be treated by mobilization rather than by immobilization. *B,* Displaced marginal fracture involving less than one-third of the articular surface for which early excision is usually indicated. *C,* Comminuted fracture of the radial head with minimal displacement for which complete excision of the radial head is indicated. *D,* Severely comminuted displaced fracture of the radial head for which excision of all of the fragments is indicated. (From Hampton, OP and Fitts, WT: Open Reduction of Common Fractures (Modern Surgical Monographs). New York, Grune & Stratton, 1959, p. 60. By permission.)

Most fractures of the radial head can be treated simply by immobilization in a padded plaster splint with the elbow at 90 degrees and the forearm in a neutral position. Immobilization is continued for 10 to 14 days, following which an arm sling is used for support as the patient regains active motion. Undisplaced fractures of the neck or proximal radial epiphysis are treated in the same manner.

Displaced fractures of the neck of the radius or proximal radial epiphysis may be reduced by manipulation using controlled pronation and supination of the forearm and direct pressure over the head of the radius. Rarely, an open reduction may be necessary.

When the head of the radius is badly comminuted and particularly when a fragment is displaced into the joint as a free body, excision of the radial head should be considered as an initial form of treatment. In other patients in whom malunion of the radial head occurs with limitation of supination, and flexion and extension of the elbow, resection of the radial head should also be considered. When the radial head is removed, the line of resection should not extend distally below the orbicular ligament that tethers the upper end of the radius to the ulna. A late complication of radial head resection may be incongruity of the distal radioulnar joint at the wrist, caused by shortening and subsidence of the radius.

Fractures of the olecranon can result from avulsion of the triceps insertion or from direct injury. Comminuted or open fractures or both are frequent. The seriousness of the injury is related directly to the amount of injury to the articular surface of the olecranon. When the fracture fragments are undisplaced, immobilization in a plaster dressing for a few weeks is sufficient. Displacement of the fracture fragments is an indication for open reduction. In many cases, the proximal fragment can be discarded and the insertion of the triceps transferred to the distal fragment. In other cases an accurate reduction and internal fixation may be carried out. Ideally in such patients, fixation should be secure enough to permit early motion of the elbow.

FRACTURE-DISLOCATION OF THE FOREARM

Fracture-dislocations of the forearm occur as the result of violent injuries. They represent complicated problems in management, the first of which is proper diagnosis. The radius and the ulna are attached at the proximal and the distal radioulnar joints. When one of the two bones is broken and the fracture is angulated and displaced, the other bone must also be fractured and displaced or there must be an associated dislocation of one of the radioulnar joints. The roentgenograms must show the entire length of the bones so that the relationship of the radioulnar joints can be seen. *Beware the single-bone fracture of the forearm.* Two varieties of these fracture dislocations of the forearm are seen.

The *Monteggia fracture* (Fig. 21–14) is a fracture of the ulna, usually at the junction of the upper and middle thirds, with an associated dislocation of the head of the radius. In children, this injury can usually be treated by closed manipulation. The arm should be immobilized in a plaster dressing with the elbow at 90 degrees and the forearm in full supination. In adults, the best results are obtained by open reduction of the fracture of the ulna and internal fixation with a plate and screws. An open reduction of the dislocation of the head of the radius may also be required.

The *Galeazzi* or *reverse Monteggia fracture* consists of a fracture of the shaft of the radius, usually at the junction of the middle and distal thirds with an associated dislocation of the distal end of the ulna. The indications for treatment are similar to those of the Monteggia fracture. The position of immobilization should be with the elbow at 90 degrees and the forearm in full pronation. The results of the treatment are good if the condition is

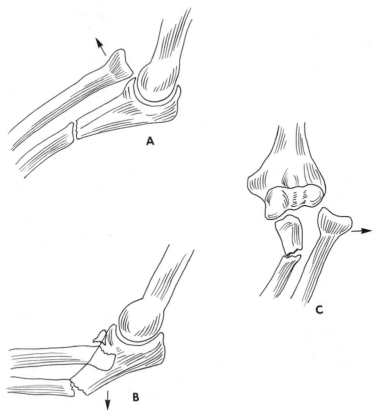

Figure 21–14. Varieties of Monteggia fractures. *A,* Fracture of ulna with apex of ulnar angulation forward and anterior dislocation of radial head. *B,* Fracture of ulna with apex of ulnar angulation posterior and posterior dislocation of radial head. Note fracture of radial head. *C,* Uncommon lateral dislocation of radial head.

recognized immediately following the injury and if an accurate reduction is obtained and maintained during the healing period.

Isolated fractures of the shaft of the radius or of the ulna are not common and usually result from direct blows, such as an impact against the steering wheel or from a falling object. The diagnosis is made only after excluding the possibility of a fracture-dislocation (Monteggia or Galeazzi) and the presence of a bowing fracture in which the bone is bent; that is, multiple subliminal fractures without roentgenographic evidence of a fracture. Single-bone fractures of the forearm are not badly displaced ordinarily because the uninjured companion acts as an effective splint through the medium of the interosseous membrane. Rotation deformities can exist and are easily overlooked. Treatment of single bone fractures in the forearm can be accomplished easily by means of above-elbow plaster dressings with the elbow at 90 degrees and the forearm in neutral position. With rotary malalignment the degree of pronation or supination or both may require adjustment.

Fractures of both bones of the forearm occur frequently both in children and adults as a direct result of falls on the outstretched arm and other violence. They can be splinted initially with a folded magazine or newspaper and the arm supported by an arm sling. Occasionally one or both fractures may be open, and the size and nature of the wounds vary greatly.

In children, bowing fractures and greenstick fractures are seen. These are incomplete fractures and although there may be considerable angulation, the continuity of the bone is not disrupted. Such fractures should be treated by completing the fracture, aligning the bones axially, and immobilizing the arm and forearm in a plaster dressing with the elbow at 90 degrees and the forearm in a neutral position. The fracture is completed by bending the fracture site in the direction opposite to the angulation. The maneuver is carried to the point of overcorrection, at which the unbroken cortex is felt or heard to break. The bones are then brought back into normal alignment. If this maneuver is carried out carefully, there should be no problem of displacement, because the periosteal tube surrounding the bone is not disrupted. Failure to complete the fracture usually results in angulation at the fracture site in spite of good initial alignment and immobilization.

Displaced fractures of both bones of the forearm in children can almost always be treated by closed reduction by manipulation (Fig. 21–15). This may be difficult if there is considerable swelling. Loss of position can occur during the first two weeks following injury, so that early follow-up roentgenography is essential. While mild to moderate angular deformities can be expected to undergo some improvement with growth, rotational deformities do not. Great care must be taken in the immediate management and follow-up care of these fractures if permanent partial loss of pronation or supination or both is to be prevented.

Displaced fractures of both bones of the forearm in adults can be reduced and immobilized in plaster dressings. However, for optimal results, open reduction and internal fixation is the method of choice in most patients.

Volkmann's ischemic contracture can occur as a complication of fractures in the forearm as a result of the trauma to bones and soft tissue or of the dressing applied to immobilize the forearm. For this reason, great care must be taken to avoid constriction, and the condition of the patient must be carefully observed during the first 48 hours following treatment.

Fractures of the lower end of the radius are very common and usually occur as the result of falls on the outstretched arm.

Separations of the distal radial epiphysis are almost always of the Type I or Type II varieties, and late deformities due to disturbance of epiphyseal

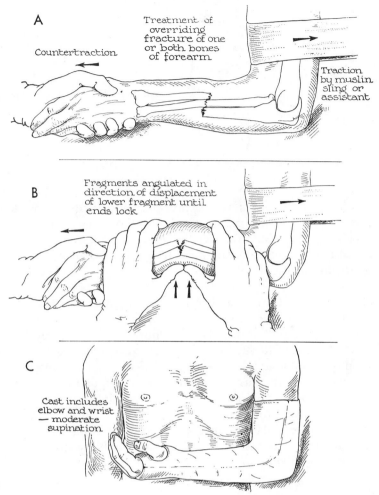

A Treatment of overriding fracture of one or both bones of forearm

Countertraction

Traction by muslin sling or assistant

B Fragments angulated in direction of displacement of lower fragment until ends lock

C Cast includes elbow and wrist — moderate supination

Figure 21–15. Closed reduction of transverse fractures of the middle part of the shafts of the bones of the forearm and immobilization in long-arm plaster cast with the forearm in supination. (Reproduced with permission from Compere EL, Banks SW, Compere CL: Pictorial Handbook of Fracture Treatment, 5th ed. Copyright © 1963 by Year Book Medical Publishers, Inc., Chicago.)

growth are unusual. The displacement of the epiphysis is posterior or dorsal and resembles that of a displaced Colles' fracture.

Treatment consists of closed reduction by manipulation and immobilization in a plaster dressing. It is important to have adequate anesthesia for the reduction. Failure to relieve pain usually leads to a less than optimal reduction.

A *Colles' fracture* is a fracture of the distal radius that is characterized by radial shortening and posterior or dorsal displacement of the distal fragment (Figs. 21–16, 21–17).

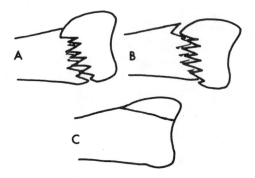

Figure 21–16. A, Colles' fracture; B, Smith's fracture; C, Barton's fracture.

A *Smith's fracture* is similar to a Colles' fracture except that the displacement of the distal fragment is anterior or volar. Colles' fractures occur very frequently; Smith's fractures are rare. In both types there may be comminution of the distal fragment by vertical fractures involving the articular surface of the distal radius.

Normally, the styloid process of the radius extends distally about a fingerbreadth beyond the styloid process of the ulna. In these fractures, the radius is shortened and the two processes are at the same level. As the radius shortens, the pull of the triangular fibrocartilage avulses the styloid process of the ulna. Reduction of the fracture displacement involves restoration of radial length by traction, followed by correction of dorsal or volar angulation of the distal fragment by manipulation (Fig. 21–18). Reduction is maintained by means of a plaster splint. Care must be taken not to extend the splint or dressing distally to immobilize the metacarpal phalangeal or interphalangeal joints, because resulting stiffness of the hand and fingers causes serious permanent disability. Similarly, every effort should be made to promote normal shoulder motion during

Figure 21–17. A, Colles' fracture with radial and dorsal displacement of the distal fragment. B, Following reduction, the normal inclinations of the articular surface of the radius have been restored and the styloid of the radius extends well beyond the styloid of ulna. (From Rhoads JE, Allen JG, Harkins HN, Moyer CA: Surgery, Principles and Practice, 4th ed. Philadelphia, J. B. Lippincott Co., 1970.)

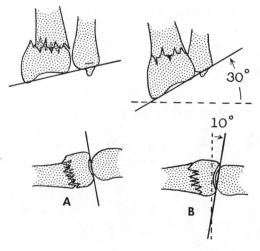

convalescence. The cast must not extend beyond the proximal palmar crease.

Fractures of the styloid process of the radius are usually not displaced. They involve the articular surface of the distal radius and when they are displaced an anatomical reduction is essential. This can be obtained by traction. If the reduction cannot be maintained by immobilization in a plaster dressing, additional fixation by means of a Kirschner wire inserted percutaneously across the fracture site is useful.

Fracture-dislocation of the radiocarpal joint (Barton's fracture) is a rare injury. Since such fractures involve the articular surface of the distal

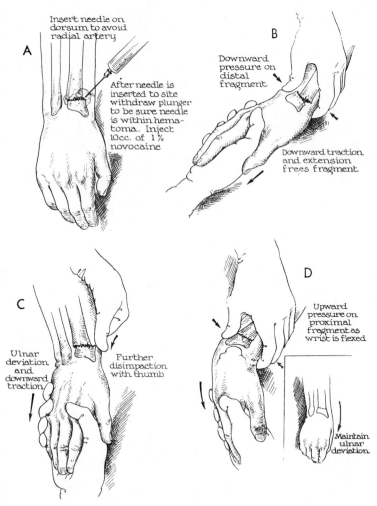

Figure 21–18. Closed reduction of Colles' fracture under local anesthesia. (Reproduced with permission from Compere EL, Banks SW, Compere CL: Pictorial Handbook of Fracture Treatment, 5th ed. Copyright © 1963 by Year Book Medical Publishers, Inc., Chicago.)

radius, an exact reduction is essential. Such a reduction can be obtained easily by traction, but it cannot be maintained without internal fixation. For this reason, open reduction and internal fixation is the treatment of choice.

FRACTURES AND DISLOCATIONS IN THE CARPUS

The several fractures and dislocations of the carpal bones are most commonly produced by falls on the outstretched hand with varying degrees of forced hyperextension of the wrist. Since these injuries may occur in combination, it is good clinical practice to consider all of them in the differential diagnosis of acute injuries. Physical examination should pinpoint areas of local tenderness to identify sites of injury and to locate possible dislocations and ligamentous disruptions that may not be apparent on roentgenograms. Areas of bruising may give an important clue to the mechanism of injury. Depending upon the mechanism of injury and physical findings, roentgenographic studies in addition to anteroposterior and lateral views may include scaphoid views, tunnel views, or stress views. Roentgenographic interpretation of the several carpal views is subtle, and significant injuries of the carpus may have minimal or no roentgenographic signs other than soft tissue swelling.

FRACTURE OF THE SCAPHOID

The most common fracture of the carpal bones is a fracture of the scaphoid. It is often misdiagnosed acutely as a "wrist sprain" in the absence of roentgenographic findings. Tenderness in the anatomical snuff box can be elicited by palpation just distal to the tip of the radial styloid as the wrist is deviated toward the ulna. Scaphoid roentgenographic views may not show an undisplaced fracture line until some bony resorption has occurred 10 to 14 days following the acute injury. Suspected scaphoid fractures should, therefore, be treated by plaster immobilization until follow-up physical examination and x-rays are reviewed. If there is displacement of a fractured scaphoid, ligamentous injury with subluxation of other carpal bones should be suspected.

The majority of undisplaced or minimally displaced fractures of the scaphoid are treated adequately in a below-elbow plaster bandage with the wrist dorsiflexed and deviated toward the radius, thumb in a position of relaxed opposition and immobilized to the interphalangeal joint, and the finger metacarpophalangeal joints freely mobile (Fig. 21–19). Healing of this fracture may require two to six months of immobilization. The plaster dressing should be changed and roentgenograms obtained out of plaster at about six-week intervals.

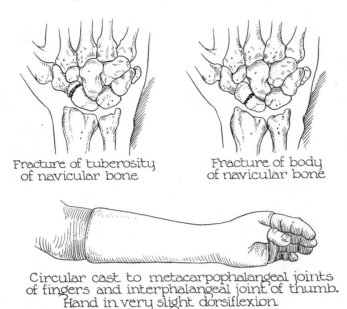

Fracture of tuberosity
of navicular bone

Fracture of body
of navicular bone

Circular cast to metacarpophalangeal joints
of fingers and interphalangeal joint of thumb.
Hand in very slight dorsiflexion

Figure 21-19. Treatment of recent fracture of the carpal navicular (scaphoid) bone. (Reproduced with permission from Compere EL, Banks SW, Compere CL: Pictorial Handbook of Fracture Treatment, 5th ed. Copyright © 1963 by Year Book Medical Publishers, Inc., Chicago.)

Open reduction and internal fixation is indicated for carpal scaphoid fractures when such fractures are displaced and irreducible or associated with displacement of other carpal bones. Nonunions and delayed unions are not uncommon and can be effectively managed by bone grafting with or without internal fixation, depending on the stability of the particular fracture. If the proximal fracture fragment of the nonunion is small, and particularly if there is evidence of aseptic necrosis, the fragment may be excised. Post-traumatic arthritis of the radiocarpal joint produces significant functional impairment following carpal scaphoid fractures, even in the absence of nonunion or avascular necrosis. In selected patients with post-traumatic arthritis, scaphoid implant arthroplasty, radiocarpal implant arthroplasty, selected carpal fusions, or wrist fusion may be necessary to reduce pain and improve position and function.

FRACTURE OF THE HOOK OF THE HAMATE

Fractures of the hook of the hamate are caused by a direct blow to the ulnar aspect of the base of the palm. A blow to the palm of the hand as with a fall or the momentum of a tightly gripped object such as a bicycle handlebar or racquet handle in several racquet sports may produce this fracture. Patients with this injury generally present days, weeks, or even months after the inciting episode with complaints of pain in the palm with power grip and local tenderness at the hook of the hamate. The latter can be palpated about one third of the distance between the wrist flexion crease and the distal palmar crease in the axis of the fourth ray. There may be symptoms and signs of ulnar neuropathy with paresthesias and hypesthesias of the small and ring fingers as well as ulnar intrinsic motor weakness. The diagnosis is confirmed by carpal tunnel roentgenograms. Immobilization with a below-elbow plaster that includes the small and ring fingers flexed over a padded splint may allow healing of this fracture. In patients with pain and neuropathy in which diagnosis has been delayed, surgical removal of the bone fragment may be necessary.

DISLOCATION OF THE SCAPHOID

The scaphoid is an elongated cuboidal bone that articulates with the trapezoid, the capitate, the lunate, and the radius. Among the complex movements of the scaphoid is one of rotation around an approximately transverse axis during flexion, extension, and radioulnar deviation. Disruption of the scapholunate ligaments may result in a fixed rotated position of the scaphoid producing local pain and limitation of wrist motion. Roentgenograms in several projections will show a fixed flexed position of the scaphoid and a widened interval between the scaphoid and the lunate. This *rotatory subluxation* of the scaphoid is frequently unstable and may require open reduction for ligamentous repair and stabilization. Complete dislocations of the scaphoid are rare.

DISLOCATIONS OF THE LUNATE

The dislocated lunate is rotated and extruded anteriorly where it entraps the median nerve and flexor tendons against the volar carpal ligament. In this position, median nerve neuropathy may be noted and there is a characteristic inability to fully extend the third and fourth digits. Roentgenograms in lateral projection show loss of articulation of the lunate with the radius and capitate while the anteroposterior views demonstrate loss of the normal trapezoidal shape of the lunate and asymmetry of the lucent spaces between the lunate and surrounding carpal bones.

In a *perilunar dislocation* the lunate remains in its anatomical location while the surrounding carpal bones dislocate dorsally. This injury may appear roentgenographically identical to the lunate dislocation if the dislocated carpal bones spontaneously reduce, forcing the lunate anteriorly. The perilunar dislocation is more likely to be associated with fractures of the scaphoid.

Both the lunate and perilunar dislocations are reduced by manipulation while longitudinal traction is placed upon the carpus. This maneuver is generally best performed under general anesthesia, utilizing finger traps for traction. Immobilization for three to four weeks in a below-elbow plaster with the wrist in a few degrees of flexion is then carried out (Fig. 21–20). Roentgenograms should be obtained immediately and as swelling decreases in order to detect evidence of carpal instability signifying ligamentous injury. Such instability may be an indication for open reduction and possibly surgical repair of ligaments.

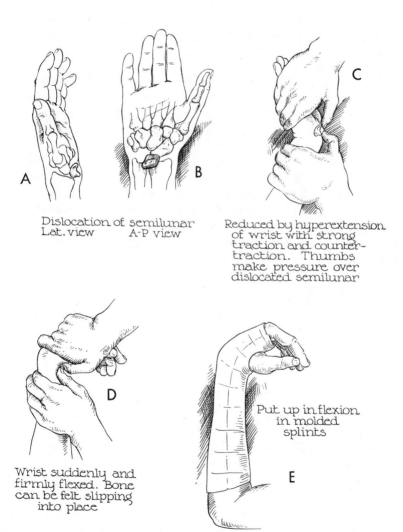

Dislocation of semilunar
Lat. view   A-P view

Reduced by hyperextension of wrist with strong traction and counter-traction. Thumbs make pressure over dislocated semilunar

Wrist suddenly and firmly flexed. Bone can be felt slipping into place

Put up in flexion in molded splints

Figure 21–20. Manipulative reduction of dislocation of lunate bone of the wrist. (Reproduced with permission from Compere EL, Banks SW, Compere CL: Pictorial Handbook of Fracture Treatment, 5th ed. Copyright © 1963 by Year Book Medical Publishers, Inc., Chicago.)

FRACTURES AND DISLOCATIONS OF THE HAND

Injuries to the bones and joints of the hand are sometimes viewed as relatively minor. This attitude may lead to suboptimal care for many patients with hand injuries. Significant functional impairment can result from subtle degrees of deformity or instability as well as from failure to orient treatment toward early rehabilitation. The initial treatment plans should incorporate principles of mobilization as well as immobilization. It is essential for the treating physician to approach patients who have suffered hand fractures with the anticipation of devoting adequate time to their management, for such injuries generally require equal or more time than similar fractures or dislocations in larger bones and joints.

A detailed physical examination should document the function of all intrinsic and extrinsic muscles of the hand, locations of wounds, detailed sensory examination, areas of local tenderness and swelling, and ligamentous instability around the joints. Roentgenographic evaluation includes anteroposterior, oblique, and lateral views initially. Subsequent roentgenographic views of individual joints with stress may be useful to demonstrate ligamentous instability. It is important to note that rotational deformity of phalanges and metacarpals is usually not apparent on x-rays and must be assessed by physical examination showing the approximate parallel orientation of the fingernail beds or the directional orientation of the flexing digits toward the scaphoid tubercle on the thenar eminence (Fig. 21–21). The rotational alignment should be checked repeatedly.

The position of immobilization of the injured hand will vary depending upon the patient's anatomy and the position of stability for the particular fracture. Judgment regarding the position of the hand can be based upon two general principles of hand anatomy. First, the position of "rest" for the hand is one in which the tensions of flexor and extensor

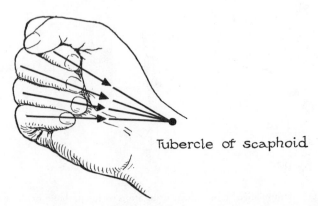

Figure 21-21. Axes of the flexed fingers do not correspond to those of the metacarpal or forearm bones but converge on the tubercle of the scaphoid. Finger splinting in flexion should be in this direction. (From McLaughlin HL: Trauma. Philadelphia, W. B. Saunders Co., 1959.)

muscle groups are equal or in balance, thereby eliminating significant deforming forces upon the fracture. This position of rest varies in the finger and thumb joints as the wrist is flexed or extended. Second, the metacarpophalangeal and interphalangeal joints exhibit a cam effect that causes the length and tension of the collateral ligaments to pass through a maximum at about 50 to 70 degrees of flexion. It is important to the ultimate rehabilitation of the hand that the finger joints be immobilized with the collateral ligaments in their elongated position, since this will minimize contracture of this most significant capsular component pending mobilization of the joint. The basic position for immobilizing the hand therefore is with the wrist in 10 to 20 degrees of extension, the metacarpophalangeal joints in 60 to 70 degrees of flexion, and the interphalangeal joints in 40 to 50 degrees of flexion. Immobilization methods that place the finger joints in full extension or full flexion, as in the use of tongue blade splints or 90–90 degree splints or casts, are to be avoided. No fixed position should be maintained for longer than absolutely necessary.

Manipulation of fractures and dislocations requires sufficient pain relief to permit the treatment. Some injuries, especially those seen close to the time of the accident, can be manipulated without analgesics. Children may require a general anesthetic if they are too young or too frightened to understand or cooperate with their treatment. Most often, regional anesthetic techniques are satisfactory.

While virtually all fractures of the hand may be treated by nonoperative means, it is a matter of increasingly sophisticated judgment to select the treatment plan that will achieve the restoration of hand function with the greatest certainty, safety, and speed. A hand that is grossly swollen in a patient whose treatment has been delayed or who gives a history of a crushing injury may be best managed by application of a bulky hand dressing and elevation for several days before definitive treatment. Patients with multiple hand fractures, intra-articular fractures, or associated soft tissue injuries may often be better served by operative reduction and stabilization of their fractures. Therefore, it is not possible to be dogmatic in the recommendation of management for individual fractures, and the methods for common injuries suggested below should be varied according to the specific needs of the patient.

Dislocation of the carpometacarpal joints of the finger metacarpals is an easily overlooked injury produced by crushing mechanisms, longitudinal forces along the metacarpals, or flexion of the palm over unyielding objects such as a handlebar. Diagnosis is readily confirmed on the lateral roentgenogram. Reduction is achieved acutely by longitudinal finger traction and manipulation, but reduction is often unstable and fixation using a percutaneous pin inserted from the base of the metacarpal into the carpal bones is recommended in addition to below-elbow immobilization. Both the plaster and pins can be removed at four weeks and protected mobilization begun.

Fractures of the finger metacarpals tend to angulate with the apex of the angle pointing dorsally. The border metacarpals, the second and fifth, may rotate significantly but can generally be maintained in correct rotational alignment by splinting with the adjacent finger. Transverse fractures allow stable reductions, but oblique or comminuted fractures are subject to unacceptable shortening and are often best managed by pin fixation. Fractures of the neck of the metacarpals (most frequently seen in the fifth) are reduced by flexing the metacarpophalangeal joint to 90 degrees and pushing in a proximal direction on the proximal phalanx to lift the head of the metacarpal into its normal position. Up to 30 degrees of angulation can be tolerated in the mobile fifth metacarpal neck provided there is no rotational deformity. Near anatomical alignment is essential for the other finger metacarpals. Reduction can be maintained by finger traction while a below-elbow plaster is applied. The fingers corresponding to the injured metacarpal, together with that of the adjacent metacarpal, are then flexed and taped over a padded malleable splint that is contoured to support the palmar aspect of the metacarpal head. The splint is incorporated in the plaster, and the fingers are stabilized to the splint using circumferential tape. Protected motion can be started in three to four weeks and immobilization discontinued at six weeks following the injury.

Fractures of the middle and distal phalanges typically show angular deformity with the apex of the angle directed volarly. It is important to visualize the fracture deformity on the lateral roentgenograms because the anteroposterior and oblique views may not reveal significant degrees of angulation or displacement when present. Reduction is carried out by increasing the angular deformity slightly, distracting the fragments while maintaining the angulated position, and then manipulating the distal fragment into proper alignment with the proximal fragment. Flexion of the digit over a volar padded malleable splint incorporated in a below-elbow plaster cast is maintained for three to four weeks before protected motion is begun (Fig. 21–22). Nail or pulp traction rarely is necessary but may be an excellent adjunct to treatment in special instances. Both

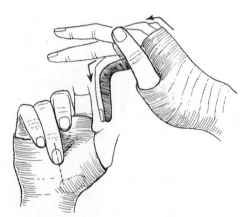

Figure 21–22. Metal splint incorporated in cast to support flexed finger that is contiguous to a fractured metacarpal shaft. (From DePalma AF: The Management of Fractures and Dislocations: An Atlas, Vol. 2. Philadelphia, W. B. Saunders Co., 1970.)

immediate and frequent follow-up documentation of angular and rotational alignment are carried out.

Avulsion fractures of the distal phalanx are significant if they disrupt the integrity of the extensor tendons producing baseball finger, mallet finger, or drop finger. If a fracture fragment is noted roentgenographically and can be reduced, the distal phalangeal joint can be splinted in hyperextension, leaving the proximal phalangeal joint freely mobile (Fig. 21–23). Disruption of the extensor tendon with no apparent bone fragment may be treated in the same fashion. A narrow padded malleable splint material can be used to construct the immobilization device that should be continued for six to eight weeks. If the bone fragment cannot be reduced, open reduction should be performed with Kirschner wire or pull-out suture fixation.

Fractures of the distal phalanx are generally produced by crushing mechanisms and are therefore comminuted and associated with soft tissue

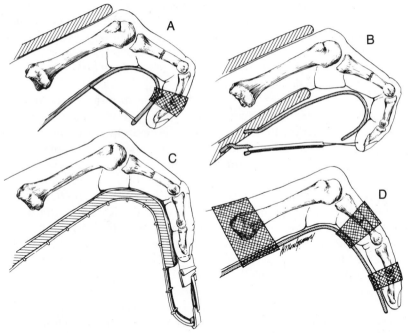

Figure 21–23. Several types of splinting have been described for treating fractures of the phalanges. *A,* Böhler described the use of a wire outrigger combined with a dorsal plaster slab which immobilized the wrist. The tip of the outrigger was wired to itself to hold the finger in rather acute flexion. *B,* Bunnell, and later Boyes, used a modified Böhler splint together with pulp traction, applying just enough tension to maintain the position obtained by manipulation. *C,* Moberg designed a padded wire ladder which is used widely in Sweden, but is not available in this country. This technique uses a specialized form of nail-pulp traction. (The illustration is slightly inaccurate, in that the wire should pass through the periosteum at the tip of the distal phalanx.) *D,* James has advocated that fingers should not be immobilized in the position of function, but rather in a position that more nearly resembles the intrinsic plus position in which the metacarpophalangeal joints are immobilized in at least 70 degrees flexion, and the interphalangeal joints in minimal flexion. (From Rockwood CA and Green DP: Fractures, Vols. 1 & 2. Philadelphia, J. B. Lippincott Co., 1975.)

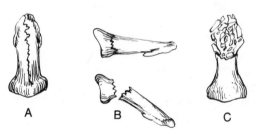

Figure 21–24. The three general types of fractures of the distal phalanx. *A,* Longitudinal fractures rarely show displacement. *B,* A transverse fracture may show a marked degree of angulation and may require internal or external splinting. *C,* The so-called crushed-egg-shell type of comminuted fracture. (From Rockwood CA and Green DP: Fractures, Vols. 1 & 2. Philadelphia, J. B. Lippincott Co., 1975.)

injury as well (Fig. 21–24). Occasionally, angulation of a single fracture may be seen. If there is deformity, manipulation with or without anesthesia may be necessary before protective splinting is applied. Splinting is continued until swelling and tenderness have subsided.

Condylar and other intra-articular fractures of the metacarpals and phalanges can sometimes be reduced and maintained by nonoperative methods. Surgical fixation with or without open reduction affords greater security of fixation and permits earlier motion, and is generally to be preferred in the presence of intra-articular injuries.

Fractures of the thumb metacarpal may be intra-articular or extra-articular. Extra-articular fractures are managed by manipulation and immobilization in a thumb spica plaster with the thumb in a position of rest. Intra-articular fractures may involve a single condylar fragment, as in *Bennett's fracture,* or more than one fragment, as in *Rolando's fracture.* Closed methods can yield excellent results provided that meticulous plaster technique with a well-molded thumb spica is used; this method is to be preferred in severely comminuted fractures of the Rolando type. If there are few fragments of adequate size to accept a Kirschner wire, an unstable fracture of the Bennett's or Rolando's type may be fixed with percutaneous fixation or internal fixation with open reduction. Protected motion is begun at three to four weeks.

Dislocations of the metacarpophalangeal joints are common in the second ray. Since the head of the metacarpal is subject to entrapment, open reduction through a palmar incision is often necessary and should follow failed attempts at closed reduction (Fig. 21–25). Closed reduction should be performed by pushing the base of the hyperextended proximal phalanx distally over the head of the metacarpal; longitudinal traction may entrap volar capsular structures within the joint (Fig. 21–26). If the reduction is successful and complete as demonstrated by stability, range of motion, and roentgenograms, the finger may be splinted in flexion or splinted to the adjacent finger using tape or Velcro straps. Protected motion can be started as soon as pain permits.

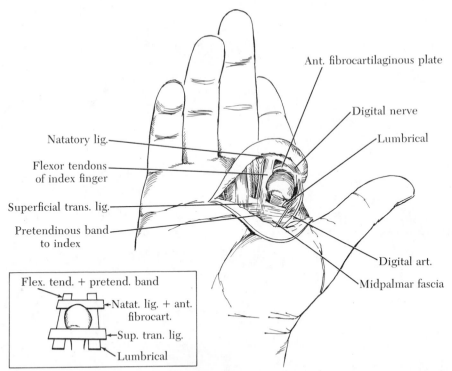

Ant. fibrocartilaginous plate

Digital nerve

Natatory lig.

Lumbrical

Flexor tendons
of index finger

Superficial trans. lig.

Pretendinous band
to index

Digital art.

Midpalmar fascia

Flex. tend. + pretend. band

Natat. lig. + ant.
fibrocart.

Sup. tran. lig.

Lumbrical

Figure 21-25. Entrapped dislocated index metacarpal head. (From Kaplan EB: Discoid lateral meniscus of the knee joint; nature, mechanism, and operative treatment. J. Bone Joint Surg. 39A:1081, 1957.)

Dislocations of the interphalangeal joints most commonly occur in a dorsal direction, with the base of the phalanx displaced dorsally to the head of the more proximal phalanx. Reduction is accomplished in the same fashion as that of the metacarpophalangeal dislocation; the base of the hyperextended dislocated phalanx is pushed distally while minimal traction is applied in the longitudinal axis of the phalanx. If the reduction and the collateral ligaments are stable, the joint may be splinted to the adjacent finger with tapes or Velcro straps for three to four weeks. If reduction is incomplete or if collateral ligament rupture is demonstrated by physical examination or by plain or stress roentgenograms or by both, open reduction for removal of interposed soft tissues and repair of disrupted volar plate or collateral ligament structures is usually indicated.

Dislocations of the thumb metacarpophalangeal joint are reduced in a manner identical to the dislocated interphalangeal joints just described, and similar criteria are applied in electing open reduction or surgical repair or both of capsular-ligamentous structures. Surgical repair of complete disruption of the ulnar collateral ligament is usually preferred,

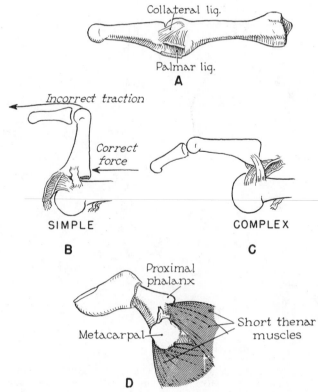

Figure 21–26. Simple and complex metacarpophalangeal dislocation. *A,* The volar aspect of a metacarpophalangeal joint capsule is reinforced with a palmar ligament or fibrocartilage. *B,* In a simple dislocation the phalanx is hyperextended and the palmar ligament hangs like a curtain over the metacarpal head. Traction may pivot the phalanx on the intact collateral ligaments and interpose the palmar ligament between the bones. The phalanx should be pushed into place. *C,* The finger is not hyperextended on, but more nearly parallel to, the metacarpal in a complex dislocation. The volar joint capsule and palmar ligament are interposed, and usually prevent reduction by manipulation. *D,* In the metacarpophalangeal joint of the thumb the short thenar muscles augment the pivot force predisposing to complex dislocation. (From McLaughlin HL: Trauma. Philadelphia, W. B. Saunders Co., 1959.)

because the adductor apponeurosis is often interposed between the avulsed ligament and its bony bed. Unlike the interphalangeal joints of the fingers, the reduced or repaired metacarpophalangeal joint is immobilized in a thumb spica for six weeks before active motion is permitted.

Chip fractures are often reported on roentgenograms of the hand. The meaning and significance of this observation is that the bony attachment of a capsular, ligamentous, or tendinous structure has been avulsed. The bone "chip" may serve as a useful marker of the site, nature, and extent of injury as well as of the adequacy of the apposition of disrupted parts.

Chapter

22

Injuries of the Lower Extremity

FRACTURES OF THE PELVIS

Fractures of the pelvis, next to head injuries, are associated with the highest mortality of any injury resulting from motor vehicle accidents. Because the bony basin of the pelvis contains a great variety of important anatomical structures, associated injuries are frequent. The greater the disruption of the basin, the greater the incidence and severity of such injuries. In addition, since pelvic fractures are the result of substantial mechanical violence, concomitant injuries of the head, trunk, and extremities are common. The successful management of patients with fractures of the pelvis requires accurate diagnosis and assessment of *all* injuries, effective resuscitation and treatment of the systemic manifestations of injury (such as shock, pulmonary insufficiency, and renal shutdown), and treatment of the individual injuries themselves.

The major cause of death in patients with fractures of the pelvis is hypovolemic shock due to bleeding from veins and arteries torn by fractures and disruption of the pelvic contents. The amount of blood loss can be life-threatening even in the absence of other injuries. One should anticipate the loss of at least one unit of blood for every pubic ramus fractured; with disruption of the pelvis, especially displaced fractures of the hemipelvis, local blood loss can exceed this by much greater amounts. When combined with additional blood loss from associated injuries in the abdomen, chest, and extremities, the resulting hypovolemic shock may be lethal.

Control of this bleeding during the period of transportation and evaluation in the emergency department can be achieved best by the use of pneumatic splints, the so-called MAST suit. The pneumatic trousers limit bleeding by compression, provide an autotransfusion from the lower extremities, and immobilize the fractures, thereby reducing further blood loss. This device should be applied at the accident scene to any patient suspected of having a pelvic fracture and especially to those patients with additional fractures of the femurs and tibiae when a lengthy period of transport is anticipated. If the MAST suit has not been applied in the field,

331

consideration should be given to putting it on the patient in the emergency department as soon as the initial clinical examination has been made in order to limit further bleeding during the period of resuscitation and special roentgenographic procedures. Before this is done, however, a careful assessment should first be made to exclude associated intra-abdominal lesions. Supraumbilical peritoneal lavage may be helpful in excluding intra-abdominal injury necessitating laparotomy. If the patient is in shock and requires an operation, the MAST suit should not be deflated until intravenous lines are in place, hypovolemia has been corrected, and the patient is in the operating room prepared for definitive treatment. Premature removal without immediately available support may easily result in death.

Retroperitoneal intrapelvic bleeding from veins is best managed by continued transfusion. If major arterial hemorrhage is suspected as evidenced by failure of continuing transfusion, arteriography followed by embolization of any demonstrated bleeding points is the treatment of choice. Exploration of the retroperitoneal intrapelvic hematoma with the hope of controlling bleeding by ligation of arteries and veins has been abandoned except in critical injuries associated with major vessels or open fractures.

Although *open fractures of the pelvis* are uncommon, the mortality rate of such injuries is greater than 50 percent. Once the retroperitoneal intrapelvic hematoma becomes infected, control of sepsis is almost impossible. For this reason, it is essential to detect such fractures at the time of the initial examination. The wound that communicates with the fractures can be in the wall of the vagina or rectum, the perineum, or the skin about the pubis. The wound may be very small, such as a puncture wound from inside out made by a sharp bony spicule, or may be large as a result of a straddle injury. Even a very small amount of bleeding from the rectum or vagina in a patient with a fracture of the pelvis raises the possibility of an open fracture. Every female patient with a pelvic fracture must have a careful rectal and vaginal examination. The roentgenograms of the pelvis in a patient with an open fracture may show gas in the soft tissues of the pelvis or even in the hip joint. This represents air aspirated into the tissue through the wound at the time of injury.

Treatment of open fractures of the pelvis consists of the early intravenous administration of antibiotic drugs, thorough irrigation, debridement, and primary closure of the wound if at all possible. If there is a wound in the rectum, colostomy is mandatory, and the distal portion of the colon must be emptied completely and cleansed. Stabilization of the pelvic fracture by means of external skeletal fixation such as the Hoffmann apparatus is important in selected cases.

The diagnosis and management of injuries of the genitourinary and intra-abdominal organs in patients with pelvic fractures is discussed in Chapters 10 and 11.

The treatment of pelvic fractures is expedited by a simple classification (Table 22–1) based upon whether or not the fractures involve a weight-bearing segment of the pelvis. If a weight-bearing segment is not involved, mobilization of the patient can progress rapidly. When a weight-bearing segment of the pelvis is fractured, treatment is more complicated and convalescence more protracted. Fortunately, only 25 to 30 percent of pelvic fractures fall into this category.

Avulsion fractures of the pelvis occur in athletes and represent detachments of a muscle origin with an associated bony fragment. Avulsion of the anterior superior iliac spine (sartorius m.), anterior inferior iliac spine (rectus femoris m.), and the ischial tuberosity (hamstring muscles) is seen in sprinters, hurdlers, and gymnasts. Failure to warm up and stretch the muscles thoroughly prior to competition predisposes to these injuries. Immediate pain aggravated by contraction of the involved muscle characterizes the injury and is followed by swelling and local hemorrhage. Rest and application of cold will limit this local reaction. Activity is slowly resumed as swelling and pain diminish. The use of local heat, diathermy, or ultrasound is to be avoided. Once healing has occurred, athletics can be resumed. Surgical reattachment of these avulsed fragments is rarely if ever indicated.

Isolated fractures of the wing of the ilium (Duverney) are the result of direct blows. Shortly after the injury, the fragment can be felt to move on palpation. However, local swelling and muscle spasm soon obscure this finding. Since the muscles of the abdominal wall are attached to the crest of the ilium, coughing and straining aggravate the pain. The abdominal muscles are tense. This rigidity may suggest peritoneal irritation caused by intra-abdominal injury, and peritoneal lavage will assist in avoiding unnecessary celiotomy. Treatment is entirely symptomatic with the encouragement of early activity.

Fractures of the pubic rami are the most frequent type of pelvic fractures. The seriousness of the injury is related directly to the number of pubic rami fractured. The fracture can be detected on clinical examination by

TABLE 22–1. CLASSIFICATION OF PELVIC FRACTURES

Fractures Not Affecting Weight Bearing
Avulsion fractures
Isolated fractures of the wing of the ilium
Fractures of the pubic rami
Some sacral fractures

Fractures Affecting Weight Bearing
Central fractures of the acetabulum
Fractures of the hemipelvis
Separation of the symphysis
Some sacral fractures

compression and distraction of the iliac crests and by direct palpation of the rami at the symphysis. On the initial anteroposterior roentgenograms of the pelvis, the fractures may not be well visualized. For this reason, additional anteroposterior roentgenograms of the pelvis taken with the pelvis tipped 45 degrees to the right and left (Judet views) are very helpful in defining the nature and extent of the fractures. In the absence of other injuries or complications, patients with fractures of the pubic rami can quickly be ambulatory on crutches with early weight bearing. Prolonged recumbency is not indicated in the treatment of these fractures.

Fractures of the sacrum fall into two groups. The first of these are caused by direct blows incurred in falls. The fractures are transverse and occur at levels below the sacroiliac joints. Weight bearing is not compromised. Local tenderness and swelling can be palpated at the site of fracture subcutaneously and on rectal examination. The fractures are seen best on lateral roentgenograms of the sacrum, and may involve only the anterior or posterior cortex of the sacrum. Initial treatment should consist of local applications of cold to inhibit swelling. Later, sitz baths are helpful. Early activity should be encouraged.

The second group of sacral fractures are caused by shearing forces and are associated with fractures of the anterior pelvic ring. The fracture lines are vertical and are adjacent to the sacroiliac joint. These fractures compromise weight bearing. The fractures may be difficult to evaluate on routine roentgenographic views because of overlying soft tissue shadows. Planigrams may be required for more accurate definition. Treatment of these fractures is related closely to treatment of associated fractures in the anterior pelvic ring.

Separations of the pubic symphysis are dramatic injuries. The defect at the symphysis can be easily palpated and visualized on the roentgenograms. What is not readily apparent is the damage to one or both sacroiliac joints. This posterior injury is always present, because it is impossible to open a ring in one place without opening it in another. The extent of the injury posteriorly is directly related to the amount of the separation anteriorly. Since the sacroiliac joints are affected, weight bearing is compromised. When the separation is greater than 1 to 2 cm, reduction and fixation by means of external skeletal fixation are indicated. This is superior to the use of slings and other suspension systems because it permits early activity and weight bearing with crutches.

Fractures of the hemipelvis (Malgaigne) are the most dangerous fractures of the pelvis — these result from violent injuries and are usually accompanied by other serious injuries. A variety of combinations occurs: separation of the pubic symphysis and dislocation of a sacroiliac joint, unilateral fractures of the pubic rami and a vertical fracture through the sacrum or ilium, and combinations of fractures and dislocations through anterior and posterior segments of the pelvic ring. The hemipelvis may be displaced laterally or superiorly, or may be rotated. Because of the immediate and urgent problems of resuscitation and treatment of associated injuries, initial treatment of fracture of the hemipelvis may have to be limited to application of skin traction to the leg on the affected side. However, as soon as the condition of the patient permits, reduction of the displacement and fixation by means of external skeletal pin fixation should be carried out.

Fractures of the acetabulum result from either central or posterior dislocation of the hip. Direct blows against the lateral aspect of the upper end of the thigh can drive the femur medially, disrupting the acetabulum. Blows to the knee, as in dashboard injuries, can produce simple posterior dislocation of the hip, posterior dislocation of the hip with a fracture of the posterior wall of the acetabulum, or central dislocation of the hip. The position of the hip at the time of impact determines the type of injury. The presence of soft tissue injuries around the knee or a fracture of the patella should raise strong suspicion regarding an associated hip injury. While a routine roentgenogram of the pelvis may indicate the diagnosis, evaluation of the injury may require oblique views, planigrams, and computerized tomography, which may be most helpful.

The initial treatment of a central fracture-dislocation of the hip consists of the application of traction to the leg. The amount and type of traction depends upon the muscularity of the patient and the degree of displacement of the hip. A posterior dislocation of the hip must be reduced immediately, after which the leg is stabilized in traction.

Displaced fractures of the acetabulum must be reduced anatomically to minimize the potential for subsequent traumatic arthritis resulting from joint incongruity. These fractures almost always require open reduction with internal fixation of the fragments. Fortunately this intervention can be delayed until the patient's condition is good and the nature of the fracture has been detailed.

DISLOCATIONS OF THE HIP

The hip joint can be dislocated either anteriorly or posteriorly (Fig. 22–1). Posterior dislocations are the most frequent, whereas anterior dislocations are rare.

Posterior dislocations of the hip result from blows on the knee while the hip is flexed and adducted. The passenger in the right front seat of an automobile, sitting with his legs crossed, is peculiarly vulnerable to this injury if his knee strikes the dashboard. The posterior capsule of the hip joint is ruptured and the head of the femur lies behind the acetabulum. In some cases there is an associated fracture of the posterior rim of the acetabulum or, rarely, a fracture of the head of the femur. The patient presents with the thigh flexed, adducted, internally rotated, and shortened. There may be associated injuries to structures surrounding the knee at the point of impact.

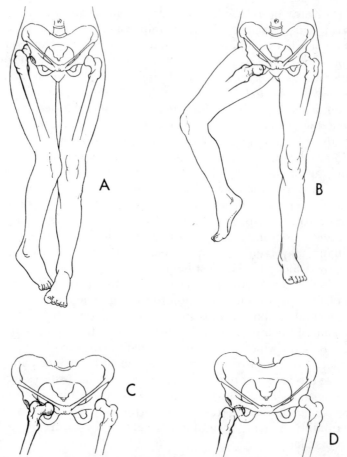

Figure 22–1. Types of dislocations of the hip. *A,* Posterior dislocation with the leg flexed, adducted, and internally rotated. *B,* Anterior dislocation with the leg flexed, abducted, and externally rotated. (Reproduced with permission from Compere EL, Banks SW, Compere CL: Pictorial Handbook of Fracture Treatment, 5th ed. Copyright © 1963 by Year Book Medical Publishers, Inc., Chicago.)

Since the sciatic nerve passes directly behind the hip joint, it can be injured by the displacement of the head of the femur posteriorly. For this reason, the sensory and motor function of this nerve should be evaluated and the results recorded before and after any attempt to reduce the dislocation. Nerve damage is rarely complete. The peroneal portion is most commonly affected. The patient is unable to dorsiflex the ankle and has no sensation on the dorsum of the foot at the base of the first and second toes.

While an anteroposterior roentgenogram of the hip will establish the diagnosis, the head of the femur may lie directly behind the acetabulum and the superimposition of the shadows may on cursory examination give the false impression of a normal relationship. However, because of the marked internal rotation of the femur, the shadow of the lesser trochanter is absent or very small, suggesting the correct diagnosis. A view of the entire pelvis with the opposite hip for comparison is very helpful.

A dislocation of the hip is an emergency and requires reduction as quickly as circumstances permit. Delay in reduction predisposes the patient to the complication of aseptic necrosis of the head of the femur. While this complication can occur in any patient with such an injury, it is more common in patients in whom reduction has been delayed 12 to 24 hours.

Reduction of a posterior dislocation of the hip can be accomplished in most cases by closed manipulation. Except in a comatose patient some form of anesthesia, spinal or general, should be used. If the patient requires other operative treatment, reduction of the hip should be carried out as the first procedure because it takes very little time and has a high priority. While closed reduction can be done with the patient on the operating table or in bed, it is done most conveniently with the patient lying supine on the floor (Fig. 22–2). The assistant kneels on the floor and anchors the pelvis by pressing down on the iliac crests. The surgeon straddles the affected leg, flexes the knee, and applies traction on the femur. The hip is gradually flexed to 90 degrees and the head of the femur is drawn forward over the posterior rim of the acetabulum. An audible sound signals that the hip has been relocated. The hip and knee are extended. The leg is examined to be sure that the deformity has disappeared. In cases complicated by a fracture of the posterior rim of the acetabulum, the hip and knee are again flexed 90 degrees and the femur is pushed posteriorly in an attempt to redislocate the hip. If the fragment of the posterior rim is insignificant, the hip does not redislocate. If the fragment is large enough to be functionally important, the hip will redislocate and must be reduced again. Such a test is

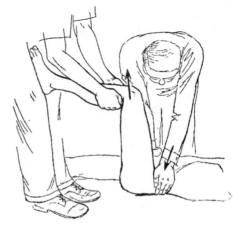

Figure 22–2. Method of reducing a posterior dislocation of the hip. (From De Palma AF: The Management of Fractures and Dislocations: An Atlas, Vol. 2. Philadelphia, W. B. Saunders Co., 1970.)

important in determining those cases requiring open reduction and internal fixation of the fragment of the acetabulum.

After the dislocation is reduced, the leg is maintained in extension in traction for a few days, after which the patient can be allowed to walk with crutches with partial weight bearing.

Anterior dislocations of the hip are the result of forces that widely abduct the hip. The patient's deformity may be quite grotesque; the thigh lies in flexion, external rotation, and wide abduction. The head of the femur may be palpated below the inguinal ligament and pressure of the femoral head may occlude the femoral artery, making prompt reduction very urgent. Reduction can be accomplished by closed manipulation in most cases. The maneuver is carried out in the same manner as for posterior dislocation, by applying traction, flexion, adduction, and internal rotation of the hip. Postreduction management is the same as for posterior dislocation of the hip.

Occasionally, dislocations of the hip cannot be reduced by closed methods, because of buttonholing of the capsule around the neck of the femur or the interposition of soft tissue or bone fragments. In such cases, immediate open reduction is required. Suspected interruption of sciatic nerve function, more likely to occur in posterior dislocations associated with a displaced fragment of bone, also may be an indication for open reduction and visualization of the sciatic nerve.

FRACTURES OF THE HIP

Fractures of the hip in young healthy patients are caused by the substantial violence accompanying falls, industrial accidents, and vehicular trauma. Multiple associated skeletal and soft tissue injuries are common. The number of complications directly related to management of these fractures is large. In contrast, fractures of the hip in the aged, infirm, and chronically ill are related to the degree of osteopenia in the upper end of the femur. In these patients, the fractures occur with minimal or minor trauma. Associated injuries are minimal. The difficulties encountered in managing these patients are related not only to the osteoporosis but also to the identification and treatment of underlying medical problems, which may be numerous.

Hip fractures can be divided into two categories based on their relationship to the insertion of the capsule of the hip joint onto the femur. Intracapsular fractures occur proximal to this insertion; extracapsular fractures, distal to this insertion. Fortunately, this relationship can be determined from the initial roentgenograms in over 95 percent of the patients. This classification has important prognostic significance. Intracapsular hip fractures have a high incidence of nonunion and aseptic necrosis of the head of the femur is also a potential complication. The local blood loss accompanying intracapsular hip fractures is small because the hematoma is confined by the capsule of the hip joint. The local loss in extracapsular hip fractures may be substantial; the hematoma is not confined by a tight fascial compartment.

Any patient suspected of having a hip fracture should be transported with the injured leg supported and stabilized in a traction splint. The presence or absence of a hip fracture can be determined with a high degree of certainty by means of auscultation, so-called osteophony (Fig. 22–3). Since sound is conducted efficiently through the solid bone medium, a break in the continuity of the bone (a fracture) is accompanied by a decrease in sound conduction. A stethoscope is applied to the symphysis pubis. First one, and then the other patella is tapped sharply with the finger. If there is a fracture, there will be a decrease in the pitch and intensity of the sound on the fractured side. Such a positive sign will be

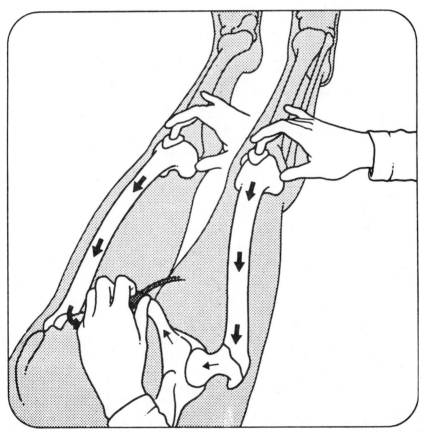

Figure 22–3. Diagnosis of a hip fracture by auscultatory percussion. (From Peltier LF: The diagnosis of fractures of the hip and femur by auscultatory percussion. Clin Orthopaed Related Res 123:9–11, 1977.)

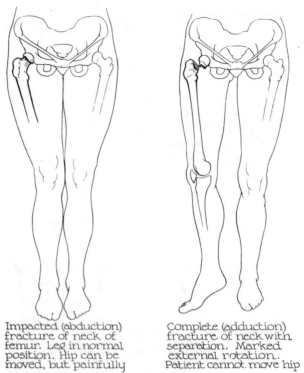

Impacted (abduction)
fracture of neck of
femur. Leg in normal
position. Hip can be
moved, but painfully

Complete (adduction)
fracture of neck with
separation. Marked
external rotation.
Patient cannot move hip

Figure 22–4.   Position of the leg following hip fracture. The leg is in external rotation and is shortened. (Reproduced with permission from Compere EL, Banks SW, Compere CL: Pictorial Handbook of Fracture Treatment, 5th ed. Copyright © 1963 by Year Book Medical Publishers, Inc., Chicago.)

present also if there is a dislocation of the hip or if there are unilateral pubic rami fractures. This maneuver can be carried out easily at the accident site as well as in the emergency department and can be done without moving the patient or removing the splint.

The classical deformity associated with fracture of the hip is shortening and external rotation of the leg (Fig. 22–4). Undisplaced or impacted fractures may be present without any deformity.

A roentgenogram of the pelvis should be obtained in any patient suspected of having a hip fracture. The advantages of this large film over a small film of the hip are several: (1) a view of the uninjured hip is available for comparison, (2) any pelvic fracture may be detected, and (3) conditions such as Paget's disease or bony metastases may be seen. To obtain a lateral view of the hip, a technique that does not require that the injured leg be moved, such as a cross-table or groin view, should be used. This avoids added pain and displacement of an impacted fracture.

Following presumptive diagnosis, the initial treatment of a fracture of the hip is the application of some form of traction to the affected limb. The fractured extremity is stabilized in this way while the patient's condition is thoroughly evaluated and any medical problems are brought under

Figure 22–5. Buck's traction. (From De Palma AF: The Management of Fractures and Dislocations: An Atlas, Vol. 1. Philadelphia, W. B. Saunders Co., 1970.)

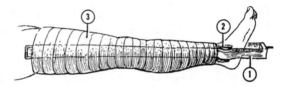

control. While in some patients traction may be the definitive treatment of choice, the majority of patients with hip fractures are treated by operation. Reduction and internal fixation or arthroplasty are carried out electively under optimal conditions.

The form of traction most appropriate for patients with hip fractures is skin traction (Fig. 22–5). This is applied to the distal two thirds of the thigh and to the leg by means of fabric-backed foam rubber strips 4 to 6 cm wide, or by means of adhesive tape of similar width if the foam strips are not available. Undue pressure over the peroneal nerve at the proximal end of the fibula and over the malleoli at the ankle is prevented by appropriate padding. After the traction strips are applied, they are held in place by wrapping with an elastic bandage. This circumferential wrap must be applied without compression or constriction. Traction then is applied by means of a cord attached to a spreader block just distal to the foot. When applied in this fashion with the leg in complete extension, it is called Buck's traction. Buck's traction does not control rotation, and the leg commonly lies in external rotation.

Flexion of the knee controls rotation and prevents an external rotation deformity. This is accomplished by the arrangement called Russell's traction; it produces its effect through the skin or through a calcaneal pin. In addition to the traction on the leg, a sling is placed under the distal thigh to elevate and flex the knee. This sling is connected by a cord through a series of pulleys to produce a balance of traction forces (Fig. 22–6).

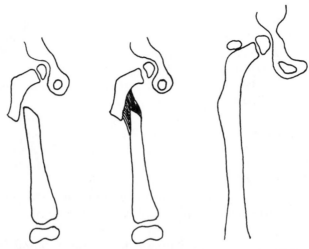

Figure 22–6. Russell's traction. (From Blount WP: Fractures in Children. Baltimore, Williams and Wilkins, 1955.)

Russell's traction, properly applied and maintained, can be used as a simple definitive form of treatment for extracapsular fractures of the hip.

The amount of traction to be applied varies with the size, weight, and muscular development of the individual patient, usually falling within the range of 4 to 5 kg. The complications to be avoided are pressure sores over the heel, malleoli, and head of the fibula, and peroneal palsy due to pressure over the peroneal nerve just below the head of the fibula. The advent of any complication is an indication to discontinue skin traction and proceed with some other form of treatment, such as skeletal traction or operation.

Skeletal traction, by means of a pin through the distal femur or proximal tibia, is indicated in the treatment of young vigorous patients requiring traction in excess of 5 kg. It also can be used in patients with leg ulcers or skin conditions in which skin traction cannot be tolerated. It is the method of choice for patients with serious arterial insufficiency. The use of skeletal traction permits good control of rotation, and all the benefits of Russell's traction.

Subcapital fractures of the hip occur at the junction of the head with the neck of the femur. These fractures are often impacted; that is, the neck is driven into the head and the two fragments remain firmly attached to one another. When such a fracture is impacted in abduction (valgus) and is not tipped posteriorly or anteriorly on lateral roentgenogram, it is stable and resists the forces tending to displace the fragments. Fractures impacted in adduction (varus) or with posterior angulation are not stable and almost always displace or come apart. Good anteroposterior and lateral roentgenograms of the hip are required to determine these relationships. The initial treatment of a stable impacted fracture consists of the application of Buck's traction. Subsequent treatment consists of a program of early walking with crutches preceded in some cases by pinning of the fracture fragments in situ.

Patients with displaced subcapital fractures of the hip should have stabilization in traction during the initial period of evaluation. Closed reduction and internal fixation is the treatment of choice in the younger age group, while removal of the femoral head and replacement with a prosthesis (hemiarthroplasty) may be the treatment of choice for the older or more debilitated patient.

Fractures through the neck of the femur are rarely impacted and are almost always displaced. The angle of the fracture through the neck is important if treatment by closed reduction and internal fixation is used. When the fracture line is vertical, the shearing force through the fracture line adversely affects fixation and healing. A more horizontal fracture line allows compression and promotes stability and healing. These features are not important if treatment by means of a prosthetic replacement is chosen.

In children, separation of the proximal femoral epiphysis can occur as the result of trauma or as the result of a process leading to gradual displacement of the head of the femur. This latter process can be accelerated at any stage by an injury that completes the disruption. The patient presents with an external rotation deformity of the leg. A roentgenogram of the pelvis with lateral views of both hips is essential to determine the position of the epiphyses and also to evaluate the asymptomatic hip, because the condition is frequently bilateral. The initial treatment of such a patient consists of the application of traction. Options for definitive treatment include pinning in situ, reduction with traction distally and internal rotation followed by pinning, and osteotomy.

The greater and lesser trochanters of the femur can be avulsed by the strong contraction of muscles inserted into them. Rarely, the greater trochanter is broken by a direct blow, as in a fall. Isolated fractures of the greater trochanter usually occur in older osteopenic patients. Isolated fractures of the lesser trochanter occur in young athletes such as sprinters or jumpers. Isolated fractures of the greater or lesser trochanters require only symptomatic treatment with the use of crutches during the painful initial period of healing.

Extracapsular fractures of the hip occur with a considerable variety of patterns from the base of the neck of the femur to below the lesser trochanter. They may be undisplaced single fractures or they may be displaced and badly comminuted. These fractures should be managed initially by the application of Buck's or Russell's traction. The blood loss associated with the comminuted fractures may be quite large and it is particularly important in the elderly patient with a chronically constricted blood volume. Such patients will require blood replacement regardless of whether or not operative treatment is planned. While most extracapsular fractures of the hip can be treated successfully in traction, open reduction and internal fixation with a variety of metallic appliances is chosen as the definitive treatment for most patients because open reduction and internal fixation should allow a shortening of the period of enforced bed rest and hospitalization. The difficulties and complications of operative treatment are directly related to the extent of the comminution of the fracture.

FRACTURES OF THE SHAFT OF THE FEMUR

Fractures of the shaft of the femur involve the tubular diaphyseal bone extending from below the lesser trochanter to about the junction of the middle and lower thirds of the femur. They occur in all age groups. Because of the strength of the bone, substantial forces are required to produce a fracture and additional associated injuries are common.

Immediately following a fracture of the shaft of the femur, the patient is threatened by the twin complications of hypovolemic shock and fat embolism. These complications can be minimized by effective prehospital care. Before the introduction of the Thomas splint during World War I, the mortality rate following open fractures of the shaft of the femur was 85

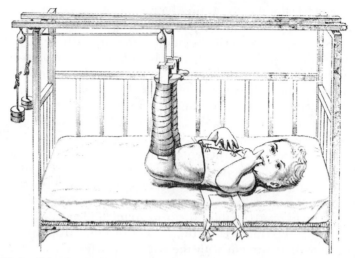

Figure 22–7. Bryant's traction. (From Blount, WP: Fractures in Children. Baltimore, Williams and Wilkins, 1955.)

percent. After this traction splint was introduced, the mortality rate for these fractures fell to 15 percent. All patients suspected of having fractures of the shaft of the femur should be treated initially at the accident scene by the application of a traction splint (e.g., Thomas, Hare) unless pneumatic trousers (MAST suit) are used. Patients admitted to the emergency department without such splints should have splints applied before roentgenograms and other diagnostic studies are obtained. The splints should not be removed until the surgeon is ready to carry out some form of definitive treatment. In patients with fractures of the shaft of the femur, it is essential to obtain roentgenograms that show the entire femur including the hip and the knee, including the tibial plateau. A pelvic film should also be taken to ensure that other associated fractures or dislocations are not overlooked.

The initial treatment of fractures of the shaft of the femur usually consists of the application of some form of traction to the leg. In children and in the elderly, skin traction may be sufficient. Skin traction can be used as the definitive form of treatment in small children (<35 kg) in the form of Bryant's traction (Fig. 22–7). In older children and some adults, Russell's traction (see Fig. 22–6) can be used effectively. Skeletal traction by means of Kirschner wires or Steinmann pins is used in healthy muscular patients. The pins are placed through the metaphyseal bone of the distal femur or proximal tibia. Care must be taken not to transgress the epiphysis or epiphyseal line if these are still present. When skeletal traction is used, the leg is supported with a balanced Thomas splint and a Pearson attachment (Fig. 22–8). Once the patient is properly aligned in traction, there are several options. The patient can be maintained in traction until (1) the

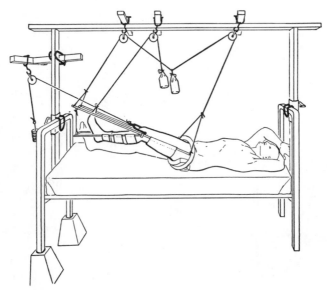

Figure 22–8. Balanced skeletal traction using a Thomas splint with a Pearson attachment. (From Rhoads JE, Allen JG, Harkins HN, Moyer CA: Surgery, Principles and Practice, 4th ed. Philadelphia, J. B. Lippincott Co., 1970.)

fracture has healed; (2) partial healing has occurred at which time a plaster spica, cast brace, or conventional brace can be used; or (3) open reduction and internal fixation of the fracture is carried out after the patient's condition has stabilized.

In patients with undisplaced fractures of the shaft of the femur, particularly small children, simple application of a plaster of Paris hip spica may suffice for treatment. Plaster immobilization of this type is used frequently as a second stage of treatment after the fracture has partially healed in traction.

The use of the cast brace as the primary or secondary form of treatment for fractures of the shaft of the femur has been used with success in the management of many patients (Fig. 22–9). The advantages of the cast brace are a shortened period of recumbency and the early resumption of joint motion and ambulation. Cast bracing is useful particularly in the older adolescent and young adult without associated injuries. Some experience in the method is required and the patients must be monitored carefully if shortening and angulation are to be avoided.

Open reduction and internal fixation of fractures of the shaft of the femur carries the risk of infection of the fracture, which can have catastrophic consequences. On the other hand, when successful, open reduction and internal fixation permit early joint motion and activity. It is valuable particularly in the patient with multiple injuries, especially in patients with fractures of the ipsilateral tibia and fibula.

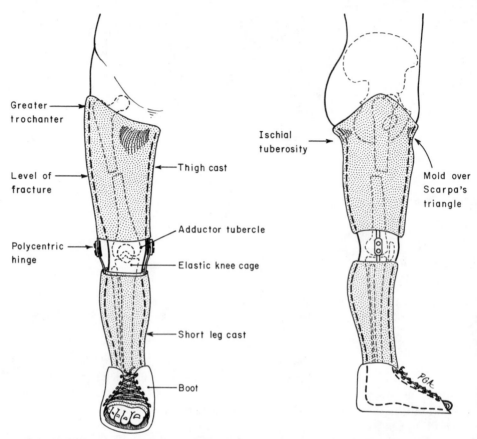

Greater trochanter

Level of fracture

Polycentric hinge

Thigh cast

Adductor tubercle

Elastic knee cage

Short leg cast

Boot

Ischial tuberosity

Mold over Scarpa's triangle

Figure 22–9.   A cast brace for the treatment of a femoral shaft fracture. (Reproduced with permission from Patel D and Brown T: Fractures of the Femoral Shaft. *In* Cave EF, Burke JB, Brown T: Trauma Management. Copyright © 1974 by Year Book Medical Publishers, Inc., Chicago.)

FRACTURES OF THE DISTAL END OF THE FEMUR

Fractures of the distal end of the femur include supracondylar fractures, isolated fractures of the femoral condyles, and separations of the distal femoral epiphysis. Many of the fractures are open fractures as the sharp edge of the proximal fragment is pushed through the anterior aspect of the thigh above the patella. Such fractures, as well as isolated fractures of the femoral condyles, are typical of dashboard injuries. This is a common area of fracture in the elderly osteopenic patient.

Fractures in this area always involve the knee joint either directly by displacement and malalignment of the articular surfaces, or indirectly because of joint stiffness resulting from the period of immobilization required for healing and the formation of scar tissue about the fracture.

For this reason, treatment is directed toward the open anatomical reduction of fractures involving the femoral condyles and fixation of the fractures to allow early joint motion.

In addition to the complications of hypovolemic shock and fat embolism, fractures of the distal end of the femur may be accompanied by injuries of the femoral or popliteal artery and vein. Emergency splinting and initial care are similar to those applied to femoral shaft fractures. While some supracondylar fractures can be treated successfully by skeletal traction, cast braces, or both, operative intervention to obtain anatomical reduction and stabilization is indicated more frequently. Displaced separations of the distal femoral epiphysis can be reduced by closed manipulation in most cases, the reduction being maintained in a cast. If a satisfactory reduction cannot be maintained in the cast, open reduction and/or percutaneous pinning of the epiphysis to the diaphysis should not be delayed.

FRACTURES OF THE PATELLA

Isolated fractures of the patella result from direct blows, such as the knee striking the dashboard. These fractures are usually stellate, comminuted, and not displaced. The fragments are contained within the fibrous structure of the quadriceps muscle. Since the structure of the muscle is in continuity, patients with these fractures may be able to lift the heel off the bed or to straighten the knee against gravity if the pain is not severe.

More commonly fractures of the patella occur in association with injuries of the quadriceps muscle. When the quadriceps muscle strongly contracts to extend the knee against a force which is flexing the knee, rupture or avulsion of the quadriceps mechanism can occur. There are several varieties of injury caused in this fashion.

Avulsion of the quadriceps muscle from the top of the patella occurs in the older age group. In such cases a defect in the substance of the quadriceps muscle at the top of the patella can be palpated. When the quadriceps muscle contracts, the patella does not move upward. On roentgenograms of the knee, the patella appears to occupy a position somewhat lower (more distal) than normal.

Transverse fractures of the patella may be undisplaced or the fragments may be separated. When the fragments are separated there must be associated tears in the quadriceps expansions on either side of the patella. The extent of these tears is related directly to the degree of separation of the fragments. These patellar fractures may be comminuted, but there is usually one large fragment, proximally or distally. If the patient is examined early, before the findings are obscured by swelling or hemorrhage into the prepatellar bursa, the fracture fragments can be palpated. Roentgenograms, especially lateral films, should establish the diagnosis. A normal bipartite or tripartite patella may be mistaken for a fracture.

Avulsions of the patellar ligament are unusual. They occur in adolescents or young adults or in chronic debilitated patients. Most commonly, the tendon is avulsed from its insertion into the tibial tubercle; rarely, the tendon is avulsed from the base of the patella. When tendons are pulled from their bony insertions, fragments of bone from the site of insertion are pulled away also. Occasionally, these bony fragments may be quite large. On roentgenograms, the patella appears to be displaced proximally.

When a fracture of the patella is suspected, the initial treatment should consist of splinting the leg with the knee in complete extension. Undisplaced fractures of the patella can be treated simply in a cylinder cast extending from the high thigh to a point 2 cm above the medial malleolus. The average period of immobilization required for healing ranges from six to ten weeks.

The majority of patients with fractures of the patella will require operative treatment to reconstitute the disrupted quadriceps apparatus and correct irregularities in the articular surface of the patella. While the repair of closed injuries may be delayed until the patient's condition is stable, open injuries must be debrided and repaired immediately.

Avulsion of the quadriceps muscle from the top of the patella is treated by direct suture. Avulsions of the patellar tendon are treated by suture or by reattachment of the bony fragment in continuity with the tendon by means of a pin or screw. The treatment of displaced comminuted or transverse fractures of the patella consists of total or partial distal patellectomy. An alternative approach favored by some is repair with circumferential and tension band wiring.

No matter which procedure is chosen, the associated soft tissue damage to the quadriceps apparatus must be repaired meticulously. The postoperative management consists of immobilization of the knee in extension in a cylinder cast for a period of eight weeks.

DISLOCATIONS OF THE PATELLA

Dislocations of the patella can result from tangential blows to the edge of the patella. More commonly, they occur as a consequence of a sudden, strong, uncoordinated contraction of the quadriceps muscle as the patient attempts to recover equilibrium after slipping or falling or during vigorous dancing. In such cases there may be predisposing factors such as a small, high-riding patella, a knock knee (valgus) deformity, hyperflexible joints, and a weak quadriceps muscle. The patient may give a history of previous subluxations or dislocations of the patella.

The patella almost always dislocates laterally over the edge of the lateral femoral condyle. The knee is held in flexion and the patella can be palpated in the abnormal position. Reduction is accomplished by extending the knee. This often occurs spontaneously before the patient is seen in the emergency department.

Roentgenograms of the knee may show the patella in the abnormal position and after reduction, a small, thick, high-riding patella. Occasionally, a small bony fragment sheared off of the patella is noted within the joint. The tangential "sunrise" view of the patella may show hypoplasia of the lateral femoral condyle and a shallow intercondylar groove.

Immediately after reduction of the dislocation, the leg should be immobilized in extension with a compression dressing to limit swelling and joint effusion. Any operative procedures to prevent recurrent dislocation can be delayed while the indications are considered and the choice of the procedure is tailored to the needs of the individual patient.

LIGAMENT AND MENISCAL INJURIES OF THE KNEE

Injuries of the ligaments and menisci of the knee occur frequently as sports injuries. However, the same mechanisms of injury also occur in the home, at work, or on the highway. When they occur as isolated injuries, diagnosis and treatment are quite straightforward. However, injuries of the ligaments and menisci occurring in association with other injuries, particularly fractures of the shaft of the femur or tibia, are quite often overlooked. It is very important to discover if a ligament is injured, because early treatment is essential if a good end result is to be obtained. For this reason, the integrity of the knee must be checked following internal fixation of the fractured femur or tibia. Treatment of a torn meniscus can be delayed for a period of weeks without affecting the end result.

The amount of swelling in the knee gives no clue to the presence or absence of a ligamentous injury. Many serious ligamentous injuries have little swelling because the hemarthrosis and effusion leak into the surrounding tissues through a rent in the capsule. Aspiration of the knee for swelling following an injury should be done *only* for the relief of pain caused by severe distention of the capsule of the joint. Aspiration should not be done routinely, as fluid reaccumulates rapidly. If the knee is aspirated, any fluid recovered should be collected in a metal basin and examined to determine if any fat droplets are present. Such fat droplets indicate the presence of a fracture communicating with the joint.

The diagnosis of a tear of a ligament or portion of the joint capsule is based upon the detection of an abnormal range of motion in the joint. For this reason, the examination should begin by an evaluation of the range of motion in the opposite normal joint. In the knee, laxity or abnormal movement can occur as a result of injury to structures in any sector of the entire circumference of the knee. Motion in the anterior or posterior sectors is tested with the knee flexed 90 degrees (Fig. 22–10). The tibia is then pulled forward or pushed backward. Excessive motion anteriorly (the anterior drawer sign) indicates a tear of the anterior cruciate ligament. Excessive motion posteriorly (the posterior drawer sign) indicates a tear of

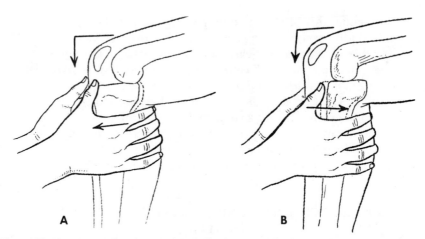

Figure 22–10. *A*, Anterior drawer sign indicating a tear in the anterior cruciate ligament. *B*, Posterior drawer sign indicating a tear in the posterior cruciate ligament. (From De Palma AF: The Management of Fractures and Dislocations: An Atlas, Vol. 2. Philadelphia, W. B. Saunders Co., 1970.)

the posterior cruciate ligament. The knee is placed in extension for evaluation of the medial and lateral collateral ligaments of the knee (Fig. 22–11). With the knee flexed about 15 degrees, a valgus stress is applied to the knee. Excessive motion indicates a tear of the medial collateral ligament. This maneuver should be repeated with the knee in full extension. If only the medial collateral ligament is torn, the knee will be stable. Excessive movement indicates an additional tear of the anterior cruciate ligament. The integrity of the lateral collateral ligament is tested by applying a varus stress with the knee in full extension. Excessive motion indicates a tear of this ligament. Excessive motion on varus or valgus stress of the knee may be found in cases in which the ligaments are intact but in

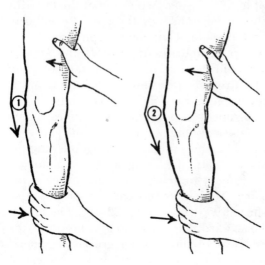

Figure 22–11. The examination for collateral ligament tears. (From DePalma AF: The Management of Fractures and Dislocations: An Atlas, Vol. 2. Philadelphia, W. B. Saunders Co., 1970.)

which depressed fractures of the medial or lateral tibial plateaus or, very rarely, the femoral condyles are present.

If the patient is examined immediately after the injury before swelling and protective muscle spasms have developed, the findings can be determined accurately. After a short time, examination may be difficult and inconclusive. An anesthetic providing full muscular relaxation may be required to assess accurately the extent and location of the ligamentous injury. If this is necessary, examination under anesthesia, followed by operative repair of any seriously damaged ligamentous structure, should be scheduled within the first 24 to 48 hours after injury. If the patient requires an anesthetic for the management of any acute associated injuries, advantage should be taken of this to carry out such an examination. Appropriate informed consent for repair should be obtained.

A torn meniscus is usually accompanied by a moderate effusion, joint line tenderness, and limitation of full extension and full flexion of the knee. When there are associated ligamentous injuries, the finding of ligamentous rupture overshadows the signs of meniscal injury. In the acute phase, it is impossible to perform the manipulation required to establish clinically the diagnosis of a torn meniscus. Such a patient should be treated by splinting of the knee to relieve pain and by compressing the knee to limit swelling. Both of these ends are achieved by using a Jones' dressing (Fig. 22–12). Repeated re-examination of the knee during the ensuing days and weeks as swelling and pain diminish will establish the diagnosis.

DISLOCATIONS OF THE KNEE

Ligaments are torn when a joint is carried through a range of motion greater than normal. For this reason, all ligamentous injuries of the knee

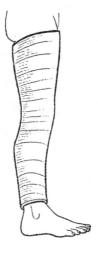

Figure 22–12. A Jones' dressing. This dressing consists of several layers of cotton batting compressed with a muslin or roller gauze bandage. Plaster or yucca splints may be incorporated for greater rigidity. (From DePalma AF: The Management of Fractures and Dislocations: An Atlas, Vol. 2. Philadelphia, W. B. Saunders Co., 1970.)

are associated with subluxations or dislocations of the tibia on the femur. In most cases displacement is small and has been reduced spontaneously by the time the patient is seen. Occasionally the displacement may be quite large and remain unreduced. Such dislocations of the knee are caused by severe trauma and are associated with a high incidence of dangerous vascular and nerve injuries. The knee can be dislocated anteriorly, posteriorly, medially, laterally, or in rotation. This last mode, rare but important because it cannot be reduced by closed manipulation, can be recognized easily because of the presence of a skin dimple or depression, 2 to 3 cm in diameter, over one of the femoral condyles. Other dislocations of the knee involve gross deformities that should suggest the diagnosis.

Like all other dislocations, dislocation of the knee is an emergency, and should be reduced as quickly as possible after evaluation of the circulation and nerve function distal to the knee and after appropriate roentgenograms are obtained. An anesthetic providing good muscular relaxation is usually required. Reduction should not be difficult and is accomplished by applying traction to the tibia and realigning the joint. At the time of the reduction, the knee should be carefully examined to determine the type and extent of the damage to the knee ligaments and capsule. The knee is then immobilized in a dressing with the foot exposed so that the posterior tibial and dorsalis pedis arteries can be palpated and the sensation and motor function in the foot can be tested. When any vascular injury has been ruled out, operative repair of the torn ligaments and capsule should be carried out without further delay.

Damage to the popliteal artery occurs in a substantial number of patients with dislocations of the knee. When this damage is not diagnosed promptly and treated effectively, a potentially avoidable amputation may subsequently become necessary. The evaluation of the distal circulation by clinical observation and by the use of flow meters can be confusing and may sometimes lead to delay in diagnosis. For this reason, when any question regarding the possibility of arterial injury arises, a femoral artery arteriogram should be obtained promptly. Many believe that this should be routinely done, certainly in anterior dislocations. In addition, the need for a fasciotomy after repair of an injured popliteal artery should always be considered, especially when a delay or more than a few hours between injury and repair has occurred.

The peroneal nerve is particularly vulnerable to stretch injury. This occurs frequently with knee injuries, particularly with dislocations. Injury to the popliteal nerve is less common. In evaluating nerve function, it is important to be aware that loss of sensation and impairment of motor function can also result from vascular injury. Treatment of any nerve injury is accomplished initially by the splinting and support of the leg and foot.

FRACTURES OF THE UPPER END OF THE TIBIA

Fractures of the tibial spines occur occasionally, usually in children, as a result of a hyperextension injury of the knee. The patient will present with a swollen, painful knee that cannot be fully extended. The fracture is best visualized on the lateral roentgenogram of the knee. While it is the displacement of the spine that is seen, the fracture itself actually involves moderate to large fragments of the upper surface of the tibia. During the initial traumatic displacement, the anterior horn of the medial meniscus can become interposed between the fragments, making closed reduction impossible. An anesthetic is usually required for reduction. Preparations for open reduction should be made if closed reduction fails. The knee is fully extended and another lateral roentgenogram of the knee is taken. If this shows a satisfactory reduction, a cylinder plaster is applied and the patient is allowed to bear weight on the extremity with crutches. If the fracture is not reduced, arthrotomy, repositioning of the interposed meniscus (it need not be removed), and reduction of the displaced fragment are carried out. In selected cases, internal fixation of the fragment with a wire may be added. Postoperative management is the same as following a closed reduction.

Dislocations of the head of the fibula are rare injuries, usually caused by direct trauma. A contusion of the peroneal nerve may be associated with this type of injury. When recognized early, the dislocations usually can be reduced by direct pressure on the head of the fibula. Dislocation of the head of the fibula also can occur in association with displaced fractures of the tibia. In such cases, the mechanism is similar to the fracture-dislocations of the forearm. The tibia breaks and shortens and the unbroken fibula dislocates at the proximal tibiofibular joint. In these patients the chief concern is the treatment of the tibial fracture.

Fractures of the tibial plateau result from falls on the extended leg or, more frequently, from varus or valgus stress to the extended leg. These occur frequently in pedestrians struck by motor vehicles (Fig. 22–13). In the young adult such stress often produces collateral ligament injuries because the bone is stronger than the ligament. In the older adult, the ligament is stronger than the cancellous metaphyseal bone and fracture results. The patient presents with a painful, swollen knee, with or without deformity. There may be an associated injury to the peroneal nerve. Careful examination may indicate instability to varus or valgus stress similar to what is found with tears of the medial or lateral collateral ligaments. The roentgenograms establish the nature and extent of the fracture. The tibial plateau may be crushed and compacted by the pressure of the opposing femoral condyle. There may be vertical fractures resulting from shearing forces. Damage to the articular weight-bearing surface of

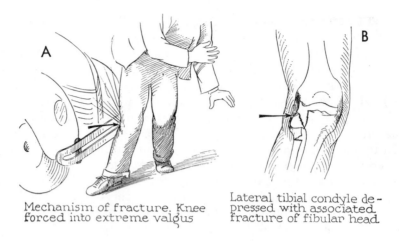

Mechanism of fracture. Knee forced into extreme valgus

Lateral tibial condyle depressed with associated fracture of fibular head.

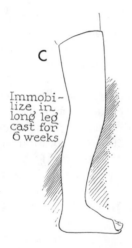

Immobilize in long leg cast for 6 weeks

Figure 22-13. A common mechanism of tibial plateau fracture. (Reproduced with permission from Compere EL, Banks SW, Compere CL: Pictorial Handbook of Fracture Treatment, 5th ed. Copyright © 1963 by Year Book Medical Publishers, Inc., Chicago.)

the tibia can be extensive. Special roentgenographic views and tomograms of the tibia are helpful in demonstrating this.

The initial treatment consists of the application of a rigid compression dressing to limit swelling and splint the fracture. Subsequent treatment depends upon the condition of the patient and the nature of the fracture, consisting of closed reduction and immobilization, a cast brace, skeletal traction through the tibia with promotion of early motion in the fracture, or open reduction and internal fixation of the fracture.

Isolated fractures of the shaft of the fibula above the distal syndesmosis are usually the result of direct blows and are transverse or comminuted in type. Roentgenograms of the ankle must always be taken to ensure that there is not an associated disruption of the ankle mortise. Treatment of these fractures consists of a compression dressing to control swelling and crutches. A below-knee walking cast may be used for a time if pain and swelling are severe.

Isolated fractures of the shaft of the tibia are also caused most often by direct blows. Roentgenograms of the entire tibia and fibula must be taken to ensure that there is not an associated fracture of the fibula at another level or a dislocation of the proximal tibiofibular joint. Rarely, an associated bending fracture of the fibula may be present. Since the tibial fragments are strongly attached to the intact fibula by means of the interosseous ligament, displacement of the fracture is usually not large and there is considerable intrinsic stability. Treatment ordinarily consists of closed reduction and alignment followed by application of a long leg plaster dressing.

Fractures of the shaft of the tibia and fibula are more serious injuries than isolated fractures of the tibia or fibula. Open fractures and vascular injuries are more frequent because of the greater displacement of the fragments. Local blood loss and swelling are greater. Associated injuries in the trunk, extremities, and head are more common. These patients will usually require admission to the hospital and some form of anesthesia for reduction. Whenever possible, closed reduction and plaster immobilization remains the treatment of choice. While some anterior bowing can be tolerated, posterior bowing is unacceptable and should be avoided if at all possible. The articular surfaces of the tibial plateau and the ankle joint (the tibial plateau) should be parallel as seen on the anteroposterior roentgenogram. Minor adjustments of the alignment can be made after the initial cast application by wedging. Open reduction and internal fixation or the use of external pin fixation in the treatment of these fractures is reserved for those cases in which a satisfactory closed reduction cannot be obtained or in those fractures complicated by loss of skin or bone or by vascular injury.

Fractures of the ankle occur frequently and are responsible for substantial temporary and permanent disability. They are seen in all age groups and are associated with a wide spectrum of activities. Since the ankle has a complex motion and is a major weight-bearing joint, fractures involving the articular surfaces must be accurately reduced and maintained in position during the healing period to avoid the late development of traumatic arthritis. While this can be accomplished by closed manipulation and plaster immobilization in many cases, open reduction and internal fixation is often required for an optimal result.

When seen initially, some patients will have few symptoms and little swelling. Others will have gross deformity. All variations between these two extremes are seen. When there is a gross deformity due to a displaced fracture-dislocation the skin may be torn, producing an open fracture, or the skin may be tightly tented over a malleolus and in danger of sloughing. In either case, immediate realignment of the ankle is indicated before splinting is done and roentgenograms obtained. The longer the gross dislocation is allowed to remain unreduced, the greater is the incidence of skin and neurovascular complications. Realignment can usually be done quite simply, especially with intravenous sedation, by bending the knee to

90 degrees and placing the foot in equinus to relax the Achilles tendon. The foot is then aligned on the tibia and a splint is applied.

The initial roentgenographic examination must include anteroposterior and lateral views of the entire tibia and fibula as well as anteroposterior, 15 degree internal rotation oblique (true anteroposterior ankle), and lateral views of the ankle. In children and adolescents, comparative views of the opposite, uninjured ankle are helpful in evaluating potential epiphyseal injuries.

In many patients with ankle injuries, the roentgenograms will show no evidence of fracture, although there may be considerable pain and swelling. These cases represent *ankle sprains*. The exact ligament involved can usually be determined by careful palpation. Ankle strapping and elastic bandaging may be sufficient for the treatment of most such injuries. If pain and swelling are severe or if the patient must be very active, the use of a below-knee walking plaster for a period of three weeks is preferred.

Fractures of the ankle can be categorized conveniently into four groups depending upon the mechanism of injury. In the order of frequency, these are fractures traceable to: (1) external rotation, (2) abduction, (3) adduction, and (4) vertical compression (Fig. 22–14). Each group has its own characteristic roentgenographic findings. Useful generalities that enable the mechanism of injury to be determined from the roentgenograms are: (1) transverse fractures of the malleoli are caused by avulsions; (2) spiral fractures of the fibula by external rotation and torque; and (3) vertical fractures of the tibia by shearing forces. Knowledge of the mechanism of injury is important because closed reduction by manipulation is accomplished by reversing the mechanism of injury.

External-rotation fractures of the ankle result from the external rotation of the talus in the ankle mortise. When the distal tibiofibular ligaments that hold the ankle mortise together are not ruptured, a spiral fracture of the distal end of the fibula results. With rupture of the anterior distal tibiofibular ligament, the spiral fracture of the fibula commonly occurs as high as the proximal third of the fibula (Maisonneuve's fracture). Sometimes the tibiofibular ligaments are completely torn with total disruption of the ankle mortise. As the talus and distal tibia continue to rotate externally, the medial malleolus is avulsed from the tibia through a transverse fracture. Continued rotation and shear produce a fracture of the posterior distal process of the fibula (the so-called posterior malleolus), resulting in a trimalleolar fracture.

Abduction fractures of the ankle are caused by eversion of the talus in the ankle mortise. The fibula is broken off transversely below the ankle mortise. As displacement continues, the medial malleolus is avulsed through a transverse fracture line.

Adduction fractures are produced by inversion of the talus in the ankle mortise. The medial superior edge of the talus shears off the medial malleolus through a vertical fracture extending into the tibial metaphysis.

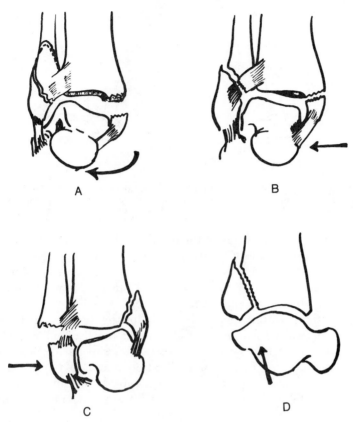

A   B

C   D

Figure 22–14.   Basic mechanisms of ankle injury with the characteristic features produced by each: *A*, external rotation, *B*, abduction, *C*, adduction, and *D*, vertical compression. (From Rockwood CA, Jr, Green DP: Fractures, Vol II. Philadelphia, J. B. Lippincott Co., 1975.)

With continuing displacement, the distal end of the fibula is avulsed through a transverse fracture line.

When the talus is driven up into the lower end of the tibia, the articular surface of the ankle joint is fractured by vertical compression. When the foot is in plantar flexion at impact, the major fragment is sheared off posteriorly; with dorsiflexion, anteriorly.

About 95 percent of all ankle fractures can be grouped into these four categories. The most serious injuries are those with disruption of the ankle mortise and those with fractures through the articular surface of the distal tibia.

The treatment of undisplaced ankle fractures consists of immobilization with the foot in a neutral position for a period of six to eight weeks in a below-knee cast. When there is a good deal of swelling initially, any cast must be replaced at intervals as the swelling recedes. Following removal of the cast, an elastic support may be required to control dependent swelling for several weeks.

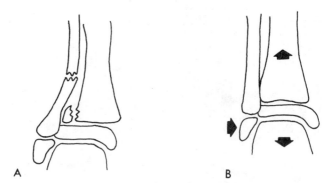

Figure 22–15. *A*, Epiphyseal separation of the distal tibia (Salter-Harris Type II) with separation and lateral displacement of the epiphysis. *B*, Treatment by closed reduction.

Many displaced fractures of the ankle can be reduced satisfactorily by manipulation. For the best results, an anesthetic is usually necessary. Good plaster technique is essential if the reduction is to be maintained. Subsequent roentgenograms of the ankle must be taken during the postreduction period to detect any change in position.

Most patients with displaced fractures of the articular surface of the distal tibia or with disruptions of the ankle mortise will require open reduction and internal fixation. Fractures that slip out of position after closed reduction and plaster immobilization may also require operative treatment. Fortunately, operation can be delayed and done as an elective procedure if the fracture is not open. In the meantime, the leg is immobilized in a below-knee plaster splint.

Fractures of the ankle in children almost always involve the epiphyses. Usually these injuries are of the Salter-Harris Type II variety and are amenable to closed reduction if displaced (Fig. 22–15). When there are injuries of the Salter-Harris III and IV varieties, careful open reduction and pinning is required if there is displacement of the fragments (Fig. 22–16). Injuries of the Salter-Harris V variety will give rise to serious later deformity that may require surgical correction (see Chapter 20).

Fractures and dislocations of the talus are uncommon injuries caused by forcible dorsiflexion of the foot, sometimes combined with inversion and rotation, such as occurs when the foot is pressed down on the brake pedal at the time of a collision. They can also result from falls from a height when the patient lands on the foot. The fracture line usually runs transversely across the neck of the talus at its junction with the body, although vertical shearing fracture of the body is seen. When the fracture is undisplaced, simple immobilization in a below-knee walking plaster is all that is required.

The treatment of displaced fractures and dislocations of the talus is more difficult. These are often open injuries with wounds on the medial side of the ankle where the skin was ruptured at the time of maximal

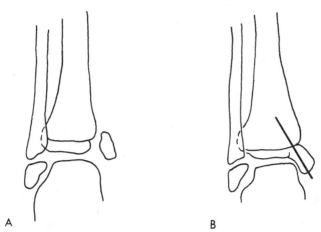

A   B

Figure 22–16. *A*, Epiphyseal fracture of the distal tibial epiphysis (Salter-Harris Type III). *B*, Open reduction and fixation with a pin.

displacement. If not torn, the skin is tented tightly over the prominence of the medial malleolus and will slough if the reduction is not accomplished quickly. Anesthesia providing good muscle relaxation is required. The knee should be flexed 90 degrees and the foot placed in full equinus (plantar flexion) to relax the pull on the Achilles tendon (Fig. 22–17). The reduction is accomplished by direct pressure on the talus. If the reduction of the fracture or dislocation is unstable, transfixion of the fragments or bones with one or two Kirschner wires is helpful. Immobilization in a plaster dressing follows. The prognosis for healing without complications is poor if there has been dislocation of the body from both the ankle and the subtalar joints, because the blood supply to the talus is poor. Late aseptic necrosis of the talus occurs frequently in such cases.

Fractures of the os calcis occur commonly in falls from a height onto the feet. Bilateral fractures can occur. Occasionally there is an associated compression fracture of the spine. Fractures of the os calcis can be very painful because of bleeding into the closed space of the heel. A well-padded plaster dressing is required and it may be extended above the knee, with the knee flexed to relieve the pull on the Achilles tendon. The leg must be kept elevated to limit swelling.

The nature of the fracture is determined by examining lateral and tangential roentgenograms of the os calcis. The fractures can be divided into two groups. The first is a small group of fractures that involve the posterior part of the body of the os calcis (Fig. 22–18). The second large group consists of comminuted fractures that involve the body and articular surfaces of the subtalar joint and sometimes even the calcaneocuboid joint. The first group of fractures has a good prognosis for healing with normal function. The second group of fractures heals well, but with permanent impairment of talar joint function. If any motion through this joint

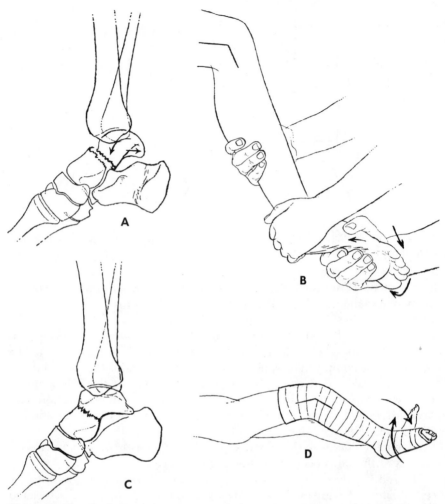

Figure 22–17. *A,* Displaced fracture through the neck of the talus. *B,* Manipulation to achieve closed reduction. *C,* The reduced fracture. *D,* Reduction is maintained in a long leg plaster dressing that holds the foot in plantar flexion and inversion and the knee bent.

remains, it is usually painful. The best result is obtained with solid ankylosis of the joint in a neutral position. The patient will have a short wide heel with loss of the normal inversion and eversion of the foot that occurs through the subtalar joint.

Dislocations of the os calcis are rare and are managed in the same manner as dislocations of the talus.

Fractures and dislocations of the mid-tarsal region are infrequent. The fracture lines may be transverse to, or in line with, the axis of the foot. Crushing injuries of the bones are common. Dislocations and subluxations may be associated with fractures. Reduction and realignment of these injuries can usually be obtained by closed manipulation followed by

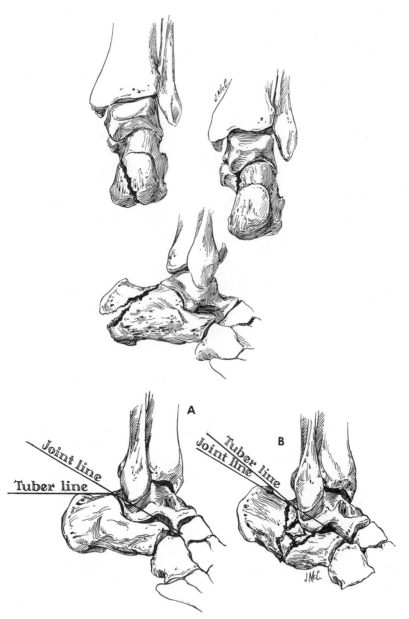

Figure 22–18. Varieties of fractures of the os calcis. *A*, Uninjured foot showing the normal tuber angle. *B*, Fracture of the body of the os calcis with marked reduction in the tuber angle. (From Davis.)

immobilization in a plaster cast. Occasionally, open reduction and fixation by transfixion pins may be required. The fractures will heal, but there will be partial or complete loss of motion in the involved joints.

Fractures and dislocations of the metatarsals often result from the dropping of heavy objects onto the dorsum of the foot. Many of these injuries as well as injuries of the toes can be avoided by wearing work shoes with steel caps over the toe.

Dislocations of the proximal ends of the metatarsals from the cuneiforms and the cuboid are usually accompanied by fractures of the articular surfaces involved and may displace easily after reduction. If this is the case, they can be held in place with transfixion pins, after which the foot is immobilized in a padded plaster dressing.

Satisfactory weight-bearing function of the forefoot is dependent upon a normal relationship of metatarsal heads to one another. For this reason, fractures of the shafts and necks of the metatarsals must be carefully aligned with preservation of normal length and angulation. Occasionally it is necessary to perform open reduction and fixation with transfixion pins to obtain satisfactory position. A below-knee walking plaster will provide immobilization.

An avulsion fracture of the base of the fifth metatarsal (Jones' fracture) is a common injury caused by forcible inversion of the foot that is resisted by a strong contraction of the *peroneus brevis*. Tenderness and swelling are well localized to the base of the fifth metatarsal and pain can be reproduced by active eversion of the foot against resistance. Initially, treatment should consist of the application of a below-knee walking plaster, although in some cases without displacement or marked pain, a stiff-soled shoe with a reverse Thomas heel and a one fourth inch lateral heel wedge will suffice.

Fractures and dislocations of the toes can be prevented by wearing work shoes with steel toe caps. Treatment of the injuries of the small toes (2 through 5) is usually quite simple and consists of manual reduction and realignment using a local anesthetic block, followed by application of a foot dressing or buddy taping. Fractures of the first toe can also be realigned or reduced by manipulation. When the articular surfaces of the metatarsophalangeal joint or interphalangeal joint are involved, late joint stiffness can be anticipated. Occasionally a patient will benefit from a closed reduction and percutaneous pinning of such a fracture. A painful subungual hematoma associated with a fracture of the distal phalanx may require drainage through a hole drilled in the nail for relief.

HUMAN-TO-HUMAN BITES

The human bite is commonly sustained during a spirited engagement, following which the victim, often in an inebriated state, fails to appreciate the serious potential hazards of such an injury and consequently delays his visit to a physician. During this crucial interval, the wound may develop serious infection characterized by purulent exudate, cellulitis, and regional lymphadenitis. Human bites are invariably contaminated with a multiplicity of pathogens including anaerobic organisms. It is therefore advisable, when the wound is first sustained, to flush the contaminated area with hydrogen peroxide, activated zinc peroxide, or sodium hypochlorite (Dakin's solution). The wound is then judiciously debrided and loosely packed with gauze so that it remains readily accessible for inspection. Threatening sequelae may be combated with catheter irrigation using a continuous drip of an organism-specific antibiotic or by the administration of systemic antibiotics. Even after the wound is clean and healing, closure by second intention or by skin grafting is often preferable to direct closure. Damaged tendons or nerves are repaired later after the skin is well healed. Human bites on the face or minor bites elsewhere can often be cleansed and closed primarily with a few sutures.

Tetanus prophylaxis is obtained with toxoid or tetanus immune globulin, depending on the severity of the wound and on the patient's immunization status. Hand infections are immobilized with the metacarpophalangeal joints in 90 degrees of flexion and the interphalangeal joints extended. Once infection has subsided, active motion is initiated. The use of chemical and thermal cauterization in the therapy of human bites is to be discouraged.

DOG BITES

About one million people in the United States are bitten by dogs each year, constituting almost 1 percent of visitors to hospital emergency departments. Most bites are trivial, however, and less than 1 percent of patients require hospitalization. Most dog bites heal well if simple principles are followed. Bites on the hand and deep puncture bites are at greatest risk of infection.

Children are the most frequent recipients of dog bites, particularly those between the ages of 2 and 15 years. As a rule, it is the child and not the dog who is responsible for the attack, but occasionally the dog is an aggressive habitual offender and the recipients are hapless passersby. The face and extremities are the commonest sites of injury.

The dog's oral bacterial flora is comparable to the human's, and the dictum "clean as a hound's tooth" should be regarded as anything but the truth. In the past dog bites were seldom closed for fear of wound contamination. This approach is still advisable when soft tissues are extensively avulsed or when the period between the bite and definitive treatment is of long duration. The treatment of dog bites is identical to that of human bites, including copious cleansing, vigorous irrigation, careful debridement of the crushed tissue, and meticulous subsequent daily care. Some dog bites cause only simple superficial lacerations that when thoroughly cleansed, debrided, closed, and possibly covered by an appropriate antibiotic prophylactically heal with a lower infection rate than if the wound were to be left open. The face constitutes a special case; with its excellent blood supply, facial wounds become infected in less than 5 percent of patients. Primary repair usually results in less disfiguration and should be made without buried sutures, with conservative debridement, and with a wound closure that is free of tension. Conversely, the hand, with an infection rate of almost 30 percent, should be treated more conservatively, with many such wounds being left open in the first place.

RABIES

Only five persons contracted rabies in the United States in 1979; no cases were reported in 1980, and only one by the summer of 1981. Nevertheless, the entity remains important, because 20,000 to 30,000 people are treated with rabies vaccine annually. The local public authorities are an invaluable source of information if the physician is suddenly called upon to treat a potential case of rabies.

Over the past few years, decisions about treatment of the patient possibly bitten by a rabid animal have been made very much easier by the availability of human diploid cell rabies vaccine (HDCV) and human rabies immune globulin (HRIG), which are effective and safe. The use of HDCV has supplanted that of the painful, hazardous, and unreliable duck embryo vaccine (DEV). Until recently DEV was the only relatively effective therapeutic agent, but it caused life-threatening reactions in about 0.6 percent of recipients, severe reactions in 10 percent, and minor transient reactions in 30 percent.

HDCV is extremely dependable in its production of antibodies and gives a response up to 20 times that of the old DEV. Furthermore, HDCV produces a much more rapid response, causes virtually no allergic or neurological complications, and is administered much more simply and less frequently. The safeness and relative comfort of HDCV have helped physicians considerably in making the clinical decision to administer vaccine in doubtful cases. The level of immunity remains high and an effective anamnestic response usually follows a booster dose.

HRIG made from the serum of immunized donors, although it dampens the effect of HDCV given simultaneously, acts effectively and rapidly. HRIG by its safety has replaced the hazardous equine antirabies serum as the desirable therapeutic agent.

The incidence of rabies in wild animals has increased, while the incidence in domestic animals has greatly decreased. Skunks, foxes, and bats are the wild animals most commonly infected and constitute the essential rabies reservoir, but 95 percent of human rabies is transmitted by dogs. Squirrels are very rarely the carriers of rabies, and it is questionable whether squirrel-to-human transmission of rabies occurs.

The incubation period of the responsible ultramicroscopic, filterable, neurotropic virus in the human recipient varies from ten days to a year. The period is shortest in the most severe wounds, especially those involving the face or neck. The unusually long incubation period provides time for effective neutralization by the rabies vaccine.

CLINICAL SEQUENCE

The victim tends to complain early of a persistent pain at the wound site and later develops generalized skin hyperesthesia and profuse perspiration. In a short time, the pupils dilate and an intolerance to sunlight and loud noise develops. An increase in lacrimation, difficulty in swallowing, and the gathering of froth in the mouth soon occurs. This increased salivation, sometimes referred to as hydrophobia, is the hallmark of the disease. As the patient's status deteriorates, skin twitchings become marked. Terminally, convulsions and Cheyne-Stokes respiration develop.

CONFIRMATION OF THE DISEASE

The diagnosis of rabies can be confirmed by several techniques. If the suspected animal does not develop signs of rabies within ten days, it is not rabid. If the animal dies within this period, however, its brain is examined for the presence of Negri bodies on direct microscopy or by immunofluorescent or transmission studies.

Treatment

Surgical Treatment

One should always consider the possibility of rabies infection following any animal bite, especially an unprovoked attack by a dog. Strange dogs are much more dangerous than domestic dogs, virtually all of which would be immunized against rabies. Any patient who has been bitten should be · instructed to wash the wound immediately and thoroughly with soap and water and to follow this with an irrigation of alcohol or some other germicide. After the patient arrives at the hospital, this is repeated, with syringe flushing of all penetrating wounds. The wounds, whether excised or not, are left open. It has been reported that only about 5 percent of patients whose rabies-infected wounds were scrubbed with soapy water subsequently developed the disease; in contrast, 90 percent of patients whose wounds were not cleansed died of rabies. If there is a distinct possibility that the animal was rabid, the area of the bite should also be excised even if 24 hours have elapsed since the incident.

Adjunctive Treatment

1. HRIG (40 IU/kg) is given once, half of the dose being infiltrated around the site of the wound and the other half given intramuscularly.
2. HDCV (1 ml) is injected intramuscularly without delay and this is repeated on days 3, 7, 14, and 28 after the first dose. It is no longer necessary to inject the vaccine in the abdominal muscles or in the thigh; the arm serves perfectly well. A previously immunized patient with demonstrated rabies antibody needs only two doses, one given immediately and the second about three days later.

All patients given HDCV should have their antibody response measured after about a month to ensure that the response has been adequate. This is absolutely essential if DEV has been used. A useful guide in the prophylaxis of patients who have been exposed to rabies has been published by the Center for Disease Control, USPHS, Atlanta. Table 23–1 is based on this publication.

SPIDER BITES

Black Widow Spider (Latrodectus) Bites

This spider is the most dangerous of American arthropods; it has an established envenomation mortality of 4 percent. The physician often misses the diagnosis during the initial examination, but a subsequent, more

TABLE 23–1. RABIES POSTEXPOSURE PROPHYLAXIS GUIDE*

Animal Species	Condition of Animal at Time of Attack	Treatment of Exposed Person
Household pets Dogs and cats	Healthy and available for 10 days of observation	None unless animal develops rabies. At first sign of rabies in animal, treat patient with RIG and HDCV. Symptomatic animal should be killed and tested as soon as possible.
	Rabid or suspect Unknown (escaped)	RIG and HDCV. Consult public health officials. If treatment indicated, give RIG and HDCV.
Wild animals Skunks, bats, foxes, coyotes, raccoons, bobcats, other carnivores	Regard as rabid unless proved negative by laboratory tests. If available, animal should be killed and tested as soon as possible.	RIG and HDCV.
Other animals Livestock, rodents, lagomorphs (e.g., rabbits, hares)	Consider individually. Local and state public health officials should be consulted on the need for prophylaxis. Bites by the following almost never call for antirabies prophylaxis: squirrels, hamsters, guinea pigs, gerbils, chipmunks, rats, mice, and other rodents, rabbits, and hares.	

*From Plotkin SA: Rabies vaccination in the 1980's. Hospital Practice November 1980: 65–72.

careful history and examination usually reveals the minute punctate red fang marks in the skin. The patient will usually then recall a sharp pricking sensation and a moment of sharp pain. A variety of problems may develop, depending upon the severity and the location of the bite. If the envenomization is severe and on the lower extremity, the pain may progress to the abdomen, where the muscles become spasmodically rigid and simulate peritonitis. Upper extremity bites cause pain and muscle spasms in the shoulder, chest, and back. These symptoms with the accompanying dyspnea may closely simulate myocardial infarction or pneumonia. Laboratory findings of leukocytosis, albuminuria, and hematuria complicate the picture. Nevertheless, most Latrodectus bites are self-limiting and need only immediate care for discomfort and possible anaphylaxis.

1. For local bite site discomfort, cold compresses (ice packs) and anti-inflammatory ointment (Diprosone 0.05 percent, Valisone 0.1 percent, Cordran 0.5 percent) are helpful.

2. For apprehension, nausea, and muscle spasms, diazepam (Valium) is given by slow intravenous infusion in doses of 1 to 5 mg for infants and toddlers and up to 10 mg for older children and adults.

3. For continuous and severe muscular spasms, 10 ml of methocarbamol (Robaxin) given very slowly intravenously is helpful.

4. For distressing pain in adults, acetaminophen may be used initially.

If this is insufficient to relieve the pain, meperidine (Demerol) or morphine sulfate may be given cautiously.

5. For neutralizing the venom and reducing the muscular tightness in the abdominal and chest walls, 10 ml of 10 percent calcium gluconate by slow intravenous infusion is of benefit, and may be repeated at four-hour intervals.

6. Antivenin, the only specific therapy, is used only in critical envenomation or in highly susceptible persons. As antivenin is a horse serum product, sensitivity testing must be conducted as indicated on the package insert. The usual dose is 2.5 ml intramuscularly (not intravenously) and may be repeated. In severe cases, prompt excision of the bite site is also advocated. For allergic sequelae, antihistamines and corticosteroids should be used.

BROWN RECLUSE SPIDER (LOXOSCELES) BITES

Little attention was given to the bite of the brown recluse spider before 1950. Since then this problem has been increasingly recognized and has now been documented in all the southern states from Florida to California, and in Utah. This is partly due to spread of the spider by truck, train, air, and ship freighting. The Loxosceles "fiddler" has a dark-brown figure resembling a violin on its back. Although the initial bite frequently goes unnoticed, in a few hours the patient often develops a cyanotic bleb, with a white ischemic periphery surrounded in turn by an erythematous halo. This early red, white, and blue patriotic configuration is pathognomonic of Loxosceles poisoning, which ulcerates and becomes tender and painful within 48 hours. If not attended, the ulceration enlarges and exudes. There are two avenues of management — medical and surgical.

1. Corticosteroids given early are effective but require adequate dosage, beginning with methylprednisolone (Solu-Medrol) 1 mg/kg of body weight intravenously, or an equivalent, repeated at six-hour intervals. This limits local necrosis and eliminates systemic sequelae. Local infiltration is of no benefit.

2. Cephalexin (Keflex) or a similar antibiotic in doses of 125 mg q 6 hours for infants and 250 mg q 6 hours for adults will inhibit secondary infection.

3. Tetanus prophylaxis should be given for nonhealing lesions.

4. Analgesics should be given as needed for pain.

5. Antivenin is available in South America and may become available in the United States.

6. Surgically, immediate excision and loose closure of the bite wound under 0.5 percent Xylocaine is often successful in preventing ulceration.

7. Late excision of the tender, exuding necrotic ulcer and subsequent closure by wound edge approximation, skin graft, or skin flap will accelerate healing and produce a more satisfactory scar.

SCORPION STINGS

All scorpions are poisonous and dangerous to humans. The *Centruroides sculpturatus* of the southwest is responsible for more envenomations than any of the other 40 species found in the United States. There are two poison glands at the ampullar tip that excrete the venom deposited in the puncture wound.

The immediate excruciating local pain and itching can be relieved by applying cold compresses, household ammonia, Valisone (0.1 percent) or Diprosone (0.05 percent) to the sting site. Epinephrine in any form should not be used for the treatment of a scorpion sting because its effects are synergistic to the venom. To counteract apprehension, fasciculations, and convulsions, one can administer diazepam (Valium) intravenously up to 5 mg for infants and 5 to 10 mg for adults, or methocarbamol (Robaxin) 10 ml intravenously slowly. Calcium gluconate 10 ml of 10 percent solution given intravenously slowly may also be helpful. Hypersalivation can be reduced by atropine sulfate in intramuscular doses of 0.3 mg.

HYMENOPTERA STINGS

More humans die of insect bites (about 25 yearly in the United States) than from snake envenomations, and over 25 percent of the world's inhabitants are hypersensitive to hymenoptera venoms. Luckily, the stings of these insects are usually more of an aggravation than a disaster. Only the females of this arthropoda order (which comprises the bees, wasps, hornets, ants, and membranous-winged insects) are capable of stinging. The female is endowed with a canalized ovipositor (stinger) that has the double function of egg deposition and venom injection. Some ovipositors that are barbed detach from the insect's body when the sting is inflicted, resulting in the insect's death. The retained stinger causes a soft tissue reaction where it is buried. Other ovipositors are smooth, permitting the insect to sting repeatedly and remain alive. Effects of the venoms of bees, wasps, hornets, and ants differ because of the variety of the venom components, the volume injected, patient hypersensitivity, and the site of the sting. Management also varies.

1. The small black ovipositor is retrieved with a No. 11 scalpel blade. Squeezing or tweezing the barbed stinger may force it in deeper or cause it to break off.

2. Local pain is relieved by injection of 0.5 percent Xylocaine with epinephrine 1:100,000 into the affected area and application of an ice pack. (Use no heat!)

3. Local hypersensitivity is treated by application of 0.1 percent Valisone ointment and calamine lotion p.r.n.

4. Generalized urticaria in the adult can be relieved by infusion of an intravenous solution containing 10 ml of 0.1 percent Xylocaine (without

epinephrine) diluted in 1000 ml normal saline. Ten ml of a 10 percent solution of calcium gluconate given intravenously may also help. Tub baths containing one box of baking soda may also be therapeutic and may be repeated as needed.

5. Generalized anorexia, nausea, and vomiting are treated with intravenous Benadryl (4 mg/kg of body weight) or Valium (5–10 mg).

6. Generalized arthralgia is relieved by parenteral injection of Solu-Medrol (1 mg/kg).

7. Urticaria in children is treated with 0.3 ml of 1:1000 epinephrine injected subcutaneously and repeated in 30 minutes if necessary. Oral corticosteroids and baking soda baths may also be helpful.

8. Other adjunctive therapy may include intravenous injection of aminophylline 0.25 gm in 10 ml normal saline for bronchospasm. Occasionally oxygen or even assisted ventilation may be required. Hypotension must be treated aggressively with intravenous epinephrine.

9. Preventive care is advised. Areas infested with stinging insects should be avoided. In such areas, clothing with floral prints or perfumed scents should not be worn. Shoes and clothing of only one color (preferably black, gray, or white) should be worn. For individuals prone to anaphylaxis, Center Laboratories, Port Washington, New York, vends a commercial polyvalent hymenopteran antigen kit for prophylaxis.

MARINE ANIMAL STINGS

Representative of this type of injury are stings by jellyfish, Portuguese men-of-war, sea anemones, hydras, and corals. These marine animals inject their toxins by a nematoid apparatus functioning through a tiny trigger mechanism. The thousands of nematocysts in the tentacles of the marine host are embedded on and in the victim's skin, which becomes fiery and unbearably painful upon rubbing or scratching. Treatment is effective only if begun very early.

The nematocysts should be inactivated by flushing the involved skin with alcohol followed by household ammonia. Any residual tentacles should be removed by coalescing them with flour or baking soda. Stings involving the orbital area are treated with fluocinolone acetonide (Synalar solution) 0.01 percent as a wash or irrigant, followed by local application of Synalar ointment.

AQUATIC PUNCTURE WOUNDS

Marine creatures with spines may cause double trouble, because some of the spines contain venom apparatuses, and slime and debris may also be introduced into the puncture wound. Representatives of the marine animal class capable of inflicting such wounds are segmental worms, sea urchins, conus shells, stingrays, catfish, and spiny fish.

The catfish is probably the most prevalent of the poisonous fishes, of which there are over 1000 species. The dagger-sharp dorsal and pectoral fins of catfish either have venom glands or epithelial mucous cells covering the spines, which are toxic to vascular and neural tissues of humans. Treatment consists of incision or debridement of the puncture wound and cleansing of the depths with hydrogen peroxide and Betadine solutions. The wounds are left open. A broad-spectrum antibiotic and tetanus prophylaxis as dictated by the patient's immune status, along with analgesics as adjunctive therapy, are also necessary as in all aquatic puncture wounds. The wounded area should be immobilized and inspected daily.

Stingrays are responsible for 1000 penetration wounds annually along the coasts of the United States. These marine animals have a trench in their tails where a spine reclines covered with epithelium, venom sacs, and cells. Venom is released when the spine penetrates a victim. Envenomation is evidenced by immediate intense pain, vomiting, diarrhea, and muscle spasms. If these symptoms are not treated, dyspnea, convulsions, and death may ensue.

Therapy begins by retrieval of the embedded spine. The injured area is then soaked in tepid Betadine solution every four to six hours. Symptomatic therapy is instituted, including administration of antihistamines and steroids. Prophylactic therapy with antibiotics and tetanus toxoid should be initiated.

SNAKE BITES

A bite from a snake is terrifying even if the victim is a serpentologist, researcher, or experienced woodsman. The reaction to this unexpected trauma is extremely diverse — ranging from hysteria and mania to exhaustion and syncope. These variegated reactions may be extremely perplexing to the physician inexperienced in the treatment of snake bites. Consequently, he may unknowingly administer unnecessary and possibly detrimental therapy to such patients.

Immediate information as to whether the bite was from a venomous or a nonvenomous snake is important. Human limbs and even lives have been sacrificed because of improper or delayed remedies for envenomation. Conversely, susceptible people bitten by nonvenomous snakes may suffer allergic complications caused by the unnecessary administration of horse serum antivenin. The bites of pit vipers (rattlesnakes, cottonmouth moccasins, and copperheads) cause immediate excruciating pain and rapid progressive local swelling. Neither of these reactions occurs following nonvenomous snake bites. Fang puncture wounds on the skin are visible following moderate to severe envenomation by pit vipers, whereas multiple teeth scratches on the skin usually denote mild envenomation of the bite of a nonpoisonous snake. Bites by elapid snakes (coral and cobra) are mildly painful and edema does not begin until an hour or so after the bite. None of these signs, or the sequence, is seen following bites of nonpoisonous snakes.

Signs and Symptoms of Envenomation

The three cardinal findings include:

1. The presence of *one or two fang puncture wounds*. Additional wounds may be due to the snake striking a glancing blow or inflicting numerous bites.
2. *Swelling,* which is immediate, progressive, and accompanied by discoloration of the skin.
3. *Pain,* which is usually immediate and severe.

Other findings that may be present include:

1. *Erythema and ecchymosis,* which usually appear later.
2. *Bullae,* usually appearing within 12 hours or not at all.
3. *Petechiae,* developing with more severe envenomation.
4. *Hyperesthesia-anesthesia-hyperesthesia* in a sequence of neurological changes.
5. *Paresthesias* varying from "peculiar" skin sensations, formications, and tingling to terminal causalgia.
6. *Advancing pitting and brawny edema,* progressing proximally up the limb.
7. *Cyanosis, necrosis, and tissue slough,* occurring sequentially from the action of the venom and compromised blood supply.
8. *Anorexia, nausea, and vomiting* associated with marked anxiety.
9. *Dyspnea, tachycardia, vertigo, dim vision, and pinpoint pupils,* prodromal symptoms of shock.
10. Muscle twitchings and convulsions tending to progress to paralysis, coma, and death.

Laboratory findings include:

1. Hypothrombinemia, thrombocytopenia, hypofibrinogenemia, and anemia, caused by moderate to severe envenomation.
2. Pulmonary edema and even emboli revealed in the chest roentgenogram.

Factors influencing the findings include:

1. Age and size of the patient
2. Species of venomer
3. Amount of venom injected
4. Patient's sensitivity to venom
5. Location, depth, and number of bites
6. Amount of time elapsed after the bite
7. Efficacy of initial treatment

TREATMENT

General Principles

Reactions to poisonous snake bite vary greatly but may be classified as *mild* (scratch marks, minimal pain and swelling), *moderate* (fang marks, pain, local swelling, no systemic findings), or *severe* (fang marks, severe pain, progressive local swelling, evidence of systemic reaction). For the mild envenomation, the scratches are washed with soapy water or alcohol and the wound left exposed. There is usually no need for antivenin or incisions. For the moderate reaction, a linear incision joining the fang marks is made to retrieve the venom. There is no reason to apply a tourniquet. Severe envenomation is treated vigorously by cleansing the surface wound, applying a tourniquet, and excising the puncture wounds to retrieve the venom.

Antivenin should be given only if the skin test is negative but should be withheld in the absence of systemic symptoms or signs. If given, the antivenin should be administered in a saline drip to which methyl-prednisolone has been added. Following moderate envenomation, 2 to 5 vials are given, especially in children and the elderly. When envenomation is severe, 5 to 10 vials are used. The speed of administration and amount administered are directly proportional to the severity of the symptoms and the patient's response. Any patient who receives antivenin should be hospitalized for observation. For further information on the treatment of snake bites, refer to the poster "Management of Poisonous Snake Bites," American College of Surgeons, Committee on Trauma, February 1981.

Emergency Field Treatment

1. Avoid excitement, exertion, and alcoholic beverages that may accelerate circulation and propel the venom systemically.

2. Retrieve the offender for identification if this can be done without further danger.

3. Immediately apply a flat tourniquet (belt, bandana, sock, handkerchief) proximal to an extremity bite — just snug enough to permit introducing a finger (i.e., watchband tightness). Loosen the tourniquet as swelling increases. Do not remove, reapply, and remove it intermittently, as this propels the venom into the general circulation. If swelling is already present, do not apply a tourniquet. Release the tourniquet completely when antivenin is given.

4. Cleanse the bite with soapy water or alcohol and incise from one fang mark through the other and deeply to the subcutaneous fat. Do not use cruciate (cross-hatch) incisions because these are harmful, especially on the face and hands.

5. Suction or digitally express fluid (blood and venom) gently from

the incised wound without macerating it. Such wound manipulation for more than five minutes is damaging and useless.

6. Immobilize or rest the bitten limb horizontally at heart level — not above nor below heart level because either position enhances edema and necrosis. Muscular exercise should be limited at first; this speeds circulation and spread of venom.

7. Venom neutralization should be attempted. Polyvalent Antivenin (Wyeth Laboratories) has proved to be lifesaving; it is the only available antivenom therapy in the United States. North American coral snake antivenin made by Wyeth Laboratories should be used for the bite of the *eastern* coral snake only, not for bites of western or Arizona coral snakes. Early administration is beneficial, but it has been given as late as 24 hours after the bite with good results. Since the antivenin is a horse serum product, the precautions on the package insert must be heeded.

Emergency Room Treatment

1. Identify the venomous injury (fang marks, swelling, pain) and the snake if available. Record any history of allergies (drugs, horse serum, Novocain, foods) or hay fever, asthma, or urticaria.

2. If the victim's wound falls into the category of severe envenomation, prepare one vial of Wyeth's Antivenin (Crotalidae) Polyvalent and dilute this 10 ml into 100 ml of sterile normal saline solution and 125 mg Solu-Medrol or methylprednisolone equivalent. During this interval, inject 0.02 ml of a 1:1000 dilution of the Normal Horse Serum (included in Wyeth's kit) to raise a small wheal intracutaneously to test for allergy. A control test of normal saline near the horse serum test facilitates interpretation of the findings. A negative reaction shows no local skin changes; a positive response, occurring within two to ten minutes, is a white wheal with increasing peripheral erythema, edema, and itching. If the patient has any history of allergies, the use of antivenin must be adjusted to the severity of the snake bite. A safe starting dose is 0.5 ml of 1:1000 dilution. An adverse reaction to this trial dosage is adequate warning not to use the horse antiserum. If the person has no allergies and the test response is negative, the prepared antivenin is administered intravenously. Epinephrine, corticosteroids, and antihistamines should be immediately available for treatment of any untoward reactions. Children and adults are treated alike.

3. Local treatment of the snake bite wound is as follows: If the envenomation is *mild*, incision is not necessary. If the envenomation is of a *moderate* type, a linear incision through the fang punctures to the fascia followed by suction is indicated. If the envenomation is *severe*, the fang marks are elliptically excised with an equidistant margin of 1 cm through the fat to the fascia. Bleeding is controlled with an occlusive dressing. Escharotomy is necessary when extreme edema appears to be compromis-

ing the blood supply. Fasciotomy is indicated in patients with subfascial envenomation. When used judiciously, this can save an extremity and even life. Local remedies (such as cautery, acids, alkalis, cruciate incisions, and mystical remedies, some of which destroy more tissue than does the venom) are not used. The exact role and effectiveness of cryotherapy remains undefined. The snakebitten area may be cooled but not frozen. Local hypothermia reduces pain, inhibits the spread of venom, limits edema, and decreases local metabolic needs. If not monitored carefully, however, low temperature applications will stimulate bleb formation, necrosis, and gangrene. When used on digits, cold therapy may be disastrous in patients with disease states such as diabetes, arteriosclerosis, cryoproteinemia, scleroderma, Berger's disease, Raynaud's disease, and others. Once the risks and benefits of cryotherapy, hypothermia, and freezing and cooling are carefully studied in relation to snakebite, their role in management will be more realistically defined. Pressure or tight dressings are to be condemned. Tetanus immunization, antibiotics, analgesics, oxygen, calcium, transfusions, endotracheal intubation, and hemodialysis should be given as needed and tracheostomy performed if needed. Hospitalization is advised for all victims of envenomated snakebite, because the severity of injury may not be apparent initially. The patient's relatives or a responsible party should be advised of latent sequelae.

Chapter

24

Disaster Planning for Mass Casualties

As emergency medical service systems evolve, general planning for the care of mass casualties resulting from natural and man-made disasters must change. Although the individual hospital will continue to be the most important element in the delivery of care, planning must include resuscitating at the site, alerting a network of personnel and communication systems, triage, transferring patients to appropriate hospitals, and confirming transfer agreements. The common situation in which one institution receives most of the patients while others receive none is the result of poor planning. On-site triage to institutions capable of mass care that are given maximal notification is the ideal.

Civil disturbances, riots, terrorism, mass transportation accidents, industrial explosions, earthquakes, floods, and nuclear accidents are representative of disasters that may severely test the facilities of the community. All hospitals themselves will be more or less vulnerable to each type of mishap, and planning must take local conditions into account.

Further, planners must realize that frightened citizens, even if uninjured, are likely to consider the hospital as a refuge. All health facilities should therefore make unambiguous plans to direct excessive numbers of such persons to other institutions by prior agreement.

Orientation and training of hospital employees on how to function in a disaster situation are of extreme importance. Twelve-hour shifts, the possible necessity of caring for distraught or angry citizens, additional duties, and even prolonged unavoidable confinement in the hospitals are possibilities that supervisory personnel must consider. The hospital may be targeted by those seeking revenge or by vandals, and security precautions must be taken. The standard demands on emergency department facilities are likely to change in character, but substantially the same numbers of "routine" patients may be expected, even during a disaster. Medical and obstetrical emergencies continue, and one may not assume that a decrease in the number of such patients will permit care of victims affected primarily by the crisis. Lapses in medication schedules, for example, will cause patients with cardiac disease and epilepsy to be seen in increased numbers.

376

PREPARATIONS FOR DISASTER

All plans:

1. Should involve high-level officials of local police, fire, and civil defense agencies.

2. Must be written and tested (at least twice a year) in advance.

3. Must provide for communication arrangements, taking into account the likely overtaxing of existing telephone systems. Designated telephone lines inside and outside the hospital and portable radio receivers obviate the need for routing messages through switchboards, which by the nature of the situation are almost certain to become overtaxed.

4. Must provide for storage of special equipment and supplies.

5. Must provide for routine first aid.

6. Must provide for definitive care.

7. Must prepare for transfer of casualties to other facilities by prior agreements should the location in question be overtaxed or unsafe.

8. Must consider the urgent needs of patients already hospitalized for conditions unrelated to the disaster.

Although a regional approach to planning is ideal for the management of mass casualties, circumstances may require that each hospital function with little or no outside support. Earthquakes, floods, riots, and nuclear contamination may force the individual hospital to function in isolation. The crisis may be instantaneous, as with explosion, or may develop slowly, as in most civil disturbances, malfunctions of nuclear reactors, and floods. Developments that cannot be predicted may have great influence on preventing access to designated disaster facilities.

Once a state of disaster has been declared by civil authorities or internally by the hospital director, specific hospital procedures should automatically be performed. These include:

1. Notification of personnel.

2. Preparation of treatment areas.

3. Classification system to differentiate emergency department and hospital patients.

4. Checking of supplies of blood, fluids, medications, food and potable water, and other materials essential to hospital operation.

5. Provision for decontamination procedures. (This is a high-priority procedure in nuclear accidents.)

6. Institution of security precautions.

7. Control of visitors and press.

SUPPLIES

An inventory of supplies especially earmarked for disasters and specifically labeled (including expiration dates for sterilized products and pharmaceuticals) must be maintained. Items such as intravenous fluids, dressings, chest tubes, and adequate suction devices are likely to be in great demand. Treatment of a moderate number of burns may use up all the available dressings in an entire community. At first warning, the supplies of blood, plasma expanders, and other fluid available in the hospital and in the immediate region should be checked. Obstructions to communications may later make it impossible to locate and transport the essential products once the crisis is fully developed.

Consideration must be given to the difficulty of assembling packaged disaster hospitals at disaster sites in the absence of electrical power and uncontaminated water. It must be assumed that even the basic tools for the assembly of portable power equipment and the necessary fuel supplies will not be available through normal channels. Stores of morphine, dressings, and potable water must be adequate for potential requirements. Little planning has been done in the United States for the care of the victims of chemical or biological warfare. Large supplies of atropine could offset the effects of nerve gas contamination, and gas masks and protective clothing should be available for rescue personnel at least.

SPECIAL SITUATIONS

Although the variety of special requirements for individual catastrophes is great, a few will be discussed.

AIRPORT ACCIDENTS

The approach to the airport runway is literally the terminus of an "air corridor" that extends outward some 20 miles and usually overlies small towns or even a city. Few if any individual fire companies or emergency organizations have the physical resources and jurisdiction to provide adequate care for crash victims, who might number in the hundreds. The airport fence usually determines the respective jurisdictions of the airport and community rescue service organizations. Use of a command system integrating the two systems and incorporating the concepts of "airport medicine and airport disaster" planning is highly desirable near large airports. Deceleration injuries and burns are the injuries most frequently encountered.

FLOODS

Major flooding causes serious disruptions in communications and land transportation. Flash floods and the breaking of dams produce the greatest number of casualties. Deaths from drowning may be numerous, but the number of serious injuries is usually not great. However, displacement of the population and closing of physicians' offices lead to heavy hospital emergency department traffic, adding to the hospital's burden. Flooding at one hospital in a community diverts the patient load into other institutions. As helicopter evacuation plays a major role in floods, plans should be made to care for patients at the landing pad.

EARTHQUAKES

A major earthquake occurs somewhere in the world approximately every two years. Hospitals are often completely destroyed but frequently patients congregate at the hospital site or are brought there. Tent facilities in the hospital area are very useful for administration of first aid while plans for transfer of patients to undamaged installations are being made.

Grave psychological trauma, infectious disease epidemics, and even violence stemming from instincts of self-preservation must be anticipated. Crush injuries and fractures are characteristic of injury due to the collapse of homes and public buildings in the quake itself. The Polaroid technique for roentgenography, which requires no darkroom, is desirable in situations in which disruptions of power supply and destruction of darkrooms are likely. Unfortunately Polaroid film is not commonly stocked, and when it is, expiration dates may pass during the time of storage.

RADIATION ACCIDENTS

Because of distinctive differences from most other types of mass casualty accidents, radiation accidents must be given special consideration. Nuclear weapons designed for warfare, which may also be used in terroristic acts, are intended primarily for blast effect. Radiation injury is a side effect that might prove to be as great a liability to the aggressor as to the intended victims. Such an incident, rare in civilian experience, may result in serious crush, penetration, and thermal injuries in addition to heavy gamma and beta irradiation. Nuclear power generators involve no such "bomb" threat in the same sense, but the risk of explosions due to high pressures within the containment vessels is always present. High temperatures may lead to thermal injuries as well, but the overwhelming hazard is that of radionuclide contamination of victims even many miles from the reactor.

The following guidelines were developed on the basis of our experience with the Three Mile Island, Pennsylvania, episode of March, 1979.

1. A unified command with a reliable communication system is essential. Command personnel need designated telephone (single point-to-

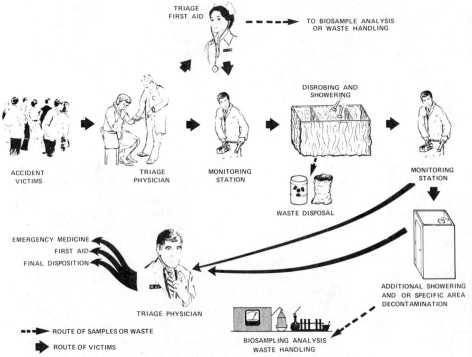

Figure 24–1. The expansion of a medical radiation emergency plan. This diagram illustrates the basic steps in triage, monitoring, showering and decontamination, biosampling, analysis and waste handling.

point) lines, conventional and two-way radio, and access to control of all television programming. Switchboards and dial telephones cannot be depended upon because of overload.

2. A regional evacuation plan for hospitals is necessary in an affected area; the plan may involve many hospitals in a wide geographic locale.

3. For affected citizens, the psychological impact may far exceed in importance the immediate physical threat. Flight because of panic may not only stall evacuation but may produce great numbers of vehicular accidents. Furthermore, emergency rescue personnel may refuse to approach an area of contamination, alleged or real.

Radiation Accident Alert. Upon notification to a hospital of a major radiation accident, a meeting of responsible physicians, nurses, and administrators should be held to plan and review procedure (Fig. 24–1). This meeting should include:

1. An explanation of the accident at the contaminating source and a list of the radioisotopes that have been released, along with their implications for public health.

2. A review of the emergency plan.

3. A review of characteristics of the acute radiation syndrome as well as low-level effects.

4. A review of basic radiation protection criteria.

5. A review of techniques of radiation detection for both patients and hospital personnel.

6. A review of contamination removal (external and internal) from patients, with techniques for disposal of contaminants.

7. Listing of emergency telephone numbers.

8. Recording of the location of supplies and sources of information.

9. The specific designation of authority to assure smooth execution of the plan and decision making should crucial decisions be required.

Initial Reception of Contaminated Victims. Ideally, the hospital will be notified to expect the victims. A health physicist should meet the ambulance (or other conveyance) for monitoring before disembarkation of any occupants; if contamination is demonstrated, hosing down of victims outside the emergency department should be carried out. Victims should then be conducted to a designated area near the entrance where further monitoring and decontamination procedures are carried out.

Detection of Radionuclide Contamination. This is the responsibility of the health physicist, usually a representative of the department of radiology, and of medical personnel. A detailed protocol should be available in the emergency department, in the department of radiology, and in the offices of generating plant health personnel, of consulting medical radiation emergency companies, and of state bureaus of radiological health. It is desirable to have such protocols in the possession of police, fire, and civil defense officials *provided* that they have been given prior indoctrination. The desirability of such wide dispersal is based on the fact that the telephone system will likely be saturated to one or more points at any given time. It is critical that this document be realistic for the hospital and personnel who will use it. It should include a list of specific supplies required for this unique situation, important sequences of the decontamination procedure, steps in the procedure for disposal of recovered contaminated materials, and methods for disposition of victims and personnel. Such a document has been formulated and a similar protocol should be adopted and provided to responsible personnel.

Initial Care of Radionuclide-Contaminated Wounds. The principles of wound care apply as in the uncontaminated patient. If the surrounding body area is contaminated, the wound must be considered contaminated. A sterile, moistened, cotton-tipped applicator is wiped over the wound prior to treatment and placed in an individually labeled envelope for counting. Identifying data including type of wound are attached. All persons having a contaminated wound or one suspected of being contaminated are instructed to collect the next 24-hour output of urine for analysis of radioactive materials in a plastic container provided.

A quick Geiger-Mueller survey or alpha survey or both are done on the patient's whole body while clothing remains in place. If radioactivity is detected, the clothing is removed and a survey is done again. Areas of radioactivity are marked and if necessary are covered with plastic sheeting to prevent spread of contamination. Special care should be taken to survey areas under nails, ear lobes, and between skin folds (axilla, inguinal area, buttocks, between toes).

Foreign bodies and tissue removed in debridement should be saved and labeled for further study.

Great care should be taken to avoid abrading undamaged skin, because systemic contamination can occur via abrasions. Flushing with sterile water and saline along with gentle washing markedly reduces contamination.

General Discussion.   There is a natural tendency to bring all persons suspected of being contaminated to the hospital. The possibility exists that thousands may arrive; plans should be considered to hose down and shower such persons in other locations — in their homes, in fire houses and in other public buildings. Weather permitting, an outside hose facility should be available near the hospital emergency entrance and shower facilities should be designated in areas adjacent to decontamination rooms. In instances of atmospheric contamination, the low level of contamination of the effluent waste water is of no more concern than the contamination that already exists, and this water may be put down existing drains. Outside hose lines serve the same purpose. For individuals highly contaminated by radioactive materials, the ideal is a special shower adjacent to the emergency facility. Effluent from this shower should be collected in an outside holding tank for future disposal. Hot water, soap, and scrub brushes should be available; monitoring should determine if there is need for further cleansing. A spray arrangement in which waste is collected in a receptacle to be disposed of later is a less desirable alternative. Several 55-gallon drums and plastic bags are useful in collecting contaminated floor coverings and personal items such as clothing, jewelry, and pocketbooks. Prior planning is required to avoid widespread contamination of the institution with very serious and costly consequences.

The responsibility for reporting the accident belongs to the licensee of the nuclear reactor, and it must be done within 24 hours. Although the hospital is not likely to be the licensee involved, contact points are listed in Table 24–1.

The acute radiation syndrome will be unfamiliar to most physicians. A careful history is crucial in determining the character and extent of exposure that usually indicates the course and prognosis. The interval to onset of symptoms is also very helpful in determining the outcome (Table 24–2).

**TABLE 24-1. UNITED STATES NUCLEAR REGULATORY
COMMISSION
INSPECTION AND ENFORCEMENT REGIONAL OFFICES**

Region	Address	Telephone No.
I		
Connecticut, Delaware, District of Columbia, Maine, Maryland, Massachusetts, New Hampshire, New Jersey, New York, Pennsylvania, Rhode Island, Vermont	Region I, USNRC Office of Inspection and Enforcement 631 Park Ave. King of Prussia, PA 19406	(215) 337–5000
II		
Alabama, Florida, Georgia, Kentucky, Mississippi, North Carolina, Panama Canal Zone, Puerto Rico, South Carolina, Tennessee, Virginia, Virgin Islands, West Virginia	Region II, USNRC Office of Inspection and Enforcement 101 Marietta St. Suite 3100 Atlanta, GA 30303	(404) 221–4503
III		
Illinois, Indiana, Iowa, Michigan, Minnesota, Missouri, Ohio, Wisconsin	Region III, USNRC Office of Inspection and Enforcement 799 Roosevelt Rd. Glen Ellyn, IL 60137	(312) 858–2660
IV		
Arkansas, Colorado, Idaho, Kansas, Louisiana, Montana, Nebraska, New Mexico, North Dakota, Oklahoma, South Dakota, Texas, Utah, Wyoming	Region IV, USNRC Office of Inspection and Enforcement 611 Ryan Plaza Dr. Suite 1000 Arlington, TX 76012	(817) 334–2841
V		
Alaska, Arizona, California, Hawaii, Nevada, Oregon, Washington, and U.S. territories and possessions in the Pacific	Region V, USNRC Office of Inspection and Enforcement 1990 N. California Blvd. Suite 202 Walnut Creek, CA 94596	(415) 943-3700

TABLE 24–2.   DOSE EFFECT OF ACUTE WHOLE BODY
RADIATION (X-RAYS, GAMMA)

Whole Body (rads)	Clinical	Laboratory
0–75	Asymptomatic	Minor depressions of WBC and platelets in a few victims
75–125	Fatigue, nausea and vomiting, anorexia within 2 days in up to 20% of victims	Mild depression of WBC and platelets in some victims
125–200	Symptomatic, transient disability	Lymphocyte depression of about 50% in 48 hours in most patients
250–350	50% mortality if untreated	75% lymphocyte depression within 48 hours
400–600	GI complications, bleeding and death in most exposed victims within 2 weeks	Profound depression of WBC and platelets
10,000 rads ± 50%	Fulminating course with GI, CNS and cardiovascular complications and death within 24–72 hours	

RECOMMENDED READINGS

1. Standards for protection against radiation. Rules and Regulations United States Nuclear Regulatory Commission (Part 20), November 10, 1978, pp. 20–11.
2. Whittaker R, Fareed D, Green P, Barry P, Borge A, Fletes-Barrios R: Earthquake disaster in Nicaragua. J Trauma 14:37, 1974.
3. Walt AJ, Wilson RF: Disaster Planning: A Modern Reality. *In* Walt AJ, Wilson RF (eds), Management of Trauma. Philadelphia, Lea & Febiger, 1975, pp. 13–24.
4. NCRP Report 65, Management of Persons Accidentally Contaminated With Radionuclides. National Council on Radiation Protection and Measurements, Washington, D.C., 1980.

Chapter

25

Legal Aspects

The purpose of this chapter is to impart a basic understanding, and to dispel misunderstandings, of the law that applies to the physician-patient relationship in the emergency department situation. It is not intended as a guide to the laws of any particular state, and it is recommended that for particular information a local attorney should be consulted.

In the emergency department there are certain medical-legal relationships that have caused concern and, at times, have affected patient care. These include doctrines of consent, standards of care for physicians in emergency situations, duty to care for patients in the emergency department, liability for the acts of others, Good Samaritan laws, and physician's duties and responsibilities in connection with the death of patients. Each of these issues is discussed in this chapter.

THE REQUIREMENT OF CONSENT

It is generally true in law that the patient has the right to decide what should be done with his body, and that patients have the right not to be treated without their consent. However, in the emergency department the requirement of consent is significantly less important than in situations in which elective procedures are being considered. In many emergency situations the law presumes or implies consent for treatment. An unconscious patient brought to the emergency department in need of treatment is presumed to have given his consent on the theory that a conscious patient in need of treatment would consent to it. The same rule may be applied in any other situation in which the patient is mentally unable to understand the consequences of either consenting or refusing to consent to treatment. In order for any consent to be effective, it must be a *competent* consent, which means that it must be given freely and voluntarily, and based on sufficient factual information so that it is intelligently granted by a person who, at the time of consenting, is a "sane, sober adult."

In *emergencies* the following guidelines should be observed:

1. Never delay life-saving treatment in order to obtain a consent.

2. It is better to treat without a signed consent than to withhold treatment for lack of one.

3. The doctrine of informed consent rarely applies in emergency situations.

4. The physician is more likely to be challenged in emergency situations for failing to treat than for treating without consent.

5. Many patients with serious illnesses or injuries lack the mental capacity to either consent or refuse to consent. In the words of one author, "no patient should be allowed to die in the emergency room . . . because there isn't someone available to sign a form."[1]

6. When a patient is legally incapable (i.e., a minor or incompetent) or factually incapable of giving consent, the physician should attempt to secure the parent's or a relative's consent if possible. But if time is too short to accommodate discussion and treatment is needed, obviously the physician should proceed with the treatment.

REQUIREMENTS FOR EFFECTIVE CONSENT

ORAL VERSUS WRITTEN CONSENT

Despite the general rule that in emergency situations it is better to treat a patient than to wait for consent, when possible, it is still desirable to obtain some form of written consent for treatment in situations in which time allows and the patient appears to have reasonable mental capacity to understand what he has signed. The majority of patients that are served in the emergency department have minor or other moderate problems, and these patients, if sane, sober adults, have the right to decide for themselves whether they should receive treatment. In the situations in which consent can be obtained, it is desirable that the consent be given in written form and that a *witnessed* notation in the emergency department record be made to the effect that the patient did consent to the treatment.

SPECIFIC VERSUS GENERAL CONSENT

The so-called general consent form — that is, the form permitting the surgeon to "do anything necessary" — has been considered by most courts to be of little or no legal significance.[2] When a specific treatment is indicated, a specific consent form for that treatment should be obtained.

It must be remembered that the term "informed consent" is used to describe two separate and distinct legal concepts. First, and most impor-

---

[1]Bergen R.: Informed Consent 13, April 23, 1963 (AMA Monograph). (*Note:* The cases and texts cited are not those most authoritative or best reasoned on the point discussed, but are those that fully explain the principle involved.)

[2]*Kennedy v. Parrot*, 243 N.C. 355, 90 SE2d 754 (1956).

tantly, it includes a "relationship" whereby a patient is adequately informed about the risks associated with a future operation or procedure. Any form used, therefore, should convey information in a manner that bolsters the appropriate relationship between physician and patient rather than disrupting it by requiring a waiver of rights, or a disclaimer of guarantee through complicated legal terminology.

Secondly, the informed consent form serves as a tangible documentation as to what information was conveyed by the physician to the patient. Here again a shorter, simpler and more easily read form is more likely to be read and understood by the patient than is a longer, more complicated form written in legal terminology.

A straightforward form that conveys the message "we thought you would like to know" can best accomplish the legal function of documentation, without disruption of the physician-patient relationship. An example of such a form is included in this chapter as the Appendix.

SCOPE OF THE PATIENT'S AUTHORIZATION

In true emergency situations when there is an immediate threat to life or health, it is not necessary to obtain additional consent for the correction of an unexpected condition discovered during surgery. However, when the unexpected condition discovered during surgery does not pose a threat to life or health and the patient has neither expressly consented nor prohibited extension of the operation, the extended operation probably should not be done. An example might be a patient who had consented to removal of one ovary and tube, but not to sterilization. Removal of a normal ovary with consequent sterilization should not be done without the patient's informed consent.[3] On the other hand, for a patient who has consented to surgical exploration for a suspected rupture of the spleen and is found at operation to have an infarcted bowel, bowel resection and colostomy should be done without obtaining additional consent from the patient. It is a good idea to obtain consent from the patient before surgery to remedy any abnormal or diseased condition found at the time of surgery. This rule applies when no one with authority to consent for the patient is immediately available and the extension does not involve the removal of a second organ. This problem illustrates the wisdom of advising patients or their families before surgery of the uncertainty in diagnosis and the possible risks and results of a contemplated extension. When possible, the consent form should reflect the possibility of extended surgery.

INFORMED CONSENT

As has been previously indicated, in life-threatening emergency situations consent is of little or no importance. However, in those situations in

---

[3]*Thimatariga v. Chambers,* 416 A.2d 1326 (46 Md. App. 260) July 11, 1980.

which consent is required, it must be an *informed consent*. While the laws in various states differ to some extent as to the requirements for an effective informed consent, probably the best general statement of the law is that a consent is effective only if the patient is given enough factual information in lay language so that any ordinarily prudent person could make an intelligent decision as to whether to have the treatment.[4] This law requires that patients be told: (1) inherent and potential hazards or "risks" of the proposed treatment; (2) alternatives to that treatment, if any; and (3) results likely if the patient remains untreated (see Appendix 1).

Many states, however, maintain less stringent legal standards for disclosure and require that these explanations be made only in accordance with the prevailing practice within the medical community. Some have measured the disclosure by "good medical practice," others by what a reasonable practitioner would have disclosed under the circumstances, and still others by what medical custom in the community would demand.

In order for any consent to be valid, it must be given by a patient who at the time of the consent is competent. Thus, a patient who is under sedation or has already been in some way medicated for surgery is probably not competent to consent. Furthermore, it is probably good practice to obtain informed consent before the patient's admission to the hospital, and it is strongly recommended that consent to *elective* surgery be obtained in the office, or at a time before the patient has already committed himself to have the operation. Thus, the patient should be given the opportunity and sufficient time to discuss the proposed operation with his family if he wishes to do so, and to reconsider his decision, if necessary. Most importantly he should be given every opportunity to arrive at a decision without pressure from the surgeon.

REQUIREMENTS OF CONSENT FOR ADULT AND CHILD PATIENTS

ADULTS

Sane, Sober, Conscious Adults. An adult who is capable of giving informed consent is the sole judge of whether he is to be given medical or surgical treatment. The husband's consent need not be given for the treatment of the wife nor the wife's for the husband.[5] In other words, consent is personal to the patient. It is sometimes wise, however, to obtain the spouse's consent or the consent of a relative when the proposed surgery involves danger to life, sterilization or impairment of sexual function, or the risk of death of an unborn child.[6]

---

[4]*Canterbury v. Spence*, 464 F.2d 722 (D.C. Cir. 1972).

[5]*Kritzer v Citron*, 101 Cal. App.2d 33, 224 P.2d 808 (1950). American Medical Association.

[6]Medicolegal Forms with Legal Analysis 14–15 (1961).

Unconscious or Incompetent Adults.   In emergencies, these patients may be treated without any expressed consent at all. What constitutes an emergency rests largely with the judgment of the treating physician. However, a physician should seek medical consultation before the procedure is begun, and the evidence indicating an emergency situation that threatens life or health should be noted in the medical record.

In instances in which the adult is unable to give consent (either for temporary reasons such as unconsciousness due to accident or sedation, or for permanent reasons such as mental illness), and the illness or injury is not one that threatens the life or health of the patient, consent should be obtained from any other person authorized either expressly or by implication to consent for the unconscious or incompetent adult.

MINORS

In General.   Minors can neither consent to nor refuse medical care; the decision is the responsibility of the parents or guardian. Here again, the parents' consent should be an *informed consent.*[7]

Age of Majority.   Many states have enacted laws establishing the age of 18 as sufficient for the purpose of consenting to medical or dental care.[8] The age is even lower when the minor is emancipated. Emancipation is a situation that ordinarily exists when a child is living apart from the parents and is outside of the parents' control. Factors that establish emancipation include marriage, the earning of one's own living, the maintenance of a home separate from one's parents, and psychological maturity.[9] An emancipated minor, whether male or female, may be treated as an adult, although some states have imposed minimal ages for emancipation.[10]

Emergencies.   If a parent or guardian cannot be reached, the usual rules for emergency care apply. Treatment for a child should *never* be delayed in order to obtain consent when an emergency situation exists. When time is important, the child brought to the emergency department in need of care should be treated *immediately* and consent obtained later. When time is not a factor, or when an emergency situation does not exist, consent should be obtained before treatment is begun.

When Treatment is Refused.   Occasionally, a minor in need of treatment will arrive at an emergency department but the parents or guardian will refuse to give their consent and attempt to remove the child from the emergency department without treatment. When the child's life is endangered, the child should be taken from the parents' custody and treated. While treatment is in progress, the hospital administrator should notify the appropriate court for the purpose of obtaining the court's

---

[7]*Brown v. Wood,*, 202 So.2d 125 (Fla. App. 1967).

[8]See e.g. *Colorado Revised Statute* §13-22-103 1973 (1979 Cum. Supp.).

[9]*Bach v. Long Island Jewish Hospital,* 49 Misc.2d 207, 267 N.Y.S.2d 289 (N.Y. City Ct. 1966).

[10]Note 7, loc. cit.

consent for treatment. The court can later issue a "nunc pro tunc" (now for then) order authorizing the treatment that has already been given.

Religious Convictions. It is ethically desirable in the practice of medicine to observe the religious beliefs of one's patients. However, a surgeon must not permit a parent's religious beliefs to interfere with the life-saving treatment of a child. The courts will not tolerate a situation in which a child's life is endangered simply because his parent has a religious conviction that the treatment should not be given. Therefore, in the case of a child in need of life-saving treatment, the treatment should be begun (this includes giving blood tranfusions), and the administrator should notify the appropriate judicial authority and obtain the court order needed to authorize the treatment.

EXTENT OF DUTY TO CARE FOR THE PATIENT

Given expressed or implied consent, the physician has a duty to care for the patient from the initial diagnosis until he withdraws from the case or properly discharges the patient. In an emergency department, there is a duty to treat a patient if an emergency exists.[11] The physician who initially treats a patient is responsible to see that the patient subsequently receives adequate medical care. Surgeons, for example, are generally held responsible for seeing that their instructions concerning postoperative care are carried out.[12] Withdrawal from a case is permissible, but in so doing the physician must give the patient sufficient time to procure other medical attention.[13] A discharged patient should be informed of any further medical care that may be necessary. The follow-up instructions given to the patient should be noted in his medical record.

Transfer of Patients to Other Hospitals. In general, it is medically and legally risky to transfer an emergency patient from one hospital to another. The medical hazards are obvious — chest pain, gastrointestinal hemorrhage, septic meningitis, intra-abdominal hemorrhage, intracranial trauma, etc. The legal problem is that the physician who transfers the patient retains legal responsibility for him until he arrives into the care of another qualified physician or medical facility. A patient whose condition worsens en route is ordinarily the responsibility of the transferring physician, unless there is an expressed understanding with the receiving physician whereby that physician agrees to accept responsibility beginning at the time of departure. Furthermore, one physician may be liable for transferring a patient to another physician if the first physician knows that the second physician is not capable of managing the patient's particular problem. Therefore, transferring emergency patients to other hospitals

---

[11]*Willington General Hospital v. Manlove,* 54 Del. 15, 174 A.2d 135 (1961).
[12]*Levy v. Kirk,* 187 So.2d 401 (Fla. App. 1966).
[13]*McManus v. Donlin,* 23 Wis.2d 289, 127 N.W.2d 22 (1964).

should be done *only* in those situations in which it is absolutely clear that the transfer will not have any adverse effects on the health of the patient and that the transfer is being made to a place at which the patient can receive quality physician and hospital care, appropriate to the illness or injury.

CONTRACTUAL LIABILITY

A physician does not have a duty to cure, but is instead held to certain professional standards discussed later in the section on malpractice. A physician may, however, *establish* a duty to cure if he contracts with a patient by assuring him that a certain result will be achieved or that a specific treatment will be given. A physician does not enter into a contract if he gives such reassurances as "You'll be all right," but he may be bound in contract by specific words of commitment. For example, the words "I guarantee to make you well," have been interpreted as establishing a contractual obligation to cure, and if cure is not achieved, damages may be recovered, even though the physician exercised due care and skill.

MALPRACTICE

In all areas of medicine and surgery, physicians are held to a standard of practice required of them by other physicians in either the same (or similar) locality or in the nation. In emergency situations in which there is little or no time for calm reflection, the law may not require the same performance as it does when the physician is not acting in an emergency. This is not to say that emergency department physicians can practice medicine of lower quality than physicians in other areas of specialization. Each physician is judged by what other reasonably careful physicians would or would not have done in the particular situation. Although there may be slight variations from state to state, in general a physician is required to practice the same quality of medicine or surgery as other physicians would practice under the same circumstances. Stated another way, if a community of physicians agrees that a particular physician's practice was substandard, his actions are considered malpractice.

LIABILITY FOR THE MALPRACTICE OR NEGLIGENCE OF OTHERS (VICARIOUS LIABILITY)

In certain instances, a physician may be liable for the acts or omissions of others. In some states, the "captain of the ship" rule applies to surgeons in the operating room. This doctrine holds the principal surgeon liable for the negligence of every other person in the operating room. The rule stems from basic common law considerations, which provide that the person who has the right of direction or control over others is liable for the negligence of his employees, agents, partners, and servants. While a surgeon may not be liable for the anesthesiologist, he *is* liable for the negligence of a nurse-anesthetist unless the nurse is working under the direction and supervision of an anesthesiologist. Under those circumstances, the surgeon would probably not be liable for the nurse-anesthetist.

GOOD SAMARITAN LEGISLATION[14]

Many states have enacted "Good Samaritan" statutes. In general, these laws grant immunity from damages to licensed physicians and to others who gratuitously render emergency care at the roadside or in public places — except in cases in which the person has been guilty of willful or wanton misconduct in providing such care. The benefit to the public from such legislation is that it encourages trained medical persons to assist in emergencies. There are no reported cases of emergency patients suing the "Good Samaritan" physician, and the passage of such legislation does not in any way change the usual rules that apply to physicians performing medical or surgical services in the emergency department of hospitals.

DUTY TO INFORM THE NEXT OF KIN OF THE DEATH OF A PATIENT

The method by which hospital staff and physicians handle all aspects relating to a deceased patient has recently resulted in increased litigation. Suffice it to say that all communication relating in any way to death, disposal of tissue, or autopsies should be handled with the utmost care and concern for the feelings of relatives and others close to the deceased.[15]

Most state statutes require that the attending physician complete a certificate upon the death of a patient,[16] and that the next of kin be notified of the death of a relative. Liability has been imposed for preventing a family from viewing the deceased's burial.[17] Autopsies should not be performed without the permission of the nearest relative or without authority from the appropriate public official.[18]

---

[14]For a comparison of good samaritan statutes on a state-by-state basis, see Louisell and Williams, Medical Malpractice, Vol. 2, Chap. XXI at 594.1 (1980).

[15]See e.g. *Muniz v. United Hospital Medical Center,* 370 A.2d 76 (N.J. 1976); *Johnson v. Woman's Hospital,* 527 SW.2d 133 (Tenn. App. 1975).

[16]See e.g. Ill. Ann. Stat. (1970 Supp.) Ch. 111-1/2 §73-18(2); Calif. Health and Safety Code (§10200).

[17]*Spiegel v. Evergreen Cemetery Co.,* 117 N.J.L. 90, 186 A. 585 (1936).

[18]*French v. Ochsner Clinic,* 200 So.2d 371 (La. App. 1967).

DUTY TO PRESERVE EVIDENCE IN THE EMERGENCY DEPARTMENT

Emergency department physicians should observe, preserve, and record items and information that are important in the prosecution and defense of crimes. Obviously the rights of victims, the rights of accused persons, the rights of injured persons, and indeed the rights of society are intertwined with the preservation of information that is important in the trying of both criminal and civil cases. The physician should be aware of the consequence of the outright loss or destruction of evidence, the failure to accumulate evidence, or the destruction of the chain of custody of evidence. Before clothing is removed or bullet holes, powder burns, blood stains, and other important evidence is destroyed, a comment should be made or photographs taken to preserve this evidence. Wounds should be identified as traumatically incurred or surgically placed, needle marks should be identified as either medical or nonmedical, missile tracks should be described, entrance and exit paths of bullets should be noted, gastric contents should be preserved, and fetal and placental tissue should be preserved for the pathologist.

RECORD KEEPING

The importance of keeping good records cannot be overemphasized. The new rules of evidence applicable to federal courts, which are followed by a great many state courts, make most medical records admissible as evidence. Good records are important both for medical reasons and for use in civil and criminal trials. Distressingly, all too often emergency department records are incomplete, illegible, and inaccurate. There can be no excuse for such records. *A significant factor in the defense of malpractice claims relates to good documentation.*

TREATMENT OF RAPE VICTIM[19]

Treatment of the rape victim is an area in which the physician in the emergency department has duties to both patient and to society. It is the obligation of the physician and hospital to care for the physical and emotional needs of the rape victim, while at the same time preserving necessary evidence.

Treatment should include a detailed history, a complete physical examination, the repair of any injury, and steps to prevent venereal disease

---

[19]See generally Schiff AF: How to handle the rape victim. South Med J 71:509–511, 1978; Enos WF: Management of the rape victim. American Family Physician 18:97–102, 1978; and Schaeffer JL: Counseling sexual abuse victims. American Family Physician 18:85–91, 1978.

and pregnancy. The psychological condition of the victim should not be ignored. Family and friends should be advised of the importance of support and sympathy. If available, a community "rape crisis" center with specialized personnel should be contacted for advice. Long-term treatment and follow-up care should also be encouraged in coordination with a local or family physician.

The preservation of evidence is discussed in detail in Chapter 11. The process can be enhanced by the careful notation of signs of recent trauma or violence, by preserving all foreign materials obtained from the body of the victim, and by the taking and preserving of secretions from the oral cavity and vaginal canal for serologic typing. To assist in this responsibility, "rape kits" should be available in the emergency department that include materials for vaginal smears, sampling of vaginal fluids, blood typing, and sampling of saliva and hairs, and vaginal swabs and supplies for blood grouping.

LEGAL PROBLEMS IN ORGAN DONATIONS[20]

The legal problems involved in organ donations and transplants is another area in which social needs must be balanced against the individual rights. Generally, the transplant surgeon's standard of care will be determined under traditional malpractice principles that would include ensuring that the organ is in good state prior to transplant and that the donor's age and antemortem condition are no contraindications to transplantation.[21] Other common problem areas include compliance with the Uniform Anatomical Gift Act in the form adopted by local state statutes, problems of informed consent, and the limitations on legal capacity of donors.

On July 30, 1968, the National Conference of Commissioners on Uniform State Laws gave final approval to a proposed Uniform Anatomical Gift Act.[22] Since that date 21 states have enacted the Act in some form and all but two states have passed law legislation dealing with the disposition of the human body or its parts after death.[23]

The Act has attempted to resolve some of the areas of legal uncertainty, while at the same time reducing the risk confronting transplant surgeons. It provides:

A person who acts in good faith in accord with the terms of this Act or with the Anatomical Gift laws of another state (or a foreign country) is not liable for damages in any civil action or subject to prosecution in any criminal proceedings for his act.

---

[20]See generally Jeddeloh NP: Legal problems in organ donation. Leavell J: Legal problems in organ transplants. Mississippi LJ 44:865–899, 1973.

[21]*Ravenis v. Detroit General Hospital,* 63 Mich. App. 79, 234 N.W.2d 411 (1975).

[22]For a detailed comparison of the various state statutes see Louisell and Williams, loc. cit., at 582.13 (1979 Cum. Supp.).

[23]Idem.

Thus, if a physician proceeds in good faith and in accord with the terms of the Act, he most often can avoid legal liability. Any surgeon who expects to become involved in transplant operations should become familiar with both the Uniform Anatomical Gift Act generally and its form as adopted in his state.

The problem of removal of an organ from a living donor for transplantation is basically one of informed consent. As long as a sane, sober, adult patient consents to the removal and that consent is properly obtained, the transplant surgeon should not be exposed to any more risk of liability than with any other routine medical procedure.

Problem areas do occur when a question exists as to the legal capacity of a minor or incompetent to consent to an organ transplant. The complex and inconsistent nature of legal opinions in this area makes donations of organs from minors and adult incompetents a difficult area. If a situation arises in which organs from this type of donor must be used, it should be done only after a well-documented informed consent is obtained from someone authorized to speak for the minor or incompetent by virtue of a court order.

ETHICAL AND LEGAL CONSIDERATIONS OF EXPERIMENTAL PROTOCOL[24]

Informed consent required in the experimenter-subject relationship encompasses all requirements of informed consent in the doctor-patient therapeutic relationship but to a far greater degree. The administration of experimental drugs or procedures should be based on a balance of harm and benefit, with the degree of risk never exceeding the humanitarian importance of the problem.

By statute, research done for the federal government must meet the following requirements in regard to informed consent:

1. A fair explanation of the procedures to be followed, and their purposes, including identification of any procedures that are experimental;

2. A description of any attendant discomforts and risks reasonably to be expected;

3. A description of any benefits reasonably to be expected;

4. A disclosure of any appropriate alternative procedures that might be advantageous for the subject;

5. An offer to answer any inquiries concerning the procedures;

---

[24]See generally Levine RJ and Lebacqz K: Some ethical considerations in clinical trials. Clinical Pharmacology and Therapeutics 25: 728–741, 1979; Check WA: Protecting and informing human research subjects. JAMA 243:1985–1986, 1980; Silva MC: Informed consent in human experimentation—the scientist's responsibility, the subject's right. Trial 16:37–41, 1980.

6. An instruction that the person is free to withdraw his consent and to discontinue participation in the project or activity at any time without prejudice to the subject; and

7. With respect to biomedical or behavioral research that may result in physical injury, an explanation as to whether compensation and medical treatment is available if physical injury occurs and, if so, what it consists of or where more information may be obtained.[25]

Institutions receiving federal funds are also required by the FDA to have groups such as the Institutional Review Board (IRB) review human research proposals to ensure that the subject's rights are protected.

In addition to these requirements, it is essential that the subject have the legal capacity to consent (the ability to understand the choice involved), and that the consent be truly voluntary and not the result of either real or perceived coercion. Even the subtle use of moral persuasion, position, or the promise of large monetary rewards should be avoided if it could possibly interfere with the voluntary requirement. Researchers must also be aware that subjects of experiments are always free to change their minds and verbally rescind any written agreement at any time.

Documentation is also very important. The *AMA Ethical Guidelines for Clinical Investigation* states that in regard to clinical investigation for scientific knowledge, without exception, consent should be in writing, either from the subject or a legally authorized representative.[26]

A final area of concern is whether any legal obligation exists to compensate the subject if unforeseen side effects or injuries occur. To date no code or regulation specifically requires compensation to injured research subjects; however, if the institution assumes medical responsibility, the issue of insurance coverage must be addressed.[27]

---

[25]Protection of Human Subjects, Code of Federal Regulations, 45 CFR 46.103, US Dept. of HEW, Washington, D.C., Revised 1979.

[26]American Medical Association: Ethical Guidelines for Clinical Investigation. Proceedings of the House of Delegates: 123rd Annual Convention, Chicago, Ill., 1974, pp. 271–272.

[27]Cooper PJ: Compensation for human research subjects: Reform ahead of its time? Journal of Legal Medicine 2:1–13, 1980.

FORM FOR PATIENT INFORMED CONSENT
(OPERATION AND OTHER MEDICAL SERVICES)

1. OPERATION OR PROCEDURE AND ALTERNATIVES:

I, _____ (patient or patient's guardian),

authorize Dr. _____ to perform the following operation

or procedure:_____. I understand the reason for the procedure is:

_____.

I understand alternative procedures include: _____

_____.

2. RISKS: This authorization is given with the understanding that any operation or procedure involves some risks and hazards. The more common risks include infection, bleeding, nerve injury, blood clots, heart attack, allergic reactions and pneumonia. These risks can be serious and possibly fatal. The significant and substantial risks of this particular operation are:

_____.

3. ANESTHESIA: The administration of anesthesia also involves risks, most importantly a rare risk of reaction to medications causing death. I consent to the use of such anesthetics as may be considered necessary by the physician responsible for these services. Other risks particular to this anesthesia procedure include:

_____.

4. ADDITIONAL PROCEDURES: If my physician discovers a different, unsuspected condition at the time of surgery, I authorize him to perform such treatment as necessary.

5. I understand that no guarantee or assurance has been made as to the results of the procedure and that it *may not cure the condition*

6. PATIENT'S CONSENT. I have read and fully understand this consent form, and understand I should not sign this form if all items, including all my questions, have not been explained or answered to my satisfaction.

Date: _____   Time: _____

_____   _____
Witness   Patient or person with authority
                                       to consent for patient

7. PHYSICIAN DECLARATION: I have explained the contents of this document to the patient and have answered all the patient's questions, and to the best of my knowledge, I feel the patient has been adequately informed and has consented.

_____
Physician's Signature

WARNING:

IF YOU HAVE ANY QUESTIONS AS TO THE RISKS OR HAZARDS OF THE PROPOSED SURGERY OR TREATMENT, OR ANY QUESTIONS WHATEVER CONCERNING THE PROPOSED SURGERY OR TREATMENT, ASK YOUR SURGEON NOW *BEFORE SIGNING THIS CONSENT FORM.*

Index

Page numbers in *italics* indicate illustrations; those followed by "t" indicate tables.

PRIMARY ASSESSMENT AND MANAGEMENT OF THE INJURED

In managing an injured patient admitted to an emergency department, the following should be carried out:

1. Make a rapid assessment of the patient's condition with emphasis on the functions of respiration, circulation, cerebration, and the possibility of injury to the cervical spine.
2. Evaluate airway and ensure its continued patency.
3. Ensure effective respiratory exchange—seal open wounds of chest, temporarily immobilize flail segments, perform thoracocentesis or tube thoracostomy when need is apparent.
4. Maintain or restore effective circulation by establishing a large bore intravenous line, obtain blood for the laboratory, and initiate volume replacement with lactated Ringer's solution.
5. Perform a rapid, but complete physical examination avoiding excessive movement of the patient, especially if spinal injury may exist.
6. Record important observations such as level of consciousness, pupil size and vital signs.
7. Obtain history of injury and of the events prior to and following the accident. Inquire as to allergies, medications, past illness, and last meal.
8. Cover open wounds using pressure to control bleeding where necessary.
9. Splint obvious or suspected fractures and the cervical spine in patients with head injuries.
10. Obtain immediate portable chest x-ray in patients with thoracic injuries or cardio-respiratory distress (shock, venous distention, hypoxia, cyanosis, dyspnea). Obtain portable anteroposterior and lateral views of the cervical spine in patients suspected of cervical spine injury. Arrange for definitive x-rays to be accomplished promptly during a single visit to the radiology suite.

IMMEDIATE TREATMENT OF SHOCK

1. Establish an adequate airway.

2. Obtain initial vital signs and start a chronologic record or flow sheet.

3. Elevate the legs to 45° to obtain a rapid return of venous blood to the heart.

4. Start a rapid infusion of electrolyte solution via one or more large bore catheters.

5. Obtain a venous blood sample for type, crossmatch, hematocrit determination, and other appropriate laboratory studies, and arterial blood for pH, pO_2, and pCO_2.

6. Insert an indwelling catheter; record urinary output every 30 to 60 minutes. Analyze urine.

7. If vital signs do not respond quickly, insert a central venous catheter and measure central venous pressure (C.V.P.) at intervals of 15 to 30 minutes.

8. If there is evidence of continued bleeding start transfusing crossmatched blood as soon as it is available.

9. A satisfactory response to fluid or blood replacement is apparent when: pulse rate decreases; arterial blood pressure increases; signs of peripheral vasoconstriction diminish or disappear; C.V.P. rises; urinary output exceeds 30 ml/hr; and metabolic acidosis improves.

10. If oliguria persists despite an improvement in other indices consider hypovolemia.

11. A satisfactory but transient response to fluid replacement in a patient with hemorrhage suggests continuing blood loss, which may require surgical intervention.